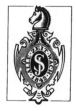

Hypertrophic Cardiomyopathy

The Therapeutic Role of
Calcium Antagonists

Edited by
M. Kaltenbach and S. E. Epstein

With 172 Figures

Springer-Verlag
Berlin Heidelberg New York 1982

Professor Dr. med. M. KALTENBACH, Zentrum der Inneren Medizin, Abteilung für Kardiologie, Klinikum der Johann-Wolfgang-von-Goethe-Universität, Theodor-Stern-Kai 7, D-6000 Frankfurt 70

S. E. EPSTEIN, M. D., Cardiology Branch, National Heart, Lung, and Blood Institute, National Institutes of Health, Bethesda, MD 20205/USA

ISBN-13:978-3-642-68284-1   e-ISBN-13:978-3-642-68282-7
DOI: 10.1007/978-3-642-68282-7

Library of Congress Cataloging in Publication Data. Main entry under title: Hypertrophic cardiomyopathy. Bibliography: p. Includes index. 1. Heart–Hypertrophy–Chemotherapy. 2. Verapamil. 3. Calcium–Antagonists–Therapeutic use. I. Kaltenbach, Martin. II. Epstein, S. E. (Stephen E.) [DNLM: 1. Myocardia diseases–Drug therapy. 2. Calcium–Antagonists and inhibitors. 3. Iproveratril–Therapeutic use. WG 280 H998] RC685.H9H957. 616.1′24. 81-16665. ISBN-13:978-3-642-68284-1(U.S.). A-ACR2

This work is subject to copyright. All rights are reserved, whether the whole or part of the material is concerned, specifically those of translation, reprinting, re-use of illustrations, broadcasting, reproduction by photocopying machine or similar means and storage in data banks. Under § 54 of the German Copyright Law where copies are made for other than private use a fee is payable to "Verwertungsgesellschaft Wort", Munich.

© by Springer-Verlag Berlin Heidelberg 1982

Softcover reprint of the hardcover 1st edition 1982

The use of registered names, trademarks, etc. in this publication does not imply, even in the absence of a specific statement, that such names are exempt from the relevant protective laws and regulations and therefore free for general use.

2127/3130-543210

Preface

First described in 1907 by Schicke but recognized as a clinical entity only as recently as 1958, when Teare published the pathologic findings in patients with hypertrophic cardiomyopathy (HCM), an explosion of knowledge about this fascinating disease has occurred, which has caused a profound evolution of our understanding of its broad pathophysiologic and clinical spectrum. Progress has been particularly rapid in the past few years when M-mode echocardiography, and more recently 2-dimensional echocardiography have been applied to the study of HCM.

In addition to new insights as to what the disease is, there has been enormous progress concerning its treatment, with the application of beta-adrenergic blocking agents and surgical relief of left ventricular outflow tract obstruction. Although these approaches have led to great strides in the symptomatic control of the disease, many patients' symptoms have remained refractory to medical and surgical therapy. Most discouragingly, sudden death still occurs, even in patients on large doses of beta-blocking agents and in patients who have had surgical relief of left ventricular outflow tract obstruction.

Therapy of HCM with calcium antagonists was initiated in 1973 in Frankfurt/Main. Independently, several years later, the group in Bethesda started with the same therapeutical approach. Many assumptions had to be made to justify this new form of treatment, e.g.:

- High doses of verapamil can be given over a long period of time without severe side effects
- Cardiomyopathy or its clinical effects relates to calcium ion overload or increased intramyocardial availability of calcium
- The negative inotropic action of verapamil is not of major clinical importance.

In the meantime our understanding of the disease as well as of the basic principle of calcium antagonism as defined by Fleckenstein has considerably increased. Most importantly, therapeutic experience with the use of verapamil in treating patients with HCM has increased markedly, and data relating to its effects have been collected at different institutions throughout the world.

This volume is aimed to represent our up-to-date knowledge of the topic. It offers for the first time an international overview on a new therapeutic approach to HCM.

MARTIN KALTENBACH · STEPHEN E. EPSTEIN

Contents

Clinical and Anatomical Characterization of Hypertrophic Cardiomyopathy

Synopsis. J. F. GOODWIN 3
Hypertrophic Cardiomyopathy: An Overview. S. E. EPSTEIN and B. J. MARON.
    With 7 Figures 5
Echocardiographic Identification of Patterns of Left Ventricular Hyper-
    trophy in Hypertrophic Cardiomyopathy. B. J. MARON, J. S. GOTT-
    DIENER, and S. E. EPSTEIN. With 17 Figures 18
Distribution and Significance of Cardiac Muscle Cell Disorganization
    in the Left Ventricle of Patients with Hypertrophic Cardiomyopathy:
    Evidence of a Diffuse Cardiomyopathic Process. B. J. MARON and
    W. C. ROBERTS. With 12 Figures 38
Left Ventricular Biopsy in Hypertrophic Cardiomyopathy: Light and
    Electron Microscopic Evaluations. B. KUNKEL, M. SCHNEIDER, R. HOPF,
    G. KOBER, K. HÜBNER, and M. KALTENBACH. With 3 Figures 58

Cardiomyopathy in Animals and Therapeutic Interventions

Synopsis. B. J. MARON 72
Spontaneously Occurring Hypertrophic Cardiomyopathy in Dogs and Cats:
    A Potential Animal Model of a Human Disease. B. J. MARON,
    S.-K. LIU, and L. P. TILLEY. With 9 Figures 73
Cardiac Effects of Nerve Growth Factor in Dogs. M. P. KAYE,
    D. J. WITZKE, D. J. WELLS, and V. FUSTER. With 7 Figures 88
Prevention of Myocardial Cell Necrosis in the Syrian Hamster – Results
    of Long-Term Treatment. K. LOSSNITZER, A. KONRAD, D. ZEYER,
    and W. MOHR. With 4 Figures 99
Prevention by Verapamil of Isoproterenol-Induced Hypertrophic Cardio-
    myopathy in Rats. A. FLECKENSTEIN, M. FREY, and J. KEIDEL.
    With 4 Figures 115

**Effects of Acute Administration of Verapamil in Patients with Hypertrophic
Cardiomyopathy**

Synopsis. S. E. EPSTEIN 122
Acute Hemodynamic Effects of Verapamil in Hypertrophic Cardiomyo-
    pathy. D. R. ROSING, K. M. KENT, R. O. BONOW, and S. E. EPSTEIN.
    With 9 Figures 124

Hemodynamics and Contractility After Oral, Intravenous, and Intracoronary Application of Calcium Antagonists. W.-D. BUSSMANN, R. HOPF, A. TROMPLER, and M. KALTENBACH. With 9 Figures 138

Effect of Verapamil on Left Ventricular Isovolumic Relaxation Time and Regional Left Ventricular Filling in Hypertrophic Cardiomyopathy. P. HANRATH, D. G. MATHEY, P. KREMER, F. SONNTAG, and W. BLEIFELD. With 5 Figures 148

Treatment of Hypertrophic Cardiomyopathy with Verapamil

Synopsis. H. KUHN 160

Verapamil Treatment of Hypertrophic Cardiomyopathy. R. HOPF and M. KALTENBACH. With 13 Figures 163

Volume Parameters of the Heart During Long-Term Verapamil Treatment in Patients with Hypertrophic Cardiomyopathy. M. KALTENBACH and R. HOPF. With 7 Figures 179

Long-Term Clinical Effects of Verapamil in Patients with Hypertrophic Cardiomyopathy. D. R. ROSING, J. R. CONDIT, B. J. MARON, K. M. KENT, M. B. LEON, R. O. BONOW, L. C. LIPSON, and S. E. EPSTEIN. With 4 Figures 187

Effects of Verapamil on Ventricular Wall Thickness of Patients with Hypertrophic Cardiomyopathy. H. O. HIRZEL, M. P. TROESCH, R. JENNI, and H. P. KRAYENBUEHL. With 6 Figures 203

Long-Term Verapamil Treatment in Patients with Hypertrophic Nonobstructive Cardiomyopathy. H. KUHN, U. THELEN, C. LEUNER, E. KÖHLER, V. BLUSCHKE, and F. LOOGEN. With 10 Figures 214

Verapamil: Its Potential for Causing Serious Complications in Patients with Hypertrophic Cardiomyopathy. S. E. EPSTEIN and D. R. ROSING. With 3 Figures 225

Long-Term Results of Different Therapeutic Interventions in Comparison with Verapamil

Synopsis. R. HOPF 236

Efficacy of Operation for Obstructive Hypertrophic Cardiomyopathy: A 20-Year Experience with Ventricular Septal Myotomy and Myectomy. B. J. MARON, J.-P. KOCH, S. E. EPSTEIN, and A. G. MORROW. With 10 Figures 238

Functional Results in Medically and Surgically Treated Patients with Hypertrophic Obstructive Cardiomyopathy. B. LÖSSE, H. KUHN, and F. LOOGEN. With 3 Figures 251

Long-Term Treatment of Hypertrophic Cardiomyopathy with Verapamil or Propranolol. Preliminary Results of a Multicenter Study. G. KOBER, R. HOPF, A. SCHMIDT, M. KALTENBACH, G. BIAMINO, R. SCHRÖDER, P. BUBENHEIMER, H. ROSKAMM, P. HANRATH, F. SONNTAG, K.-E. V. OLSHAUSEN, H. ZEBE, W. KÜBLER, W. SCHÖNUNG, A. MÜLLER, and M. SCHLEPPER. With 3 Figures 261

Contents IX

Effects of Different Calcium Blockers and Implications Regarding Therapy of Hypertrophic Cardiomyopathy

Synopsis. G. KOBER 268
The Antianginal Efficacy of Seven Different Calcium Antagonists.
   H.-J. BECKER, R. HOPF, G. KOBER, and M. KALTENBACH. With 2 Figures   269
Differentiation of Calcium-Antagonistic Drugs with Respect to Their
   Myocardial Effects. R. KAUFMANN, R. BAYER, R. RODENKIRCHEN,
   and R. MANNHOLD. With 4 Figures 276
The Concept of Calcium Antagonist Therapy in Cardiac Hypertrophy.
   Different Calcium Antagonists with Respect to Therapeutic Efficacy
   in Hypertrophic Cardiomyopathy. Combined Therapy with
   Calcium Antagonists and Other Drugs? M. KALTENBACH, G. KOBER,
   and R. HOPF. With 1 Figure 285

Clinical Pharmacology of Verapamil in Hypertrophic Cardiomyopathy

Synopsis. R. G. McALLISTER, Jr. 290
Pharmacokinetics, Bioavailability, and ECG Response of Verapamil in Man.
   M. EICHELBAUM and A. SOMOGYI. With 3 Figures 291
Verapamil Plasma Concentrations and Indices of Heart Size in Hyper-
   trophic Obstructive Cardiomyopathy – Evidence for the Existence
   of a Therapeutic Range. B. G. WOODCOCK, R. HOPF,
   and R. KIRSTEN. With 8 Figures 298
Plasma Verapamil Levels in Patients with Hypertrophic Cardiomyopathy:
   Interpatient Variability and Clinical Usefulness. M. B. LEON,
   D. R. ROSING, and S. E. EPSTEIN. With 6 Figures 309
Correlation of Verapamil Plasma Levels with Electrocardiographic and
   Hemodynamic Effects. R. G. McALLISTER, Jr. With 3 Figures 322

Subject Index 332

List of Contributors

BAYER, R., Physiologisches Institut der Universität Düsseldorf, Moorenstraße 5, D-4000 Düsseldorf

BECKER, H.-J., Medizinische Klinik I des Stadtkrankenhauses Hanau, Leimenstraße 20, D-6450 Hanau 1

BIAMINO, G., Medizinische Klinik und Poliklinik, Klinikum Steglitz, Freie Universität Berlin, Hindenburgdamm 30, D-1000 Berlin

BLEIFELD,W., II. Medizinische Klinik und Poliklinik, Kardiologische Abteilung, Universitäts-Krankenhaus Eppendorf, Martinistraße 52, D-2000 Hamburg 20

BLUSCHKE, V., Medizinische Klinik und Poliklinik, Klinik B (Schwerpunkt Kardiologie), Universität Düsseldorf, Moorenstraße 5, D-4000 Düsseldorf

BONOW, R. O., Cardiology Branch, National Heart, Lung, and Blood Institute, National Institutes of Health, Bethesda, MD 20205/USA

BUBENHEIMER, P., Benedikt-Kreutz-Rehabilitationszentrum für Herz- und Kreislaufkranke e.V., Südring 15, D-7812 Bad Krozingen

BUSSMANN, W.-D., Zentrum der Inneren Medizin, Abteilung für Kardiologie, Klinikum der Johann-Wolfgang-Goethe-Universität, Theodor-Stern-Kai 7, D-6000 Frankfurt/Main 70

CONDIT, J. R., Cardiology Branch, National Heart, Lung, and Blood Institute, National Institutes of Health, Bethesda, MD 20205/USA

EICHELBAUM, M., Medizinische Klinik der Universität Bonn, Siegmund-Freud-Str. 25, D-5300 Bonn

EPSTEIN, S. E., Cardiology Branch, National Heart, Lung, and Blood Institute, National Institutes of Health, Bethesda, MD 20205/USA

FLECKENSTEIN, A., Physiologisches Institut der Universität Freiburg, Hermann-Herder-Straße 7, D-7800 Freiburg i. Br.

FREY, M., Physiologisches Institut der Universität Freiburg, Hermann-Herder-Str. 7, D-7800 Freiburg i. Br.

FUSTER, V., Section of Cardiovascular Surgical Research, Mayo Clinic, 200 First Street SW, MN 55901/USA

GOODWIN, J. F., Royal Postgraduate Medical School, Hammersmith Hospital, Ducane Road, GB-London W12 OHS

GOTTDIENER, J. S., Cardiology Branch, National Heart, Lung, and Blood Institute, National Institutes of Health, Bethesda, MD 20205/USA

HANRATH, P., II. Medizinische Klinik und Poliklinik, Kardiologische Abteilung, Universitäts-Krankenhaus Eppendorf, Martinistraße 52, D-2000 Hamburg 20

HIRZEL, H. O., Medizinische Poliklinik, Departement für Innere Medizin, Universität Zürich, Rämistraße 100, CH-8091 Zürich

HOPF, R., Zentrum der Inneren Medizin, Abteilung für Kardiologie, Klinikum der Johann-Wolfgang-Goethe-Universität, Theodor-Stern-Kai 7, D-6000 Frankfurt/Main 70

HÜBNER, K., Zentrum der Pathologie, Klinikum der Johann-Wolfgang-Goethe-Universität, Theodor-Stern-Kai 7, D-6000 Frankfurt/Main 70

JENNI, R., Medizinische Poliklinik, Departement für Innere Medizin, Universität Zürich, Rämistraße 100, CH-8091 Zürich

KALTENBACH, M., Zentrum der Inneren Medizin, Abteilung für Kardiologie, Klinikum der Johann-Wolfgang-Goethe-Universität, Theodor-Stern-Kai 7, D-6000 Frankfurt/Main 70

KAUFMANN, R., Physiologisches Institut der Universität Düsseldorf, Moorenstraße 5, D-4000 Düsseldorf

KAYE, M. P., Section of Cardiovascular Surgical Research, Mayo Clinic, 200 First Street SW, Rochester, MS 55901/USA

KEIDEL, I., Physiologisches Institut der Universität Freiburg, Hermann-Herder-Str. 7, D-7800 Freiburg i. Br.

KENT, K. M., Cardiology Branch, National Heart, Lung, and Blood Institute, National Institutes of Health, Bethesda, MD 20205/USA

KIRSTEN, R., Abteilung für Klinische Pharmakologie, Klinikum der Johann-Wolfgang-von-Goethe-Universität, Sandhofstraße 74, D-6000 Frankfurt/Main

KOBER, G., Zentrum der Inneren Medizin, Abteilung für Kardiologie, Klinikum der Johann-Wolfgang-Goethe-Universität, Theodor-Stern-Kai 7, D-6000 Frankfurt/Main 70

KOCH, J.-P., National Heart, Lung, and Blood Institute, National Institutes of Health, Bethesda, MD 20205/USA

KÖHLER, E., Medizinische Klinik und Poliklinik, Klinik B (Schwerpunkt Kardiologie), Universität Düsseldorf, Moorenstraße 5, D-4000 Düsseldorf

KONRAD, A., Medizinische Klinik der Bundesknappschaft, Akademisches Lehrkrankenhaus der Universität des Saarlandes, Lazarettstr. 4 D-6603 Sulzbach

KRAYENBUEHL, H. P., Medizinische Poliklinik, Departement für Innere Medizin, Universität Zürich, Rämistraße 100, CH-8091 Zürich

KREMER, P., II. Medizinische Klinik und Poliklinik, Kardiologische Abteilung, Universitäts-Krankenhaus Eppendorf, Martinistraße 52, D-2000 Hamburg 20

List of Contributors

KÜBLER, W., Abteilung Innere Medizin III, Medizinische Klinik der Universität Heidelberg, Bergheimer Straße 58, D-6900 Heidelberg

KUHN, H., Medizinische Klinik und Poliklinik, Klinik B (Schwerpunkt Kardiologie), Universität Düsseldorf, Moorenstraße 5, D-4000 Düsseldorf

KUNKEL, B., Zentrum der Inneren Medizin, Abteilung für Kardiologie, Klinikum der Johann-Wolfgang-Goethe-Universität, Theodor-Stern-Kai 7, D-6000 Frankfurt/Main 70

LEON, M. B., Cardiology Branch, National Heart, Lung, and Blood Institute, National Institutes of Health, Bethesda, MD 20205/USA

LEUNER, C., Medizinische Klinik und Poliklinik, Klinik B (Schwerpunkt Kardiologie), Universität Düsseldorf, Moorenstraße 5, D-4000 Düsseldorf

LIPSON, L. C., Cardiology Branch, National Heart, Lung, and Blood Institute, National Institutes of Health, Bethesda, MD 20205/USA

LIU, S.-K., Departments of Pathology and Medicine, The Animal Medical Center, New York, NY/USA

LÖSSE, B., Medizinische Klinik und Poliklinik, Klinik B (Schwerpunkt Kardiologie), Universität Düsseldorf, Moorenstraße 5, D-4000 Düsseldorf

LOOGEN, F., Medizinische Klinik und Poliklinik, Klinik B (Schwerpunkt Kardiologie), Universität Düsseldorf, Moorenstraße 5, D-4000 Düsseldorf

LOSSNITZER, K., Medizinische Klinik der Bundesknappschaft Sulzbach/Saar, Akademisches Lehrkrankenhaus der Universität des Saarlandes, Lazarettstr. 4 D-6603 Sulzbach

MANNHOLD, R., Physiologisches Institut der Universität Düsseldorf, Moorenstraße 5, D-4000 Düsseldorf

MARON, B. J., Cardiology Branch, National Heart, Lung, and Blood Institute, National Institutes of Health, Bethesda, MD 20205/USA

MATHEY, D. G., II. Medizinische Klinik und Poliklinik, Kardiologische Abteilung, Universitäts-Krankenhaus Eppendorf, Martinistraße 52, D-2000 Hamburg

MCALLISTER, Jr., R. G., Veterans Administrations Medical Center, Lexington, Kentucky, KY 40507/USA

MOHR, W., Abteilung Pathologie der Universität Ulm, Oberer Eselsberg, M 23, D-7900 Ulm

MORROW, A. G., National Heart, Lung, and Blood Institute, National Institutes of Health, Bethesda, MD 20205/USA

MÜLLER, A., Kerckhoff-Klinik der Max-Planck-Gesellschaft, Benekestraße 6 – 8, D-6350 Bad Nauheim

VON OLSHAUSEN, K.-E., Abteilung Innere Medizin III, Medizinische Klinik der Universität Heidelberg, Bergheimer Straße 58, D-6900 Heidelberg

ROBERTS, W. C., Pathology Branch, National Heart, Lung, and Blood Institute, National Institutes of Health, Bethesda, MD 20205/USA

RODENKIRCHEN, R., Physiologisches Institut der Universität Düsseldorf, Moorenstraße 5, D-4000 Düsseldorf

ROSING, D. R., Cardiology Branch, National Heart, Lung, and Blood Institute, National Institutes of Health, Bethesda, MD 20205/USA

ROSKAMM, H., Benedikt-Kreutz-Rehabilitationszentrum für Herz- und Kreislaufkranke e.V., Südring 15, D-7812 Bad Krozingen

SCHLEPPER, M., Kerckhoff-Klinik der Max-Planck-Gesellschaft, Benekestraße 6 – 8, D-6350 Bad Nauheim

SCHMIDT, A., Zentrum der Inneren Medizin, Abteilung für Kardiologie, Klinikum der Johann-Wolfgang-Goethe-Universität, Theodor-Stern-Kai 7, D-6000 Frankfurt/Main 70

SCHNEIDER, M., Zentrum der Pathologie, Klinikum der Johann-Wolfgang-Goethe-Universität, Theodor-Stern-Kai 7, D-6000 Frankfurt/Main 70

SCHÖNUNG, W., Kerckhoff-Klinik der Max-Planck-Gesellschaft, Benekestraße 6 – 8, D-6350 Bad Nauheim

SCHRÖDER, R., Medizinische Klinik und Poliklinik, Klinikum Steglitz, Freie Universität Berlin, Hindenburgdamm 30, D-1000 Berlin 45

SOMOGYI, A., Medizinische Klinik der Universität Bonn, Siegmund-Freud-Str. 25, D-5300 Bonn

SONNTAG, F., II. Medizinische Klinik und Poliklinik, Kardiologische Abteilung, Universitäts-Krankenhaus Eppendorf, Martinistraße 52, D-2000 Hamburg 20

THELEN, U., Medizinische Klinik und Poliklinik, Klinik B (Schwerpunkt Kardiologie), Universität Düsseldorf, Moorenstraße 5, D-4000 Düsseldorf

TILLEY, L. P., Departments of Pathology and Medicine, The Animal Medical Center, New York, NY/USA

TROESCH, M. P., Medizinische Poliklinik, Departement für Innere Medizin, Universität Zürich, Rämistraße 100, CH-8091 Zürich

TROMPLER, A., Zentrum der Inneren Medizin, Abteilung für Kardiologie, Klinikum der Johann-Wolfgang-Goethe-Universität, Theodor-Stern-Kai 7, D-6000 Frankfurt/Main 70

WELLS, D. J., Section of Cardiovascular Surgical Research, Mayo Clinic, 200 First Street SW, Rochester, MS 55901/USA

WITZKE, D. J., Section of Cardiovascular Surgical Research, Mayo Clinic, 200 First Street SW, Rochester, MN 55901/USA

WOODCOCK, B. G., Zentrum der Pharmakologie, Abteilung für Klinische Pharmakologie, Klinikum der Johann-Wolfgang-von-Goethe-Universität, Sandhofstraße 74, D-6000 Frankfurt/Main

ZEBE, H., Abteilung Innere Medizin III, Medizinische Klinik der Universität Heidelberg, Bergheimerstraße 58, D-6900 Heidelberg

ZEYER, D., Medizinische Klinik der Bundesknappschaft Sulzbach/Saar, Akademisches Lehrkrankenhaus der Universität des Saarlandes, D-6603 Sulzbach

Clinical and Anatomical Characterization of Hypertrophic Cardiomyopathy

Synopsis

J. F. GOODWIN

Epstein and colleagues comment on terminology (listing 58 names that have been given to hypertrophic cardiomyopathy) and emphasize the importance of abnormalities of diastolic function and reinforce the view that "obstruction" to outflow is only one aspect of this disease. The spectrum of hypertrophic cardiomyopathy is broader than originally suspected.

Echocardiographic studies have shown that hypertrophy can occur in all parts of the ventricle and may be found throughout the length of the ventricular septum, or in its upper or in its lower portions only. Hypertrophy, though usually asymmetrical, can be symmetrical. These variations have led to suggestions that hypertrophic cardiomyopathy is not one but many diseases or is even a nonspecific reaction of the myocardium with hypertrophy. This is not true: Hypertrophic cardiomyopathy is undoubtedly a major disease entity but with many forms and variations.

Sudden death is the most common type of death. Neither hemodynamic nor electrocardiographic findings are helpful in identifying the patient destined to die; nor does any type of ventricular morphology appear to be predictive. However, there may be a trend relating septal thickness to sudden death. A strong family history, young age, and massive cardiomegaly would suggest a poor prognosis, while one subset of hypertrophic cardiomyopathy is the so-called malignant familial type alluded to by Epstein and Maron.

The identification of occult arrhythmias by ambulatory ECG monitoring has greatly added to our knowledge. The experience of Maron and Epstein, supported by our own experience at the Royal Postgraduate Medical School, indicates that ventricular arrhythmias are common, and a direct relationship has been demonstrated between ventricular tachycardia and sudden death.

Cellular disorganization can be found in hypertrophic cardiomyopathy but also in a variety of cardiac diseases and even in healthy persons. In contrast to these cases with only small foci of cellular disorganization, patients with hypertrophic cardiomyopathy show large areas of the ventricular septum and also of the free left ventricular wall with cellular disorganization. It is not the finding itself but the widespread occurrence that is considered characteristic for hypertrophic cardiomyopathy. In the study of Maron et al. the most widespread cellular abnormalities were found in patients dying suddenly without prior functional limitations. It is therefore speculated that widespread cellular disorganization could provide a substrate for malignant ectopy.

The careful studies by Kunkel and colleagues show the value of endomyocardial biopsy in assessing the severity of the disease but less so in making a diagnosis. The patchy nature of the myofibrillar disarray in hypertrophic cardiomyopathy and the presence of similar lesions in other forms of ventricular hypertrophy secondary to other cardiac disorders make diagnosis by endomyocardial biopsy extremely difficult. It is suggested that the severity of hypertrophy in the biopsy from the left ventricular free wall of patients with hypertrophic cardiomyopathy may provide information concerning the stage and progress of the disease and also the response of the myocardium to the abnormal anatomical and functional situation. Thus, although endomyocardial biopsy may provide additional information about this disease, it should not be used to diagnose hypertrophic cardiomyopathy.

Hypertrophic Cardiomyopathy: An Overview *

STEPHEN E. EPSTEIN and BARRY J. MARON

Hypertrophic cardiomyopathy presents extraordinary challenges to the investigator, partly because of the extreme diversity in its clinical, hemodynamic, and anatomical presentation, and partly because of the rapid changes that have occurred in our understanding of its pathophysiology, natural history, and treatment since it was first recognized as a clinical entity in 1958 [1]. The profound changes that have occurred in our concepts of the disease are reflected in Table 1, which lists the names that have been appended to this entity at one time or another over the years.

The multiplicity of descriptive names given to this disease relate primarily to several factors. First, several centers were involved more or less simultaneously in the pioneering studies that characterized the disease and each, understandably, developed names for this newly discovered clinical entity based on those aspects of the disease that were most impressive to the individual investigators. Second, as additional information accumulated, concepts of the disease changed, with important new insights often leading to new names.

Characteristic Features of Hypertrophic Cardiomyopathy

Initially, this disease was viewed primarily as one characterized by obstruction to left ventricular outflow; hence, the disease acquired such names as "idiopathic hypertrophic subaortic stenosis", or IHSS, [2] "muscular subaortic stenosis" [3], and "hypertrophic obstructive cardiomyopathy", or HOCM [4].

The widespread application of M-mode echocardiography to cardiac diagnosis in the early 1970s confirmed the hypertrophic nature of the disease [5–8]. Echocardiographic studies also demonstrated that outflow obstruction was absent in a large proportion of patients with hypertrophic cardiomyopathy [9], that it was often transmitted as an autosomal dominant trait [9, 10], and that an hypertrophied ventricular septum, measuring at least 1.3 times the thickness of the left ventricular free wall, was invariable. These echocardiographic observations led to the introduction of the term "asymmetric septal hypertrophy" and its acronym "ASH" to describe the *disease* hypertrophic cardiomyopathy [5]. However, recent observations have indicated the inadequacy of this concept of the disease [11]. In particular, extensive two-dimensional echocardiographic studies [11 a, 12], demonstrated that while most of the patients have septal hypertrophy, the majority also have considerable thickening of the left ventricular free wall, which not infrequently is equal to or

---

* This paper is revised and updated from that published in Clinical and Investigative Medicine 3: 185–193, 1980

Table 1. Terms used to describe hypertrophic cardiomyopathy

Asymmetrical hypertrophic cardiomyopathy	1972
Asymmetrical hypertrophy of the heart	1958
Asymmetrical septal hypertrophy	1973
Brock's disease	1977
Diffuse muscular subaortic stenosis	1973
Diffuse subvalvular aortic stenosis	1961
Dynamic hypertrophic subaortic stenosis	1971
Dynamic muscular subaortic stenosis	1966
Familial hypertrophic subaortic stenosis	1961
Familial muscular subaortic stenosis	1959
Familial myocardial disease	1967
Functional aortic stenosis	1959
Functional hypertrophic subaortic stenosis	1969
Functional obstructive cardiomyopathy	1973
Functional obstruction of the left ventricle	1957
Functional obstructive subvalvular aortic stenosis	1968
Functional subaortic stenosis	1960
Hereditary cardiovascular dysplasia	1961
Hypertrophic cardiomyopathy	1970
Hypertrophic constrictive cardiomyopathy	1972
Hypertrophic hyperkinetic cardiomyopathy	1965
Hypertrophic infundibular aortic stenosis	1971
Hypertrophic nonobstructive cardiomyopathy	1975
Hypertrophic obstructive cardiomyopathy	1964
Hypertrophic stenosing cardiomyopathy	1972
Hypertrophic subaortic stenosis	1962
Idiopathic hypertrophic cardiomyopathy	1972
Idiopathic hypertrophic obstructive cardiomyopathy	1966
Idiopathic hypertrophic subaortic stenosis	1960
Idiopathic hypertrophic subvalvular stenosis	1966
Idiopathic muscular hypertrophic subaortic stenosis	1966
Idiopathic muscular stenosis of the left ventricle	1969
Idiopathic myocardial hypertrophy	1963
Idiopathic stenosis of the flushing chamber of the left ventricle	1964
Idiopathic ventricular septal hypertrophy	1962
Irregular hypertrophic cardiomyopathy	1968
Left ventricular muscular stenosis	1968
Low subvalvular aortic stenosis	1962
Muscular aortic stenosis	1969
Muscular hypertrophic stenosis of the left ventricle	1966
Muscular stenosis of the left ventricle	1961
Muscular subaortic stenosis	1966
Muscular subvalvular aortic stenosis	1964
Non-dilated cardiomyopathy	1974
Nonobstructive hypertrophic cardiomyopathy	1975
Obstructive cardiomyopathy	1960
Obstructive hypertrophic aortic stenosis	1967
Obstructive hypertrophic cardiomyopathy	1968
Obstructive hypertrophic myocardiopathy	1968

Hypertrophic Cardiomyopathy: An Overview

Table 1. (Continued)

Obstructive myocardiopathy	1968
Pseudoaortic stenosis	1958
Stenosing hypertrophy of the left ventricle	1966
Stenosis of the ejection chamber of the left ventricle	1966
Subaortic hypertrophic stenosis	1964
Subaortic idiopathic stenosis	1968
Subaortic muscular stenosis	1964
Subvalvular aortic stenosis of the muscular type	1962
Teare's disease	1977

Dates indicate the year that the term was first published.

greater than that of the septum. Moreover, in some patients the basal, anterior portion of the septum is of normal thickness, while portions of the anteriolateral left ventricular free wall, or posterior portion of the septum, are considerably thickened. Other patients have concentric hypertrophy, and still others have hypertrophy confined mainly to the cardiac apex [11 a, 13].

Our echocardiographic and necropsy studies conducted over the past several years in more than 500 patients also revealed that a disproportionately thickened ventricular septum could occur in association with a variety of congenital or acquired heart diseases [14–17]. When disproportionate septal hypertrophy occurred in such patients, the septal thickening was usually secondary to the patients' underlying lesion and not a manifestation of a coexistent primary cardiomyopathy [14–17].

Given these findings, we now consider that the single most consistent and characteristic feature of this disease is a hypertrophied nondilated left ventricle. When this abnormality is detected in the absence of a cardiac or systemic disease that itself can produce left ventricular hypertrophy, the diagnosis of hypertrophic cardiomyopathy is established. It would therefore seem most reasonable to refer to this disease as *hypertrophic cardiomyopathy*.

Hypertrophic cardiomyopathy also presents characteristic histological findings. Microscopic examination of the hearts of patients dying of the disease revealed malaligned myocardial cells in the ventricular septum [1, 18–22]. Subsequent quantitative studies indicated these cells occupy 5% or more (average about 30%) of the ventricular septum [22], and are also present, with somewhat less frequency, in the left ventricular free wall [23]. Although such abnormal myocardial cellular disarray can be found in other diseases, it is much less common and, when it appears, only small portions (i.e., less than 5%) of the myocardium are involved [24].

Natural History

Natural history studies of patients with hypertrophic cardiomyopathy suggest that overall annual mortality from the disease is about 3% per year [25, 26], with the majority of patients dying suddenly [26]. However, virtually all patients included in these studies were evaluated in the 1960s, prior to the general application of echocardiography. This technique, employed in the study of hypertrophic cardiomyopathy with increasing frequency since the early 1970s, has demonstrated that the disease spectrum of hypertrophic cardiomyopathy is considerably broader than previously suspected [8]. Hence, a comprehensive understanding of the natural history of this disease, and the precise incidence of sudden death in the many subgroups of patients with hypertrophic cardiomyopathy, is as yet unknown. Nonetheless, the fact remains that sudden death occurs not uncommonly.

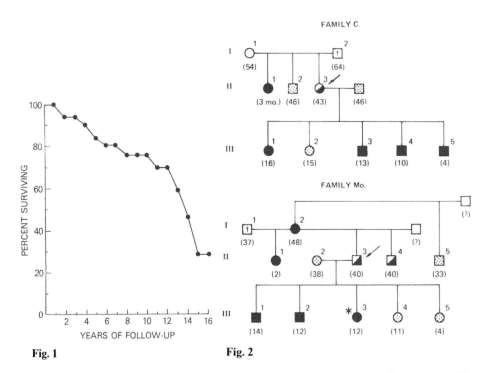

Fig. 1. Percent survival with time of the 35 children with hypertrophic cardiomyopathy. The marked decrease in survival occurring after the 12th year is due to the small numbers of patients who were followed for 13 or more years. [27]

Fig. 2. Pedigrees of "malignant" families C. and Mo. *Arrow*, propositus; *solid symbols*, death probably or due to hypertrophic cardiomyopathy; *half-filled* symbols, alive with an echocardiogram that was diagnostic of hypertrophic cardiomyopathy; *clear symbols*, echocardiogram not obtained. †, dead of noncardiac cause or cardiac disease other than hypertrophic cardiomyopathy; *stippled symbols*, alive but hypertrophic cardiomyopathy not evident in the echocardiogram; *circle*, female subjects; *squares*, male subjects. Only first degree relatives of the propositus are shown. Patients ages (yrs) are shown in parenthesis below the symbols. *, episode of cardiac arrest but has survived to date. [29]

Characteristics of Patients Experiencing Sudden Death

Although sudden death is frequently observed in adults with hypertrophic cardio-myopathy, it occurs commonly during childhood as well. We followed 35 children ranging in age from 4 to 18 years at the time of initial diagnosis [27]. In these patients the diagnosis of hypertrophic cardiomyopathy was established prior to the general availability of echocardiography. Over the course of 1 to 16 years (average 7½ years) 11 (31%) of the 35 patients died suddenly, yielding an annual mortality of approximately 4% per year (Fig. 1).

We have also identified and studied eight families in which at least two first de-gree relatives died prematurely (before 50 years of age) from hypertrophic cardio-myopathy [28]. We have termed these "malignant" families. A total of 69 first de-gree relatives in the eight malignant families were identified. Of these, 41 relatives had evidence of hypertrophic cardiomyopathy and 32 (78%) died of heart disease. Death was sudden and unexpected in 23 of the 31 patients. Two typical family trees are depicted in Fig. 2.

Symptomatic status was of no help in identifying patients at risk of sudden death. Of the 11 deaths that occurred in children with hypertrophic cardiomyopathy, three were asymptomatic and six were in New York Heart Association functional class II prior to sudden death [27]. Likewise, of the 23 patients from malignant families who died suddenly, 15 died without previously experiencing any symptoms whatsoever [28]. Finally, we have recently reported 26 patients (17 of whom were not from the malignant families) whose *first* manifestation of hypertrophic cardio-myopathy was sudden death [29], and have investigated the symptomatic status of 78 subjects who had hypertrophic cardiomyopathy and who died suddenly [29a]. The large majority of the latter had either no functional limitation or had mild symp-toms just prior to death (Table 2).

Table 2. 75 patients with sudden death[a]

Symptomatic status	Number of patients
No functional limitations	54%
Mild symptoms	31%
Severe symptoms	15%

[a] Excluding competitive athletes.

Hemodynamic Findings

Analysis of the three studies of patients who died suddenly [27–29a] yielded no hemodynamic findings that were predictive of sudden death. Fig. 3 illustrates the magnitude of the left ventricular outflow tract gradient in those patients who died and who had hemodynamic investigations prior to death [27–29a]. The data demon-strate that sudden death occurs both in patients with as well as in those without left ventricular outflow tract obstruction.

Likewise, left ventricular end diastolic pressure is not a good predictor of sudden death. Of the 12 patients who were studied and in whom sudden death was the first manifestation of disease [29], left ventricular end diastolic pressure was elevated (greater than 12 mmHg) in nine, but normal in three others. Moreover, while left ventricular end-diastolic pressure at initial study was elevated in 9 of the 11 (82%) children who subsequently died [27], it was also elevated in 16 of 21 (76%) who did not die (Fig. 4).

Ventricular Septal Thickness

Echocardiographic and necropsy measurements of ventricular septal thickness may provide some prognostic information in patients with hypertrophic cardiomyopathy [27–29a]. When ventricular septal thickness of patients with hypertrophic cardiomyopathy who died suddenly were compared to those of an age-matched group of living patients with the disease, no differences were observed. However, ventricular septal thickness of 20 mm or more were observed in 48 of the 62 patients (77%) we evaluated who died suddenly. It is perhaps of significance that in 7 of our 14 patients who had septal thick-

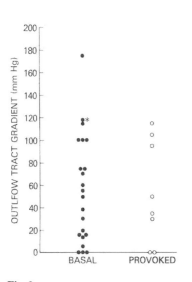 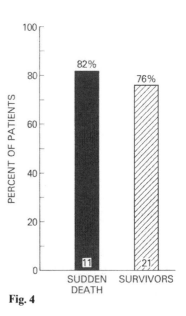

Fig. 3   **Fig. 4**

Fig. 3. Composite diagram of the left ventricular outflow tract gradient of all patients who died but were studied hemodynamically in three investigations [27–29a]. Asterisk indicates gradient across right ventricular outflow tract

Fig. 4. Percent of patients 4–18 years of age with left ventricular end diastolic pressure >12 mmHg

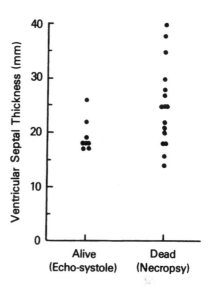

Fig. 5. Ventricular septal thicknesses obtained in eight surviving affected family members by echocardiography (echo) compared to those obtained at necropsy in 16 relatives who had died. Echocardiographic measurements shown were obtained in systole to permit comparison with necropsy measurements

ness of < 20 mm, other factors were present that could have contributed to the occurrence of a premature cardiac catastrophe in the presence of a relatively thin ventricular septum; i.e., a family history of "malignant" hypertrophic cardiomyopathy, or a competitive athletic life-style. Therefore, while absolute ventricular septal thickness cannot be used as a predictor of sudden death in a population of patients with hypertrophic cardiomyopathy, the finding of a ventricular septal thickness <20 mm in a patient who is not a competitive athlete or a member of a "malignant" family, suggests that individual is probably at low risk for sudden death.

That marked septal hypertrophy portends a greater tendency to sudden death is also reflected in our studies of malignant families [28]. The average ventricular septal thickness of those family members who died was greater than that of the surviving member (25 mm vs 19 mm). In particular, nine of ten subjects (90%) with a ventricular septal thickness ≥ 25 mm died, while only 7 of 14 relatives (50%) with septal thickness less than 25 mm died (Fig. 5). Thus, there appears to be a trend relating septal thickness and sudden death, although a relatively thin septum does not preclude the possibility of sudden death (Fig. 5).

Electrocardiographic Findings

Of the patients we studied who died suddenly, 53 had had a standard 12-lead ECG obtained, which was distinctly abnormal in all but two patients. The most common abnormalities (alone or in combination) were left ventricular hypertrophy, ST segment and T wave abnormalities, or abnormal Q waves. Although the vast majority of patients with hypertrophic cardiomyopathy and obstruction to left ventricular outflow have an abnormal ECG, it is normal in about one-quarter of asymptomatic patients without obstruction [30]. Such subjects may be at lower risk of sudden death. On the other hand, because the large majority of patients with hypertrophic cardiomyopathy have abnormal electrocardiograms, the mere *presence* of this sign cannot be employed as a specific predictor of sudden death.

Identification of Arrhythmias

Ambulatory ECG monitoring revealed that patients with hypertrophic cardiomyopathy have an alarming frequency of arrhythmias, including high-grade ventricular arrhythmias [30–32]. In a study from our laboratory [30], 100 patients with hypertrophic cardiomyopathy were studied with 24-h ambulatory monitoring. Grading of VPBs was performed according to the method of Lown (Table 3). Ventricu-

Table 3. Grading of ventricular premature beats

Grade 0	= no VPBs in 24 h
Grade 1	= occasional VPBs, but not more than 30 in any hour of monitoring
Grade 2	= more than 30 VPBs in any hour of monitoring
Grade 3	= multiform VPBs
Grade 4a	= Couplets (two consecutive VPBs)
Grade 4b	= ventricular tachycardia (3 or more VPBs in succession)

lar arrhythmias were documented in 83% of the 100 patients. Only 35% had no or low grade ($\leqq$ VPB grade II) ventricular arrhythmia; 60% had multiform VPBs, 32% had pairs of VPBs (couplets), and 19% had ventricular tachycardia with a rate equivalent to 100 beats/min or more. High-grade VPBs (grade III or higher) occurred in more than 50% of each of the subgroups of patients, i.e., regardless of whether or not symptoms or left ventricular outflow tract obstruction were present (Fig. 6).

No significant correlation between left ventricular outflow gradient and maximum VPB grade was found. However, patients with septal thickness of at least 20 mm had a greater frequency of high grade VPBs than those with septal thickness less than 20 mm (Fig. 7). Thus, while 78% of patients (52 of 67) with septal thickness $\geqq$ 20 mm had grade III VPBs or higher, only 39% (13 of 33) of patients with septal thickness of less than 20 mm had such arrhythmias ($P<0.005$).

We followed the patients who were monitored for arrhythmias over the ensuing 3 years [33a]. Of the 84 patients who did not undergo ventricular septal myotomy-myectomy, six died suddenly or experienced cardiac arrest, one died of progressive congestive heart failure, and the other 77 survived without a cardiac catastrophe. The prevalence of sudden death or cardiac arrest during the follow-up period was the same in patients with high-grade arrhythmias other than ventricular tachycardia (1 of 37 or 3%) as in those with no or low-grade arrhythmias (1 of 29 or 3%). However, the occurrence of sudden cardiac catastrophe was significantly more common in those patients with asymptomatic ventricular tachycardia of brief duration on their 24-h electrocardiogram (4 of 17 or 24%) than in those patients without ventricular tachycardia (2 of 66 or 3%; $P<0.02$).

These results lead to the following conclusions: 1) high-grade ventricular arrhythmias are commonly found in patients with hypertrophic cardiomyopathy by

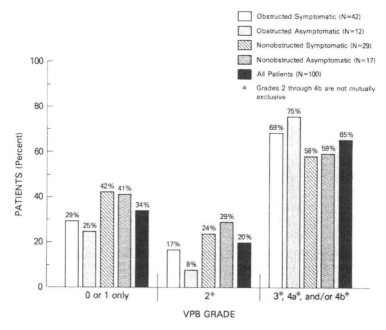

Fig. 6. Prevalence of different grades of ventricular premature beats (VPB) during 24-h in subgroups of patients with hypertrophic cardiomyopathy. [31]

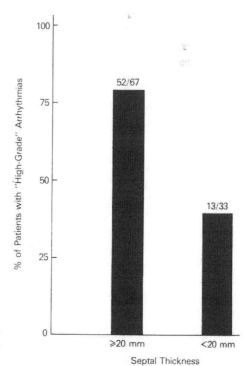

Fig. 7. Relation of septal thickness to prevalence of high-grade ventricular arrhythmias

14 Stephen E. Epstein and Barry J. Maron

continuous 24-h electrocardiographic monitoring; and (2) while sudden death is relatively uncommon in patients with high-grade ventricular arrhythmias other than ventricular tachycardia (annual mortality 1%), the finding of ventricular tachycardia on 24-h electrocardiogram identifies a subgroup of patients at high-risk for sudden death (annual mortality 8.6%).

Ventricular Function

Although it has long been known that patients with hypertrophic cardiomyopathy have hypercontractile ventricles, a complete assessment of ventricular systolic function at rest and during exercise, as well as of ventricular diastolic function, has only recently been initiated [34–38]. Most patients demonstrate normal or supernormal ejection fraction under resting conditions. However, there are a few patients who manifest impairment of systolic function during the terminal phase of their disease such that ejection fraction is reduced [34, 35]. Although data are incomplete, it appears as though a minority of patients experience this clinical course. We have also found in preliminary studies that while most patients with hypertrophic cardiomyopathy demonstrate normal or supernormal systolic function both at rest *and* during exercise, a relatively high percentage of symptomatic patients with the nonobstructive form of the disease manifest impaired systolic function during exercise [35]. The relation of impaired systolic function during exercise in patients with nonobstructive hypertrophic cardiomyopathy to clinical course is at this time uncertain.

It has been appreciated for many years [34, 36] that a major abnormality present in patients with hypertrophic cardiomyopathy is a diminution in left ventricular compliance with resultant increased resistance to left ventricular filling; this causes an increase in left ventricular filling pressures and the symptoms associated with pulmonary venous congestion. However, sensitive techniques capable of reliably and noninvasively quantitating this abnormality have only recently been developed. Based on such techniques, it has been found that abnormalities in diastolic function are common [37–38 a]. In particular, we found in a series of 50 patients with hypertrophic cardiomyopathy that 70% exhibited impaired diastolic filling [38 a]. This abnormality is characterized by a diminished maximal rate of left ventricular filling, as well as a prolongation of the time from end systole to time of maximal filling rate. Although it is uncertain how important this abnormality is to the symptomatic condition of the patients, preliminary studies indicate that while propranolol does not improve the abnormality in left ventricular filling, administration of verapamil often normalizes or considerably improves left ventricular filling characteristics [38, 38 a].

Therapy

Beta-adrenergic receptor blockade has been the major medical approach to therapy of patients with hypertrophic cardiomyopathy. Propranolol improves exercise capacity, alleviates symptoms of lightheadedness and syncope, and diminishes the frequency of angina pectoris [8, 39, 40]. The drug is usually successful in patients with the obstructive form of the disease, but less successful in those patients without obstruction. Until recently, when patients with obstruction did not experience adequate

Hypertrophic Cardiomyopathy: An Overview   15

symptomatic relief with propranolol, no other definitive form of medical therapy was available, and we therefore recommended operation. The operative procedure consists of removing a portion of the hypertrophied ventricular septal muscle that lies opposite the anterior leaflet of the mitral valve and which, together with the anterior leaflet, impinges on the left ventricular outflow tract in systole [41]. Operation results in abolition or substantial amelioration of left ventricular outflow obstruction, and marked symptomatic improvement in the large majority of patients [42].

Despite the availability of beta-adrenergic blockade and operative intervention, there are many patients who have not experienced therapeutic success. Thus, some patients who die suddenly or from progressive congestive symptoms, die or deteriorate despite large doses of propranolol. Moreover, although operation almost invariably leads to relief of left ventricular outflow obstruction, annual mortality following operation is still almost 2% [42]. Hence, considerably more remains to be accomplished in terms of (1) the recognition of factors that are predictive of sudden death and (2) the development of therapeutic modalities that can more successfully control symptoms and that can favorably alter the primary disease process. Whether slow channel calcium inhibitors will provide one such modality remains to be determined. It is the purpose of this symposium to review the results of the initial studies relating to the theoretical rationale and practical utility of slow channel calcium inhibitors in the therapy of hypertrophic cardiomyopathy.

References

1. Teare RD (1958) Asymmetrical hypertrophy of the heart in young adults. Br Heart J 20: 1–8
2. Braunwald E, Morrow AG, Cornell WP, Aygen MM, Hillbish TF (1960) Idiopathic hypertrophic subaortic stenosis: hemodynamic and angiographic manifestations. Am J Med 29: 924–945
3. Wigle ED, Heimbecker RO, Gunton RW (1962) Idiopathic ventricular septal hypertrophy causing muscular subaortic stenosis. Circulation 26: 325–340
4. Cohen J, Effat H, Goodwin JF, Oakley CM, Steiner RE (1964) Hypertrophic obstructive cardiomyopathy. Br Heart J 26: 16–32
5. Henry WL, Clark CE, Epstein SE (1973) Asymmetric septal hypertrophy (ASH): echocardiographic identification of the pathognomonic anatomic abnormality of IHSS. Circulation 47: 225–233
6. Abbasi AS, MacAlpin RN, Eber LM, Pearce ML (1972) Echocardiographic diagnosis of idiopathic hypertrophic cardiomyopathy without outflow obstruction. Circulation 46: 897–904
7. Abbasi AS, MacAlpin RN, Eber LM, Pearce ML (1973) Left ventricular hypertrophy diagnosed by echocardiography. N Engl J Med 289: 118–121
8. Epstein SE, Henry WL, Clark CE, Roberts WC, Maron BJ, Ferrans VJ, Redwood DR, Morrow AG (1974) Asymmetric septal hypertrophy. Ann Intern Med 81: 650–680
9. Clark CE, Henry WL, Epstein SE (1973) Familial prevalence and genetic transmission of idiopathic hypertrophic subaortic stenosis. N Engl J Med 289: 709–714
10. Van Dorp WG, Ten Cate FJ, Vletter WB, Dohmen H, Roelandt J (1976) Familial prevalence of asymmetric septal hypertrophy. Eur J Cardiol 4: 349–357
11. Maron BJ, Epstein SE (1979) Hypertrophic cardiomyopathy: A discussion of nomenclature. Am J Cardiol 43: 1242–1244

11a. Maron BJ, Gottdiener JS, Epstein SE (1981) Patterns and significance of the distribution of left ventricular hypertrophy in hypertrophic cardiomyopathy: A wide-angle two-dimensional echocardiographic study of 125 patients. J Cardiol 48:418–428

12. Maron BJ, Gottdiener JS, Bonow RO, Epstein SE (1981) Hypertrophic cardiomyopathy with unusual locations of left ventricular hypertrophy undetectable by M-mode echocardiography: Identification by wide-angle two-dimensional echocardiography. Circulation 63:409–418

13. Yamaguchi H, Ishimura T, Nishiyanna S, Nagasaki F, Nakanishi S, Takatsu F, Nishijo T, Umeda T, Machii K (1979) Hypertrophic nonobstructive cardiomyopathy with giant negative T waves (apical hypertrophy): ventriculographic and echocardiographic features in 30 patients. Am J Cardiol 44:401–412

14. Maron BJ, Clark CE, Henry WL, Fukuda T, Edwards JE, Mathews EC, Redwood DR, Epstein SE (1977) Prevalence and characteristics of disproportionate ventricular septal thickening in patients with acquired or congenital heart disease: echocardiographic and morphologic findings. Circulation 55:489–496

15. Maron BJ, Edwards JE, Epstein SE (1978) Prevalence and characteristics of disproportionate ventricular septal thickening in patients with systemic hypertension. Chest 73:466–470

16. Maron BJ, Savage DD, Clark CE, Henry WL, Vlodaver Z, Edwards JE, Epstein SE (1978) Prevalence and characteristics of disproportionate ventricular septal thickening in patients with coronary artery disease. Circulation 57:250–255

17. Maron BJ, Edwards JE, Ferrans VJ, Clark CE, Lebowitz EA, Henry WL, Epstein SE (1975) Congenital heart malformations associated with disproportionate ventricular septal thickening. Circulation 52:926–932

18. Paré JA, Fraser RG, Pirozynski WJ, Shanks JA, Stubington D (1961) Hereditary cardiovascular dysplasia: A form of familial cardiomyopathy. Am J Med 31:37–62

19. Ferrans VJ, Morrow AG, Roberts WC (1972) Myocardial ultrastructure in idiopathic hypertrophic subaortic stenosis. A study of operatively excised left ventricular outflow tract muscle in 14 patients. Circulation 45:769–792

20. Maron BJ, Ferrans VJ, Henry WL, Clark CE, Redwood DR, Roberts WC, Morrow AG, Epstein SE (1974) Differences in distribution of myocardial abnormalities in patients with obstructive and nonobstructive asymmetric septal hypertrophy (ASH): Light and electron microscopic findings. Circulation 50:436–446

21. Maron BJ, Epstein SE, Roberts WC (1978) Cardiac muscle cell disorganization in the ventricular septum: Evidence from quantitative histology that it is a highly sensitive marker of hypertrophic cardiomyopathy (Abstr). Am J Cardiol 41:435

22. Maron BJ, Epstein SE (1980) Hypertrophic cardiomyopathy: Recent observations regarding the specificity of three hallmarks of the disease: ASH, Septal Disorganization and SAM. Am J Cardiol 45:141–154

23. Maron BJ, Anan TJ, Roberts WC (to be published) Quantitative analysis of the distribution of cardiac muscle cell disorganization in the left ventricular wall of patients with hypertrophic cardiomyopathy. Circulation

24. Maron BJ, Roberts WC (1979) Quantitative analysis of cardiac muscle cell disorganization in the ventricular septum of patients with hypertrophic cardiomyopathy. Circulation 59:689–706

25. Hardarson T, De La Calzada CS, Curiel R, Goodwin JF (1973) Prognosis and mortality of hypertrophic obstructive cardiomyopathy. Lancet 2:1462–1467

26. Shah PM, Adelman AG, Wigle ED, Gobel FL, Burchell HB, Hardarson T, Curiel R, De La Calzada C, Oakley CM, Goodwin JF (1973) The natural (and unnatural) course of hypertrophic obstructive cardiomyopathy. A multicenter study. Circ Res (Suppl II) 24 and 25:179–195

27. Maron BJ, Henry WL, Clark CE, Redwood DR, Roberts WC, Epstein SE (1976) Asymmetric septal hypertrophy in childhood. Circulation 52:9–19
28. Maron BJ, Lipson LC, Roberts WC, Savage DS, Epstein SE (1978) "Malignant" hypertrophic cardiomyopathy: Identification of a subgroup of families with unusually frequent premature death. Am J Cardiol 41:1133–1140
29. Maron BJ, Roberts WC, Edwards JE, McAllister HA, Foley DD, Epstein SE (1978) Sudden death in patients with hypertrophic cardiomyopathy: characterization of 26 patients without functional limitation. Am J Cardiol 41:803–810
29a. Maron BJ, Roberts WC, Epstein SE (1982) Sudden death in hypertrophic cardiomyopathy: profile of 78 patients. Circulation (in press)
30. Savage DD, Seides SF, Clark CE, Henry WL, Maron BJ, Robinson FC, Epstein SE (1978) Electrocardiographic findings in patients with obstructive and nonobstructive hypertrophic cardiomyopathy. Circulation 58:402–408
31. Ingham RE, Rossen RM, Goodman DJ, Harrison DC (1975) Ambulatory electrocardiographic monitoring in idiopathic hypertrophic subaortic stenosis (Abstr). Circulation (Suppl II) 52:83
32. McKenna WJ, Chetty S, Oakley CM, Goodwin JF (1980) Arrhythmia in hypertrophic cardiomyopathy: Exercise and 48 hour ambulatory electrocardiographic assessment with and without beta adrenergic blocking therapy. Am J Cardiol 45:1–5
33. Maron BJ, Epstein SE, Roberts WC (1979) Hypertrophic cardiomyopathy and transmural myocardial infarction without significant atherosclerosis of the extramural coronary arteries. Am J Cardiol 43:1086–1102
33a. Maron BJ, Savage DD, Wolfson JK, Epstein SE (1981) Prognostic significance of 24-hour ambulatory electrocardiographic monitoring in patients with hypertrophic cardiomyopathy: a prospective study. Amer J Cardiol 48:252–257
34. Goodwin JF, Oakley CM (1972) The cardiomyopathies. Br Heart J 34:545–552
35. Borer JS, Bacharach SL, Green MV, Kent KM, Maron BJ, Rosing DR, Seides SF, Epstein SE (1978) Obstructive vs nonobstructive asymmetric septal hypertrophy: differences in left ventricular function with exercise (Abstr) Am J Cardiol 41:379
36. Steward S, Mason D, Braunwald E (1968) Impaired rate of left ventricular filling in idiopathic hypertrophic subaortic stenosis and valvular aortic stenosis. Circulation 37:8–14
37. St John Sutton MG, Tajik AJ, Gibson DG, Brown DJ, Seward JB, Giuliani ER (1978) Echocardiographic assessment of left ventricular filling and septal and posterior wall dynamics in idiopathic subaortic stenosis. Circulation 57:512–520
38. Hanrath P, Mathey DG, Siegert R, Bleifeld W (1980) Left ventricular relaxation and filling pattern in different forms of left ventricular hypertrophy: and echocardiographic study. Am J Cardiol 45:15–23
38a. Bonow RO, Rosing DR, Bacharach SL, Green MV, Kent KM, Lipson LC, Maron BJ, Leon MB, Epstein SE (1981) Effects of verapamil on left ventricular systolic function and diastolic filling in patients with hypertrophic cardiomyopathy. Circulation 64:787–796
39. Cohen LS, Braunwald E (1967) Amelioration of angina pectoris in idiopathic hypertrophic subaortic stenosis with beta-adrenergic blockade. Circulation 35:847–851
40. Hubner PJB, Ziady G, Lane GK, et al (1973) Double-blind trial of propranolol and practolol in hypertrophic cardiomyopathy. Br Heart J 35:1116–1123
41. Morrow AG (1978) Hypertrophic subaortic stenosis: operative methods utilized to relieve left ventricular outflow obstruction. J Thorac Cardiovasc Surg 76:423–430
42. Maron BJ, Merrill WH, Freier PA, Kent KM, Epstein SE, Morrow AG (1978) Long-term clinical course and symptomatic status of patients after operation for hypertrophic subaortic stenosis. Circulation 57:1205–1213

Echocardiographic Identification of Patterns of Left Ventricular Hypertrophy in Hypertrophic Cardiomyopathy*

BARRY J. MARON, JOHN S. GOTTDIENER, and STEPHEN E. EPSTEIN

Summary

Four patterns of distribution of left ventricular hypertrophy may be identified by wide-angle two-dimensional echocardiography in patients with hypertrophic cardiomyopathy. Most commonly (52% of 125 patients) hypertrophy involved substantial portions of both the ventricular septum and anterolateral left ventricular free wall (type III). In other patients, hypertrophy was confined to the anterior portion of ventricular septum (type I), involved the entire ventricular septum but not left ventricular free wall (type II), or was identified in regions of the septum or free wall other than the basal, anterior ventricular septum (type IV). In the latter subgroup of patients, conventional M-mode echocardiography failed to identify the presence of hypertrophy and therefore the diagnosis of hypertrophic cardiomyopathy could be established only by two-dimensional echocardiography. Therefore, the absence of asymmetric septal hypertrophy (or left ventricular hypertrophy) on the M-mode echocardiogram does not exclude the diagnosis of hypertrophic cardiomyopathy in a patient in whom other ancillary data suggest this diagnosis (such as an abnormal electrocardiogram or a family history of hypertrophic cardiomyopathy).

Compared with patients having the other patterns of distribution, those patients with the most widespread hypertrophy involving most of the ventricular septum as well as portions of the free wall (type III): (1) more commonly experienced moderate to severe functional limitation (38 of 65 or 58% vs 16 of 60 or 27%; $P<0.001$) and (2) more often demonstrated obstruction to left ventricular outflow under basal conditions (36 of 65 or 55% vs 11 of 60 or 18%; $P<0.001$).

Hence, although left ventricular hypertrophy is "asymmetric" in most patients with hypertrophic cardiomyopathy, it is usually not confined to the ventricular septum, often involves the anterolateral left ventricular free wall, but rarely involves the posterior portion of left ventricular free wall through which the M-mode beam passes. In patients with hypertrophic cardiomyopathy, wide-angle two-dimensional echocardiography is capable of detecting myocardial hypertrophy that involves a variety of patterns and may be more extensive than may be appreciated by M-mode echocardiography.

Introduction

M-mode (one-dimensional) echocardiography has shown asymmetric hypertrophy of the ventricular septum relative to the posterior left ventricular free wall to be

---

* This paper has already been published, in part, in American Journal of Cardiology and Circulation

2-D Echo in Cardiomyopathy

a characteristic anatomic feature of hypertrophic cardiomyopathy [1–7]. However, conventional M-mode echocardiography permits assessment of hypertrophy in only limited areas of the left ventricular wall. In contrast, wide-angle two-dimensional echocardiography is a technique that provides the capability of visualizing greater portions of the left ventricular wall [8–11]. Therefore, to characterize more completely the distribution of hypertrophy throughout the left ventricular wall, and to determine whether different patterns of hypertrophy are of particular clinical significance, a large population of patients with hypertrophic cardiomyopathy were studied by two-dimensional echocardiography.

Selection of Patients

Between February 1979 and November 1979, at the National Heart, Lung, and Blood Institute, 125 patients who were diagnosed or suspected clinically of having hypertrophic cardiomyopathy had a technically satisfactory M-mode and two-dimensional echocardiographic examination.

The criterion that was employed to establish the diagnosis of hypertrophic cardiomyopathy in the 125 patients was the demonstration, by M-mode and two-dimensional echocardiography, of a nondilated, hypertrophied left ventricle (in the absence of another cardiac or systemic disease which itself was capable of producing left ventricular hypertrophy) [12].

Characterization of Patients

The 125 study patients ranged in age from 5 to 64 years (mean 34). Seventy-seven (62%) patients were male and 48 (38%) were female. Thirty-nine (31%) of the 125 patients had no functional limitation (New York Heart Association class I), including nine with trivial transient symptoms. Thirty-two (26%) had mild symptoms (functional class II) and 54 (43%) had moderate to severe functional limitation (classes III and IV).

Cardiac catheterization was performed in 88 (70%) of the 125 patients. Left ventricular outflow obstruction was considered to be present if the peak systolic outflow gradient under basal conditions was ≥ 30 mmHg; outflow tract obstruction was considered to be absent if the gradient was zero or <30 mmHg. Those patients in whom catheterization had not been performed, or was carried out more than 1 year before the echocardiographic study (83 patients), were categorized with regard to the presence or absence of outflow obstruction based on the magnitude and duration of systolic anterior motion of the anterior mitral leaflet on the M-mode echocardiogram [13].

Methods

M-Mode Echocardiography

M-mode echocardiograms were performed using a 2.25 MHz, 1.25 cm diameter unfocused Aerotech transducer and a Hoffrel 201 ultrasound receiver interfaced with a

Honeywell 1856 strip chart recorder. Maximum thickness of the ventricular septum was measured just prior to atrial systole with the ultrasound beam directed slightly below the caudal margins of the mitral leaflets or through the leaflet tips. Thickness of the posterior left ventricular free wall was measured during the same phase of the cardiac cycle, with the ultrasound beam passing through the mitral leaflet tips.

Two-Dimensional Echocardiography

A Varian (V-3000) real-time, phased-array, 80° ultrasonic sector scanner with hand-held 2.25 MHz transducer was used to perform the two-dimensional echocardiographic studies [14].

The two-dimensional echocardiographic examination included the imaging of a number of cross-sectional planes through the heart [15, 16]. Serial short-axis views of the left of ventricle were obtained by initially orienting the sector plane perpendicular to the long axis of the left ventricle from a standard transducer placement on the chest. The "short-axis sweep" was performed by maintaining the transducer in a fixed location on the chest wall and slowly angling the image plane from aorta (cephalad) to apex (caudad) [15]. However, in the short-axis view, ultrasound beam angulation from a single fixed transducer location prohibits imaging multiple cross-sectional planes that are truly perpendicular to the left ventricular cephalad-caudad

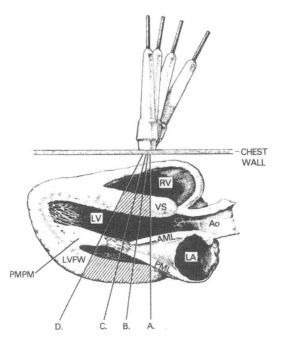

Fig. 1. Diagrammatic representation of the heart in the long-axis orientation illustrating that sequential tomographic planes (*A*–*D*) obtained from a fixed transducer site on the chest are not truly parallel to each other. Taken in sum this "short-axis scan" actually includes significantly greater portions of posterior structures (e.g., posterior left ventricular free wall) than anterior structures (e.g., anterior portion of ventricular septum)

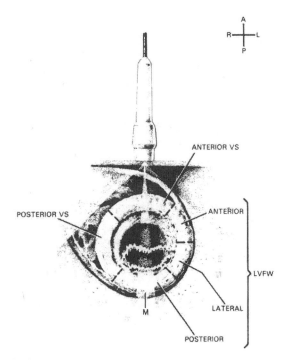

Fig. 2. Segments of left ventricular wall visualized by wide-angle (80°) two-dimensional echocardiography in the short-axis (anteroposterior) plane. Note the left mitral valve commissure is the anatomic landmark dividing the anterior from the lateral left ventricular free wall. Also shown is the expected approximate path of the conventional M-mode echo beam (*M*) through the anterior ventricular septum and posterior left ventricular free wall. *LVFW*, left ventricular free wall; *VS*, ventricular septum

axis. Therefore, apical portions of the anterior regions of the left ventricular wall (e.g. anterior ventricular septum) are not well visualized in the short-axis plane (Fig. 1); however, these regions of the left ventricle may often be visualized in the long-axis and apical views.

The long-axis view was obtained by orienting the sector plane parallel to the longitudinal axis of the left ventricle taking care to avoid improper angulation of the scan plane tangentially through the ventricle [17]. The apical four-chamber view was obtained with the transducer placed at the cardiac apex and the tomographic plane directed perpendicular to the ventricular and atrial septa and through the plane of the mitral and tricuspid valve orifices to permit simultaneous display of both atria and ventricles, atrioventricular valves, and cardiac septa [18].

The location of regions of hypertrophy was described in two cross-sectional planes. In the *anteroposterior plane*, hypertrophy was designated as involving either the ventricular septum or the left ventricular free wall. The ventricular septum was divided into two equal segments (anterior and posterior). The left ventricular free wall was divided into three approximately equal-sized segments, the anterior, lateral, and posterior (Fig. 2). In the *cephalad-caudad plane* the left ventricle was divided into two segments: the basal portion, which extends from cardiac base to

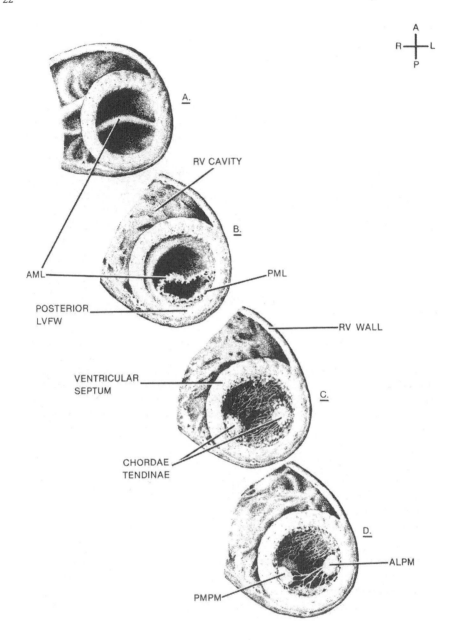

Fig. 3A–D. Artistic representation of cross-sectional planes (short-axis view) of the normal heart. (A) Level of left ventricular outflow tract. (B) Level of mitral valve leaflets. (C) Level at which the left ventricle is viewed just caudal to the tips of the mitral leaflets. (D) Level at which the papillary muscles are viewed. In subsequent figures utilizing the short-axis view, orientation of the heart is the same as shown here. *ALPM*, anterolateral papillary muscle; *AML*, anterior mitral leaflet; *A*, anterior; *L*, patient's left; *LVFW*, left ventricular free wall; *P*, posterior; *PML*, posterior mitral leaflet; *PMPM*, posteromedial papillary muscle; *R*, patient's right; *RV*, right ventricular

the inferior margins of the mitral leaflets, and the apical portion, which includes that portion of the left ventricle visualized caudal to the mitral leaflets.

For the purposes of this study, hypertrophy of the anterolateral left ventricular free wall was considered to be present if the wall was judged at two or more points to be at least 17 mm in thickness in adult patients ($\geq$ 15 mm in children younger than 16 years of age). These criteria of anterolateral free wall thickness were selected to ensure that (even assuming a potential lateral resolution error of 2–5 mm [14]) the frequency with which free wall hypertrophy was identified in our patients would not be overestimated.

For the purposes of comparison, two-dimensional echocardiograms were also performed in 30 volunteer subjects without heart disease, aged 15 to 54 years (mean 28); 16 were male and 14 were female. In none of these control subjects were regions of hypertrophy identified in the left ventricular wall (Fig. 3). In the short-axis view maximum ventricular septal thickness ranged from 7 to 10 mm (mean 9 ± 0.2 SEM.) and maximum anterolateral free wall thickness ranged from 7 to 10 mm (mean 8 ± 0.2).

Results

M-Mode Echocardiographic Findings

Ventricular septal thicknesses ranged from 6 to 41 mm (mean 21) and were particularly substantial ($\geq$ 30 mm) in 15 (12%). In 103 patients septal thickness was increased ($\geq$ 15 mm in adult patients; greater than the 95% prediction interval relative to body surface area in children less than 16 years of age [19]); in the remaining 22 (18%) patients the ventricular septal thickness was normal. Posterior left ventricular free wall thickness ranged from 6 to 19 mm (mean 12).

Asymmetric septal hypertrophy (septal to posterior free wall thickness ratio $\geq$ 1.3) was present in 98 (78%) of patients and ranged from 1.3 to 3.8, mean 1.7. Concentric (symmetric) left ventricular wall thickening (septal-free wall thickness ratio <1.3) [20] was present in 5 (4%) of the patients; the remaining 22 (18%) patients had both normal septal-free wall ratio and ventricular wall thicknesses [21] (Fig. 4).

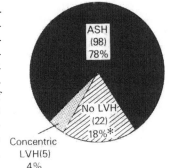

Fig. 4. M-mode echocardiographic assessment of septal-free wall ratio in 125 patients with hypertrophic cardiomyopathy*. Nine of the 22 patients without left ventricular hypertrophy (*LVH*) were specifically invited to have a two-dimensional echocardiographic study to determine the significance of an abnormal electrocardiogram (and a family history of hypertrophic cardiomyopathy) in the absence of ventricular wall thickening on the M-mode echocardiogram [21]. With these nine patients excluded from the data analysis 12% of the total study group showed absence of left ventricular hypertrophy on the M-mode echocardiogram. *ASH*, asymmetric septal hypertrophy

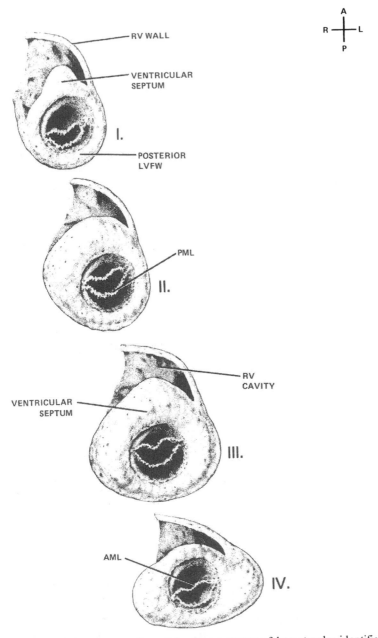

Fig. 5. Artistic representation of the four patterns of hypertrophy identified by wide-angle two-dimensional echocardiography in 125 patients with hypertrophic cardiomyopathy. Shown only are cross-sectional planes at the level of the mitral valve. *AML*, anterior mitral leaflet. *LVFW*, left ventricular free wall. *PML*, posterior mitral leaflet. *RV*, right ventricular

Two-Dimensional Echocardiographic Findings

Four basic patterns of distribution of left ventricular hypertrophy were identified by two-dimensional echocardiography (Figs. 5–11).

Type I. In 12 (10%) of the 125 patients hypertrophy was confined to the anterior portion of the ventricular septum (Figs. 5 and 6) the region of septum through which the M-mode ultrasound beam passes; the left ventricular free wall and posterior portion of ventricular septum appeared essentially normal. In 4 of these 12 patients hypertrophy in this relatively localized region was substantial and appeared (in the short-axis view) as a "mound" of myocardium on the anterior ventricular septum (Fig. 5).

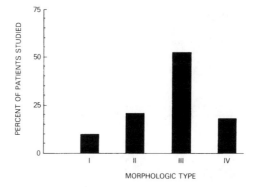

Fig. 6. Prevalence of four patterns of hypertrophy identified by wide-angle two-dimensional echocardiography in 125 patients with hypertrophic cardiomyopathy

Type II. In 25 (20%) of the 125 patients, hypertrophy involved both the anterior and posterior segments of ventricular septum; the left ventricular free wall appeared essentially normal (Figs. 5 and 6). In 18 patients the anterior and posterior regions of the septum were approximately equal in thickness or the anterior septal thickness clearly exceeded posterior septal thickness; posterior septal hypertrophy exceeded that of the anterior septum in the other seven patients.

Type III. In 65 (52%) of the 125 patients hypertrophy involved substantial portions of both the ventricular septum and the left ventricular free wall (Figs. 5–7). Most commonly (41 of 65 patients) the predominant region of left ventricular hypertrophy was in the anterior (Fig. 7A) or posterior (Fig. 7B) ventricular septum; in four other patients hypertrophy was predominant in the anterolateral free wall. In the remaining 20 patients the hypertrophied segments of septum and free wall were relatively equal in thickness.

In 60 of the 65 patients with type III, the posterior free wall segment through which the M-mode beam passes was either equal to or thinner than any other segment of the left ventricular wall (Fig. 7A). In the other five patients, however, the posterior free wall was considerably thickened (≥ 20 mm).

Type IV. In 23 (18%) of the 125 patients the anterior ventricular septum in the basal portion of the left ventricle and the posterior left ventricular free wall were normal thickness (Fig. 12). Patients with type IV hypertrophy were usually suspected clinically of having hypertrophic cardiomyopathy because of a distinctly abnor-

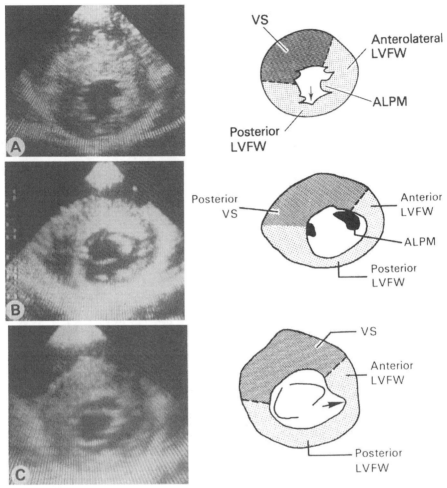

Fig. 7A–C. Stop-frames of two-dimensional echocardiograms (during diastole in short-axis view) showing anatomic variations in patients with type III distribution of hypertrophy. (A) Substantial hypertrophy of both the ventricular septum and anterolateral left ventricular free wall; a portion of the posterior free wall (*arrow*) is the thinnest region of the left ventricle; (B) Hypertrophy of the ventricular septum which is most marked in the posterior segment (but also involves the contiguous portion of posterior free wall. The anterior left ventricular free wall is hypertrophied while the lateral free wall is spared. (C) Marked hypertrophy of the ventricular septum and anterior free wall. Note "tapered" configuration of the septum and thin lateral free wall (*arrow*).

mal scalar electrocardiogram (usually showing deep Q waves, T wave alterations, or right ventricular hypertrophy) (Fig. 13) and either a family history of hypertrophic cardiomyopathy or cardiac symptoms. However, in each of these patients, M-mode echocardiography showed *no* evidence of hypertrophy (Fig. 14). Nevertheless, two-dimensional echocardiography revealed substantial hypertrophy in other regions of the left ventricular wall, inaccessible to the M-mode echo beam (Figs. 5, 9C, and

11). In 13 patients hypertrophy predominantly involved portions of the ventricular septum; in nine of these patients hypertrophy was present only in the posterior segment of septum (Fig. 11 A) and in the four other patients was confined to the septum in the apical region of the left ventricular wall (Fig. 9 C). In nine patients, hypertrophy predominantly involved portions of the anterolateral left ventricular free wall (Fig. 11 B). The remaining patient showed considerable hypertrophy of both the anterolateral free wall and posterior septum.

Comparison of M-Mode and Two-Dimensional Echocardiography

M-mode echocardiography proved to be relatively insensitive in identifying the predominant region of left ventricular hypertrophy in many patients. In 47 (37%) of the 125 patients discrepancies between M-mode and two-dimensional echocardiogra-

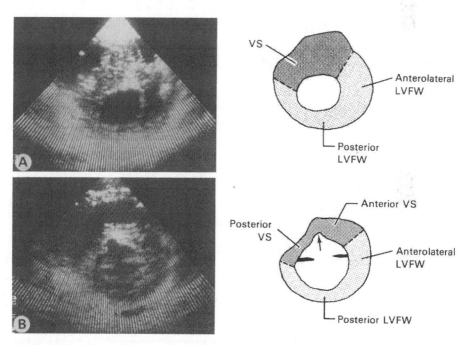

Fig. 8A, B. Unusual variations in the morphology of the anterior ventricular septum, shown in stop-frames of two-dimensional echocardiograms (obtained during diastole in the short-axis view). Each stop-frame is accompanied by a schematic illustration. (A) Bizarrely shaped region of ventricular septal hypertrophy. This substantial "mound" of septal myocardium (about 4 cm in thickness) has a "squared-off" appearance. The posterior segment of ventricular septum and anterolateral free wall were also markedly hypertrophied in this patient; (B) Hypertrophy involves only that portion of anterior ventricular septum adjacent to the thickened anterolateral free wall (shown here at the level of the chordae tendinae). Also, note the localized thinner area in the anterior ventricular septum (*arrow*). It is possible for the M-mode beam to traverse either this "notch" or the contiguous thickened area of anterior septum. *AML*, anterior mitral leaflet; *LVFW*, left ventricular free wall; *VS*, ventricular septum

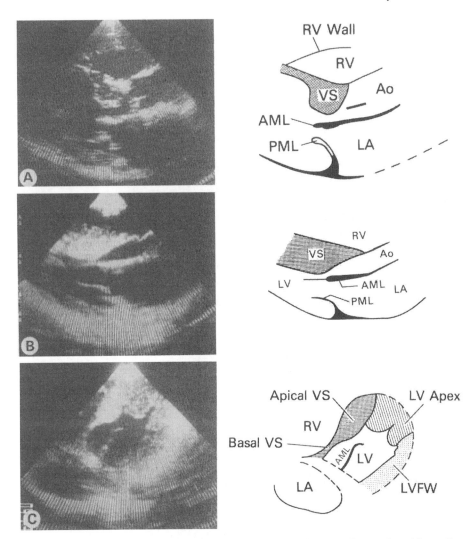

Fig. 9A–C. Spectrum of the distribution of ventricular septal hypertrophy, as viewed in cardiac base to apex planes. (A) Long-axis view showing ventricular septal hypertrophy confined to the most cephalad portion of anterior septum (in a patient with type I), producing the appearance of a prominent but localized "bump"; distal septal thickness appears normal; (B) Long-axis view showing ventricular septal hypertrophy located predominantly distal to the mitral valve leaflets; (C) Apical two-chamber view showing hypertrophy confined primarily to the apical regions of the left ventricle. The basal portion of the septum is of normal thickness. There is also marked hypertrophy of the apex and contiguous portion of left ventricular free wall. Orientation is such that the cardiac apex is to the top, the base is to the bottom and the left ventricle is to the right. *AML*, anterior mitral leaflet; *Ao*, aorta; *LA*, left atrium; *LV*, left ventricle; *LVFW*, left ventricular free wall; *PML*, posterior mitral leaflet; *RV*, right ventricle; *VS*, ventricular septum

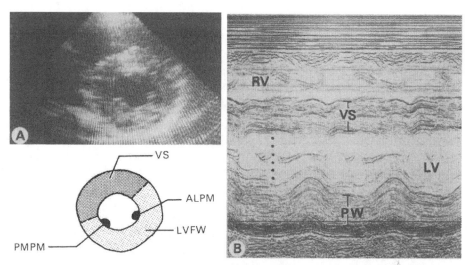

Fig. 10A, B. Two-dimensional and M-mode echocardiograms from a patient with "true" concentric (symmetric) hypertrophy. (A) Two-dimensional echocardiogram showing symmetric hypertrophy of all left ventricular wall segments. Stop-frame was obtained during diastole in the short-axis view, caudal to the mitral leaflets, and is accompanied by a schematic illustration. (B) M-mode echocardiogram recorded just caudal to the mitral leaflet tips; (anterior) ventricular septal thickness was 18 mm and posterior free wall thickness was 19 mm. Calibration marks are 5 mm apart. *ALPM*, anterolateral papillary muscle; *LV*, left ventricle; *LVFW*, left ventricular free wall; *RV*, right ventricle; *PW*, posterior left ventricular free wall; *PMPM*, posteromedial papillary muscle; *VS*, ventricular septum

phic assessment of maximum left ventricular wall thickness arose because the predominant region of hypertrophy was in a portion of the ventricle inaccessible to the M-mode echo beam.

In other patients these discrepancies appeared to be due to variations in wall thickness *within* the anterior ventricular septum, such that the M-mode echo beam did not pass through the thickest portion of that segment. These variations included: a "tapered" configuration of the septum (Fig. 7C), a diastolic "notch" in a portion of anterior septum (Fig. 7D), maximum thickness near the junction of septum and anterior free wall with less hypertrophy medially (Fig. 8B), or maximal septal thickening located distally in the left ventricle (Fig. 9B).

Of the five patients with concentric thickening on M-mode echocardiogram only one had "true" symmetric hypertrophy of the left ventricular wall on the two dimensional echocardiogram. In the other four patients the two-dimensional echocardiogram identified regions of asymmetric hypertrophy in the posterior ventricular septum or left ventricular free wall that were not appreciated by M-mode echocardiography.

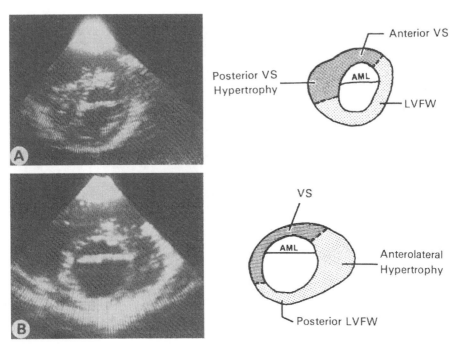

Fig. 11A, B. Stop-frames of two-dimensional echocardiograms (during diastole in short-axis view) from two patients with type IV distribution of hypertrophy. Although the cross-sectional levels shown are from the most basal portion of the ventricle, the distribution of hypertrophy was similar in the more caudal regions. (A) Hypertrophy is confined primarily to the posterior ventricular septum; (B) Selective hypertrophy of the anterolateral left ventricular free wall. Because the anterior ventricular septum was not thickened in these two patients, the M-mode echocardiograms did not suggest the diagnosis of hypertrophic cardiomyopathy. *AML*, anterior mitral leaflet; *LVFW*, left ventricular free wall, *VS*, ventricular septum

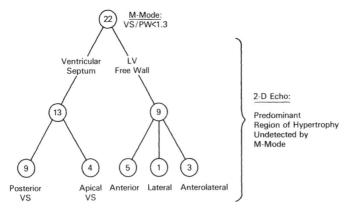

Fig. 12. Diagram summarizing two-dimensional (2-D) echocardiographic findings in 22 patients with M-mode echocardiograms that did *not* show left ventricular hypertrophy. Each of these patients had type IV distribution of hypertrophy. *LV*, left ventricular; *VS*, ventricular septum; *VS/PW*, ventricular septal to posterior left ventricular free wall thickness ratio

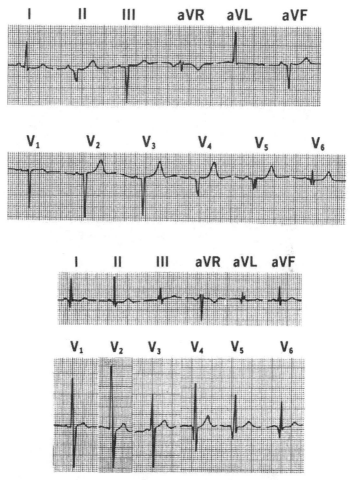

Fig. 13. Electrocardiograms from two patients with hypertrophic cardiomyopathy in whom hypertrophy was limited to the left ventricular free wall (*Top*) ECG from a 22-year-old women with anterolateral left ventricular free wall hypertrophy, showing deep QS waves in leads II, III, aV_F, and V_1–V_5 and left-axis deviation. (*Bottom*) ECG from a 12-year-old boy with lateral left ventricular free wall hypertrophy showing deep Q waves in leads V_4–V_6 and tall R wave in V_1, suggestive of right ventricular hypertrophy

Correlation of Clinical Parameters with Distribution of Left Ventricular Hypertrophy

Functional Limitation

Patients with widespread hypertrophy involving most of the ventricular septum as well as portions of the left ventricular free wall (type III) had a significantly greater prevalence of moderate to severe functional limitation (38 of 65, 58%) than did patients with the three other morphologic types combined (16 of 60 or 27%; $P<0.001$, Fig. 15). Moderate to severe symptoms were relatively uncommon in patients with type I (3 of 12, 25%) or with type IV (4 of 23 or 17%; $P<0.01$).

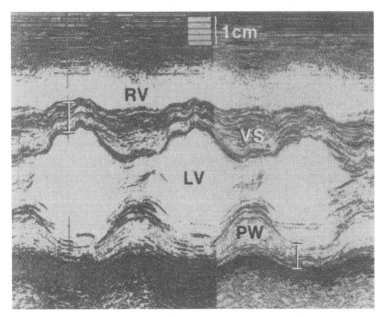

Fig. 14. M-mode echocardiogram (recorded just below the caudal margins of the mitral leaflets) from a 15-year-old girl. Note that the M-mode echocardiogram does not show hypertrophy of either the (anterior) ventricular septum (*VS*) or posterior left ventricular free wall (*PW*). Two-dimensional echocardiogram showed prominent hypertrophy of the posterior *VS*, but no hypertrophy of the anterior *VS* through which the M-mode ultrasound beam passes (see Fig. 6 and 7). *LV*, left ventricular cavity; *RV*, right ventricular cavity

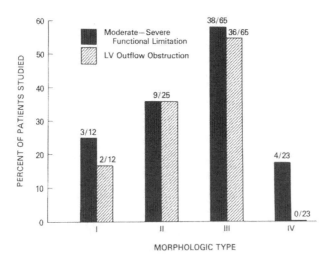

Fig. 15. Relation of distribution of hypertrophy to the presence of moderate to severe functional limitation (functional class III) or left ventricular (*LV*) outflow tract obstruction under basal conditions

Outflow Obstruction

Patients with type III distribution of hypertrophy also had a significantly greater prevalence of obstruction to left ventricular outflow under basal conditions (36 of 65, 55%) than did patients with the three other morphologic types combined (11 of 60 or 18%; $P<0.001$; Fig. 15). Outflow obstruction was uncommon in patients with type I (2 of 12 or 17%) or type IV (0 of 23; $P<0.001$). Of the 48 patients with outflow obstruction, 44 (92%) had substantial hypertrophy involving the basal portion of both the anterior and posterior segments of ventricular septum (i. e., types II or III).

Systolic Anterior Motion

Similarly, marked systolic anterior motion of the anterior mitral leaflet was significantly more common in patients with type III distribution of hypertrophy (31 of 64, 48%) than in patients with other morphologic types (11 of 60 or 18%; $P<0.001$). Of the 42 patients with marked systolic anterior motion, 40 (95%) had considerable hypertrophy involving the basal portion of both the anterior and posterior segments of the ventricular septum (i. e., types II or III).

Age

Although morphologic types II and III showed no particular predilection for age, patients with type I were significantly older (45 ± 4 years) compared to patients with the other morphologic types (33 ± 1 years; $P<0.01$). Patients with type IV were significantly younger (25 ± 3 years) compared to those with the other morphologic types (36 ± 1 years; $P<0.005$).

Discussion

This investigation, in which wide-angle two-dimensional echocardiography was employed, demonstrates that patients with hypertrophic cardiomyopathy manifest great variability in the pattern and distribution of left ventricular hypertrophy. Of the 125 patients we studied, hypertrophy was confined to the ventricular septum in 41% and to the left ventricular free wall in 7%. In the majority of patients (52%) hypertrophy involved substantial portions of both the ventricular septum and left ventricular free wall (type III) (Fig. 16). This finding of widespread distribution of left ventricular hypertrophy indicates that the cardiomyopathic process is usually diffuse in patients with hypertrophic cardiomyopathy. The extensive distribution of disorganized myocardial architecture that is characteristic of patients with hypertrophic cardiomyopathy (as described in the following manuscript) also supports the concept that the cardiomyopathic process in hypertrophic cardiomyopathy is usually diffusely distributed throughout the left ventricular wall.

Our data also suggest that the distribution of hypertrophy may provide information relevant to the clinical course and hemodynamic state of patients with hypertrophic cardiomyopathy. For example, those patients with the more extensive distribution of left ventricular hypertrophy (type III) most commonly demonstrated marked functional limitation. Conversely, marked functional limitation was less frequent in patients with localized hypertrophy (type I), or in those patients in whom hypertrophy involved portions of the left ventricular wall other than the basal, anterior ventricular septum (type IV).

Left ventricular outflow tract obstruction (and marked systolic anterior motion of the anterior mitral leaflet) under basal conditions was also most common in patients with morphologic type III. Outflow obstruction and systolic anterior motion occurred uncommonly or were absent in patients with types I or type IV, in whom

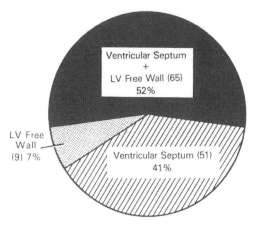

Fig. 16. Distribution of left ventricular (*LV*) hypertrophy as assessed by two-dimensional echocardiography in 125 patients with hypertrophic cardiomyopathy

ventricular septal hypertrophy was either less marked or did not substantially involve the basal, anterior septum. Hence, our data suggest that in patients with hypertrophic cardiomyopathy the presence of marked hypertrophy of the basal portion of the anterior ventricular septum is an important factor in the genesis of left ventricular outflow obstruction.

Our study also emphasizes certain limitations of M-mode echocardiography in documenting the extent of hypertrophy present. In about one-third of the patients with asymmetric septal hypertrophy or concentric wall thickening documented by M-mode echocardiography, the region of maximum left ventricular wall thickening was identified by two-dimensional echocardiography to be in areas other than the anterior ventricular septum (that were inaccessible to the M-mode beam).

Even in those patients in whom the M-mode echo beam does traverse the region of maximum left ventricular hypertrophy, *overall* left ventricular mass was often either overestimated or underestimated (Fig. 17). For example, in type I hypertrophy, the M-mode echocardiogram overestimates left ventricular mass; in these patients the septal-free wall ratio may be markedly increased even though two-dimensional echocardiography shows the hypertrophy to be confined to the anterior segment of ventricular septum. In contrast, M-mode echocardiography underestimates left ventricular mass in patients with type III because the echo beam does not visualize the thickened anterolateral free wall. Hence, ventricular wall thicknesses and septal-free wall ratios derived from the M-mode echocardiogram may be similar in patients with morphologic types I and III (or II) even though the overall distribution and magnitude of hypertrophy in those hearts differs considerably (Fig. 17).

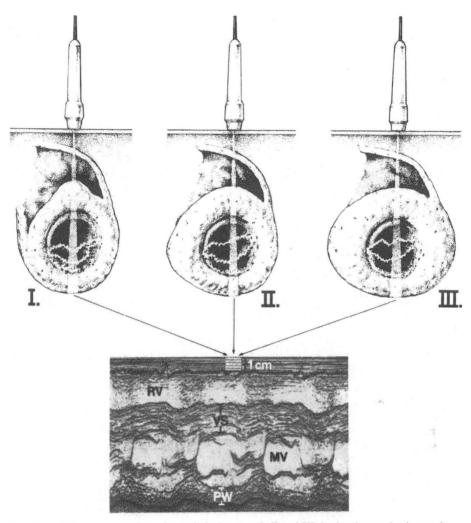

Fig. 17. Artistic representation of morphologic types I, II and III, in the short-axis view at the level of the mitral leaflets. The expected approximate path of the M-mode echo beam is shown in each heart. Note that the M-mode echocardiogram (shown below) would record identical septal thickness (20 mm), posterior free wall thickness (10 mm), and septal-free wall thickness ratio (2.0) in each of the three hearts, even though they differ substantially with regard to distribution of left ventricular hypertrophy. *VS,* ventricular septum; *PW,* posterior left ventricular wall; *MV,* mitral valve; *RV,* right ventricle

Finally, two-dimensional echocardiography proved to be essential for establishing the diagnosis of hypertrophic cardiomyopathy in those patients with morphologic type IV. These patients had represented a diagnostic dilemma; the scalar electrocardiogram was abnormal and each patient had a family history of hypertrophic cardiomyopathy, yet the M-mode echocardiogram failed to show left ventricular hypertrophy. However, wide-angle two-dimensional echocardiography demonstrated hypertrophy in regions of the left ventricular wall inaccessible to the M-mode beam, most commonly the posterior ventricular septum and anterolateral free wall. Hence, in these patients the electrocardiogram appears to be a more sensitive marker of hypertrophic cardiomyopathy than M-mode echocardiography. This subgroup also included four patients with hypertrophy virtually confined to the apical portion of ventricular septum ("apical hypertrophic cardiomyopathy" [22]).

References

1. Abbasi AS, MacAlpin RN, Eber LM, Pearce ML (1972) Echocardiographic diagnosis of idiopathic hypertrophic cardiomyopathy without outflow obstruction. Circulation 46:897–904
2. Henry WL, Clark CE, Epstein SE (1973) Asymmetric septal hypertrophy (ASH): Echocardiographic identification of the pathognomonic anatomic abnormality of IHSS. Circulation 47:225–233
3. Abbasi AS, MacAlpin RN, Eber LM, Pearce ML (1973) Left ventricular hypertrophy diagnosed by echocardiography. N Engl J Med 289:118–121
4. Tajik AJ, Giuliani ER (1974) Echocardiographic observations in idiopathic hypertrophic subaortic stenosis. Mayo Clin Proc 49:89–97
5. King JF, DeMaria AN, Reis RL, Bolton MR, Dunn MI, Mason DT (1973) Echocardiographic assessment of idiopathic hypertrophic subaortic stenosis. Chest 64:723–731
6. Chahine RA, Raizner AE, Ishimori T, Montero AC (1977) Echocardiographic, haemodynamic and angiographic correlations in hypertrophic cardiomyopathy. Br Heart J 39:945–953
7. Rossen RM, Goodman DJ, Ingham RE, Popp RL (1974) Ventricular systolic septal thickening and excursion in idiopathic hypertrophic subaortic stenosis. N Engl J Med 291:1317–1319
8. Martin RP, Rakowski H, French J, Popp RL (1979) Idiopathic hypertrophic subaortic stenosis viewed by wide-angle, phased-array echocardiography. Circulation 59:1206–1217
9. Tajik AJ, Seward JB, Hagler DJ (1979) Detailed analysis of hypertrophic obstructive cardiomyopathy by wide-angle two-dimensional sector echocardiography (Abstr). Am J Cardiol 43:348
10. Rakowski H, Gilbert BW, Drobac M, Vaughan-Neil T, Pollick C, Wigle ED (1979) Anatomic variations in subgroups of hypertrophic cardiomyopathy as assessed by wide-angle two-dimensional echocardiography (Abstr). Am J Cardiol 43:348
11. DeMaria A, Bommer W, Lee G, Mason DT (1980) Value and limitations of two dimensional echocardiography in assessment of cardiomyopathy. Am J Cardiol 46:1224–1231
12. Maron BJ, Epstein SE (1979) Hypertrophic cardiomyopathy: A discussion of nomenclature. Am J Cardiol 43:1242–1244
13. Henry WL, Clark CE, Glancy DL, Epstein SE (1973) Echocardiographic measurement of the left ventricular outflow gradient in idiopathic hypertrophic subaortic stenosis. N Engl J Med 288:989–993
14. Anderson WA, Arnold JT, Clark D, Davids WT, Hillard WJ, Lehr WJ, Zitelli LT (1977) A new real-time phased array sector scanner for imaging the entire adult human heart. In: White DN (ed) Ultrasound in medicine, vol 3 B. Plenum, New York, pp 1547–1558
15. Kisslo J, von Ramm OT, Thurstone FL (1976) Cardiac imaging using phased array ultrasound system. II. Clinical technique and application. Circulation 53:262–267
16. Tajik AJ, Seward JB, Hagler DJ, Mair DD, Lie JT (1978) Two-dimensional real-time ultrasonic imaging of the heart and great vessels. Mayo Clin Proc 53:271–303
17. Stack R, Kisslo J (1980) Evaluation of the left ventricle with two-dimensional echocardiography. Am J Cardiol 46:1117–1124

18. Silverman NH, Schiller NB (1978) Apex echocardiography. A two-dimensional technique for evaluating congenital heart disease. Circulation 57:503–511
19. Henry WL, Ware J, Gardin JM, Hepner SI, McKay J, Weiner M (1978) Echocardiographic measurements in normal subjects. Growth-related changes that occur between infancy and early adulthood. Circulation 57:278–285
20. Maron BJ, Gottdiener JS, Roberts WC, Henry WL, Epstein SE (1978) Left ventricular outflow tract obstruction due to systolic anterior motion of the anterior mitral leaflet in patients with concentric left ventricular hypertrophy. Circulation 55:527–533
21. Maron BJ, Gottdiener JS, Bonow RO, Epstein SE (1981) Hypertrophic cardiomyopathy with unusual locations of left ventricular hypertrophy undetectable by M-mode echocardiography: Identification by wide-angle, two-dimensional echocardiography. Circulation 63:409–418
22. Yamaguchi H, Ishimura T, Nishiyama S, Nagasaki F, Nakanishi S, Takatsu F, Nishijo T, Umeda T, Machii K (1979) Hypertrophic nonobstructive cardiomyopathy with giant negative T waves (apical hypertrophy): ventriculographic and echocardiographic features in 30 patients. Am J Cardiol 44:401–412

Distribution and Significance of Cardiac Muscle Cell Disorganization in the Left Ventricle of Patients with Hypertrophic Cardiomyopathy: Evidence of a Diffuse Cardiomyopathic Process *

BARRY J. MARON and WILLIAM C. ROBERTS

Summary

The distribution of cardiac muscle cell disorganization in different regions of the left ventricular wall was studied quantitatively in 52 patients with hypertrophic cardiomyopathy. Cellular disorganization was both common and extensive (mean area of tissue section disorganized $35\pm4\%$) in the ventricular septum and proved to be a highly specific and sensitive marker for hypertrophic cardiomyopathy. Disorganization was also substantial ($24\pm3\%$) in the left ventricular free wall of these patients, although less marked than in the ventricular septum ($P<0.05$). Anterior left ventricular free wall disorganization was particularly extensive ($32\pm4\%$) and did not differ significantly from that present in the ventricular septum.

Particularly marked left ventricular free wall and combined free wall and septal disorganization was present in 14 patients without functional limitation in whom sudden death occurred early in life (≤ 25 years of age) and was the initial manifestation of cardiac disease. In contrast, while abnormally arranged cardiac muscle cells were frequently identified in the left ventricular free wall of patients with heart diseases other than hypertrophic cardiomyopathy or with normal hearts (i.e., in 47%), this disorganization was usually limited in extent (mean area of section disorganized only $2\pm0.5\%$).

Hence, in a large population of patients with hypertrophic cardiomyopathy, cellular disorganization was widely distributed throughout both the ventricular septum and left ventricular free wall. In addition, our data suggest that this pattern of cellular disorganization may represent a diffuse cardiomyopathic process and be a determinant of clinical outcome by providing the substrate for malignant ventricular ectopy.

Introduction

Hypertrophic cardiomyopathy is a disease of cardiac muscle that is characterized by a hypertrophied nondilated left ventricle [1]. In most patients, the left ventricular hypertrophy is asymmetric [2–5] and diffusely involves the ventricular septum and left ventricular free wall [6], as described in the preceeding report. Marked disorganization of cardiac muscle cells in the ventricular septum [7–10] has also been

---

* This paper has already been published, in part, in Circulation

Cellular Disorganization in Hypertrophic Cardiomyopathy

shown by quantitative histologic analysis to be a highly specific and sensitive anatomic hallmark of hypertrophic cardiomyopathy [11–13]. Previous qualitative histologic studies have shown that cellular disorganization may also be present in the left ventricular free wall of patients with hypertrophic cardiomyopathy [14–19]. The present study determines: (1) in quantitative terms, the extent of cellular disorganization in both the ventricular septum and left ventricular free wall of patients with hypertrophic cardiomyopathy compared with patients having other forms of cardiac hypertrophy; and (2) whether the distribution and extent of the cellular disorganization in patients with hypertrophic cardiomyopathy has significance with regard to clinical course or hemodynamic state.

Selection of Case Material

Patients with Hypertrophic Cardiomyopathy

The cardiovascular registry of the Pathology Branch, National Heart, Lung, and Blood Institute was reviewed and 52 hearts with hypertrophic cardiomyopathy were considered to be in suitable condition for inclusion in the study.

In each, the diagnosis of hypertrophic cardiomyopathy was based on the presence of a hypertrophied, nondilated left ventricle [1]. In 41 (79%) of the 52 patients, asymmetric septal hypertrophy (septal-free wall thickness ratio $\geq$ 1.3) was present

Table 1. Clinical and hemodynamic findings in 52 patients with hypertrophic cardiomyopathy

	No. of patients		No. of patients
Functional limitation		*LVEDP (mmHg)*	
Present	36	< 12	10
Absent	16	$13 - 20$	16
		> 20	12
		Mode of death	
LVOT-PSG (mmHg)		Sudden	27
$\geq$ 30 at rest	24	Congestive heart failure	9
< 30 at rest		CVA	1
$\quad \geq$ 30 with provocation [a]	5	Suicide	2
$\quad < 30$ with provocation [b]	5	Cardiac catheterization	1
provocation not done	4	Operative	12

CVA, cerebrovascular accident; LVEDP, left ventricular end-diastolic pressure; LVOT, left ventricular outflow tract; PSG, peak systolic gradient.

[a] "Provocable outflow tract obstruction" with isoproterenol infusion, Valsalva maneuver, or amyl nitrite inhalation.

[b] "Nonobstructive hypertrophic cardiomyopathy"

at necropsy. In 40 of the 52 patients the typical clinical, hemodynamic, angiocardiographic, or operative findings of hypertrophic cardiomyopathy were also present; the 12 other patients had no cardiac evaluation during life and sudden death was the initial manifestation of cardiac disease [20].

Associated coronary heart disease (>75% cross-sectional area narrowing by atherosclerotic plaque of at least one major extramural coronary artery) was present in eight of the 52 patients; three other patients also had systemic hypertension. The 11 patients with associated cardiac lesions were included because the degree of left ventricular hypertrophy present was greater than would be expected in patients having these abnormalities alone. Clinical and hemodynamic data in the 52 patients with hypertrophic cardiomyopathy are summarized in Table 1.

Patients with Normal Hearts or with Cardiac Diseases Other than Hypertrophic Cardiomyopathy

The hearts of 83 patients were selected for study as controls. This group included 72 patients with a variety of congenital or acquired heart diseases (other than hypertrophic cardiomyopathy), as well as 11 subjects with structurally normal hearts who died of trauma (Table 2).

Table 2. Cardiac diseases in 83 control patients

Disease	No. of Patients	No. patients with marked[a] VS disorganization	No. patients with marked LVFW disorganization
Aortic valve disease	17	1	3
Coronary heart disease	15	2	1
Mitral valve disease	10	1	5
Systemic hypertension	8	1	1
Idiopathic dilated cardiomyopathy	6	0	1
Primary pulmonary hypertension	6	1	3
Pulmonic valve stenosis	3	0	0
Combined aortic and mitral valve disease	2	0	0
Supravalvular aortic stenosis	2	0	1
Ventricular septal defect	2	0	1
Discrete subaortic stenosis	1	0	0
Normal	11	1	0
Totals	83	7 (8%)	16 (19%)

LVFW, left ventricular free wall; VS, ventricular septum.
[a] Involving $\geq$ 5% of the relevant areas of the tissue section.

Materials and Methods

Tissue Preparation

In each of the 135 hearts in this study (52 with hypertrophic cardiomyopathy and 83 controls) three tissue blocks were taken from the full thickness of the ventricular wall in a plane perpendicular to the long axis of the left ventricle (i.e., transverse plane), about one-half the distance between the aortic valve and left ventricular apex. The tissue sections were obtained from three locations: (1) ventricular septum; (2) anterior left ventricular free wall about 2 cm lateral to the left anterior descending coronary artery; and (3) posterior[1] left ventricular free wall between the papillary muscles (Fig. 1). All tissue specimens were embedded in paraffin, sectioned at a thickness of 6μ and stained with hematoxylin and eosin.

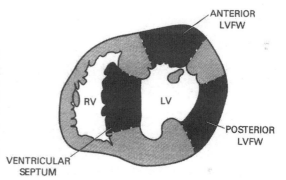

Fig. 1. Section of a heart obtained in the anteroposterior (transverse) plane about one-half the distance between left ventricular base and apex, showing the location of the three tissue sections that were analyzed quantitatively in each patient. *LV*, left ventricle; *RV*, right ventricle

Definition and Classification of Cardiac Muscle Cell Disorganization

In contrast to normal cellular arrangement, cardiac muscle cell disorganization observed in the patients in this study usually assumed four different forms [11] (Fig. 2). *Type I-A* disorganization, the most common form, consisted of areas of myocardium in which adjacent cardiac muscle cells were aligned perpendicularly or obliquely to each other, usually forming tangled masses or "pinwheel" configurations (Fig. 3). Although most of these lesions were relatively small, individual foci of Type I-A disorganization varied greatly in size and appearance (Fig. 3). In *Type I-B* disorganization, relatively broad bundles of muscle cells were oriented at oblique or perpendicular angles to each other; cells within these bundles were, however, normally arranged. Types I-A and I-B disorganization exclusively involved areas of myocardium where cardiac muscle cells were cut longitudinally, i.e., appeared to be rectangularly shaped.

---

1 The term "posterior" left ventricular wall is used to describe that region of the free wall which lies between the papillary muscles, directly behind the posterior mitral leaflet. This area is often described by pathologists as the "lateral" or "posterolateral" left ventricular free wall.

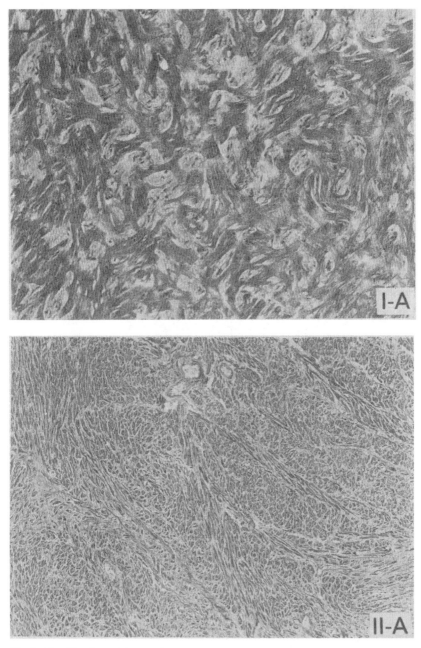

Fig. 2. Classification of four major types of cardiac muscle cell disorganization present in left ventricular myocardium. Magnifications: I–A, ×130; I–B and II–A, ×40; II–B ×80. All sections were stained with hematoxylin and eosin

Cellular Disorganization in Hypertrophic Cardiomyopathy

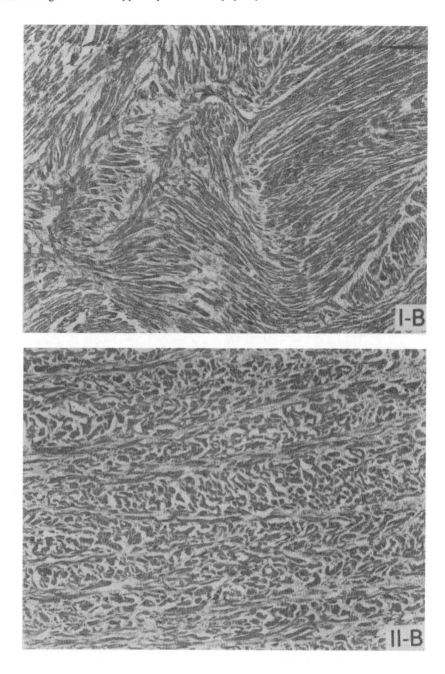

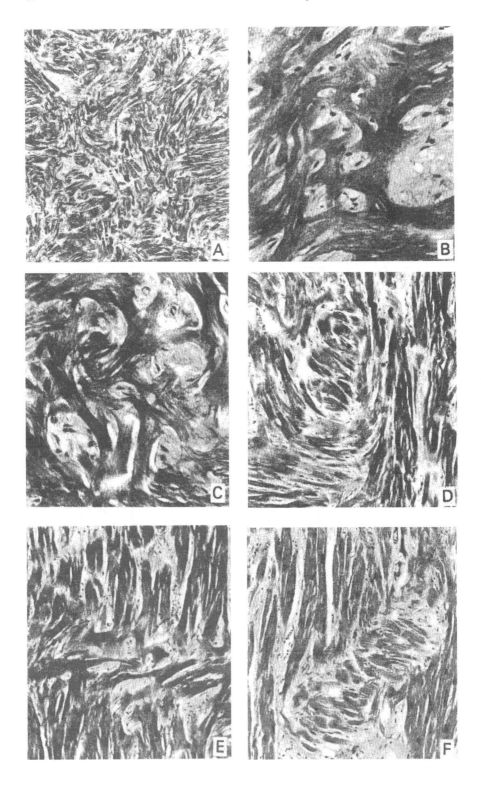

Cellular Disorganization in Hypertrophic Cardiomyopathy

Type II-A disorganization consisted of relatively narrow (usually one or two cells wide) longitudinally cut bundles that were interlaced in varous directions among larger groups of transversely cut cells (i.e., which appeared circular). This type of disorganization gave the myocardium a "swirled" appearance. *Type II-B* was similar to Type II-A disorganization, except that the narrow, longitudinally cut bundles of cells were more linear. Types II-A and II-B disorganization involved areas of myocardium which included both longitudinally and transversely cut cardiac muscle cells.

Quantitation of Cardiac Muscle Cell Disorganization

A technique [11], was employed to quantitatively assess the extent of cardiac muscle cell disorganization in the 405 tissue sections studied. Transverse plane tissue sections were used exclusively because this orientation is most appropriate for identifying cardiac muscle cell disorganization [11]. Tissue sections were photographed and the images enlarged to occupy $30'' \times 40''$ positive prints, resulting in a magnification of about 2000 times the original tissue section. A transparent cellulose overlay was then placed over the print, and the areas of myocardium occupied by disorganized cardiac muscle cells were outlined with a marking pen (Fig. 4). Areas in which cardiac muscle cells were either cut longitudinally or transversely were also demarcated. Large areas of fibrosis, artifacts of tissue preparation or large interstitial spaces containing blood vessels were excluded from the analysis. The transparent overlay was then removed from the print, photographed and the image reproduced (with substantial reduction) as a 5×7 inch positive print. Each area into which the tissue section had been divided was outlined separately with a fine-point marking pen on ordinary tablet paper, and quantitated using a video planimetry system.

The formulas used to calculate the percentage of the tissue section occupied by disorganized cardiac muscle cells are given below; the area of myocardium "at risk" for disorganization appears in the denominator of both equations:

$$\% \text{ area of type I (I-A + I-B) disorganization} = \frac{D_{\mathrm{I}}}{L + D_{\mathrm{I}}} \times 100;$$

$$\% \text{ area of type II (II-A + II-B) disorganization} = \frac{D_{\mathrm{II}}}{L + T + D_{\mathrm{II}}} \times 100;$$

where L = area occupied by longitudinally cut, but normally arranged cells; T = area occupied by transversely cut cells (excluding those incorporated into areas of type II disorganization); D_{I} = area occupied by type I disorganization; and D_{II} = area occupied by type II disorganization.

Fig. 3A–F. Several examples of type I-A disorganization which illustrate the wide morphologic spectrum of this lesion. (A) "Chaotic" pattern in which adjacent cells are arranged at perpendicular and oblique angles to each other (also, see upper left panel in Fig. 2 for similar example); magnification $\times 55$; (B) "Swiss cheese" appearance that results when adjacent cells are oriented at particularly acute angles; $\times 350$; (C) Tangled arrangement of cardiac muscle cells in whorled configurations; $\times 350$; (D) Whorl pattern in which some cells are oriented circumferentially to other cells; $\times 130$; (E) and (F) Patterns in which small groups of cells are oriented at extremely acute angles to larger groups of cells; $\times 130$

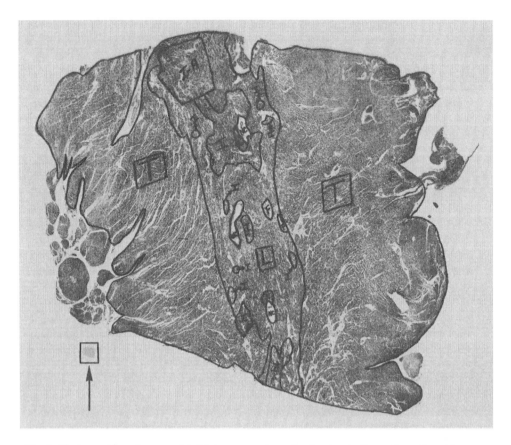

Fig. 4. Photographic enlargement (with transparent overlay in place) of a section of ventricular septum from a patient with hypertrophic cardiomyopathy. Actual size of tissue section is shown at lower left (arrow) for comparison. Magnification of the print relative to the original tissue section was ×2000

For the purposes of certain analyses, quantitative data regarding cellular arrangement in the anterior and posterior left ventricular free wall sections were combined and the sum expressed as representing the "left ventricular free wall." Ventricular septal and left ventricular free wall tissue sections were also combined for an analysis of "total left ventricular wall" disorganization.

Results

Quantitative Histologic Findings in the Ventricular Septum

Cardiac muscle cell disorganization was common and extensive in the ventricular septum of patients with hypertrophic cardiomyopathy (Figs. 5, 6). Of the 52 patients with hypertrophic cardiomyopathy, 50 (96%) had some septal disorganization, 45

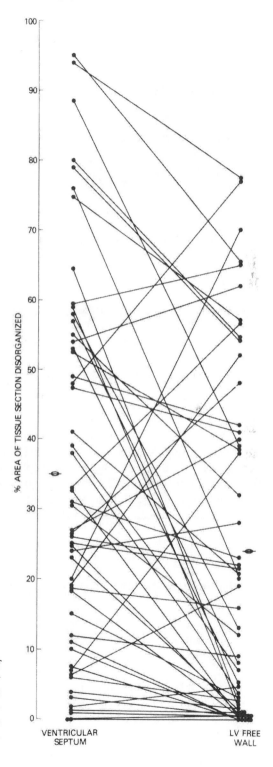

Fig. 5. Comparison of the extent of ventricular septal and left ventricular (*LV*) free wall disorganization in 52 patients with hypertrophic cardiomyopathy. Values for each patient are connected by a solid line. -θ- = Mean values

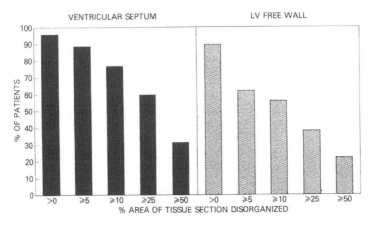

Fig. 6. Extent of cardiac muscle cell disorganization in the ventricular septum and in left ventricular (*LV*) free wall of 52 patients with hypertrophic cardiomyopathy

(87%) had disorganization comprising 5% or more of the relevant areas of the tissue section, 31 (60%) had disorganization comprising 25% or more of the section, and 16 (31%) had particularly extensive disorganization involving 50% or more of the section (Figs. 5, 6). In the patients with hypertrophic cardiomyopathy the mean percent area of ventricular septum disorganized was substantial (35% ± 4 SEM; range 0–95%).

In contrast, septal disorganization was much less common and extensive in control patients. While 25 (30%) of the 83 controls showed some septal disorganization only 7 (8%) had areas of disorganization comprising 5% or more of the tissue section and just one patient (a 43-year-old woman with mitral regurgitation) had more than 25% of the section involved. The mean area of ventricular septal tissue section disorganized in control patients (2 ± 1%) was significantly less than in patients with hypertrophic cardiomyopathy (35 ± 4%; $P<0.001$). Type I (particularly type I–A) was most often the predominant form of disorganization in a given ventricular septal tissue section, i.e., was present in 72 (95%) of the 76 patients with hypertrophic cardiomyopathy or control patients who showed septal disorganization.

Quantitative Histologic Findings in the Left Ventricular Free Wall

Cardiac muscle cell disorganization was also common and extensive in the left ventricular free wall of patients with hypertrophic cardiomyopathy (Figs. 5–10). Of the 52 patients with hypertrophic cardiomyopathy, 47 (90%) had some disorganization in the left ventricular free wall (i.e., in the combined anterior and posterior free wall sections); 33 (63%) had disorganization comprising 5% or more of the free wall sections, 20 (39%) had disorganization comprising 25% or more of the sections and 11 (21%) had particularly extensive disorganization involving 50% or more of the sections (Figs. 6, 7). In these patients with hypertrophic cardiomyopathy the mean percent area of left ventricular free wall disorganized was substantial (24 ± 3%; range 0–77%), although significantly less than the ventricular septal disorganization pres-

Cellular Disorganization in Hypertrophic Cardiomyopathy

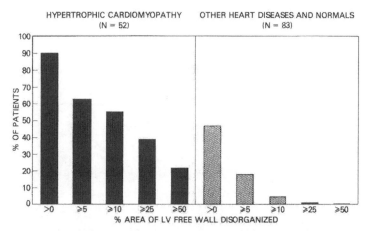

Fig. 7. Extent of left ventricular (*LV*) free wall disorganization in 52 patients with hypertrophic cardiomyopathy and in 83 controls. Comparisons of the respective bars from patients with hypertrophic cardiomyopathy and control patients each achieved high statistical significance ($P<0.001$)

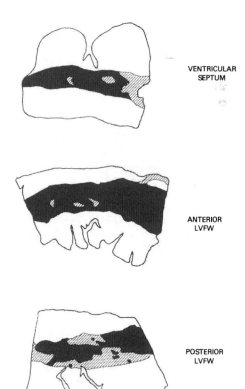

Fig. 8. Histologic "maps" of sections of left ventricular wall from a 12-year-old boy with hypertrophic cardiomyopathy, in whom sudden death was the initial manifestation of cardiac disease. Particularly marked and diffuse disorganization is present in the three tissue sections. Solid areas contain type I cellular disorganization. Striped areas represent normally arranged cardiac muscle cells that have been cut longitudinally. Clear areas contain cells cut transversely. Tissue sections are oriented with the left ventricular endocardium directed toward the bottom of the page. *LVFW*, left ventricular free wall

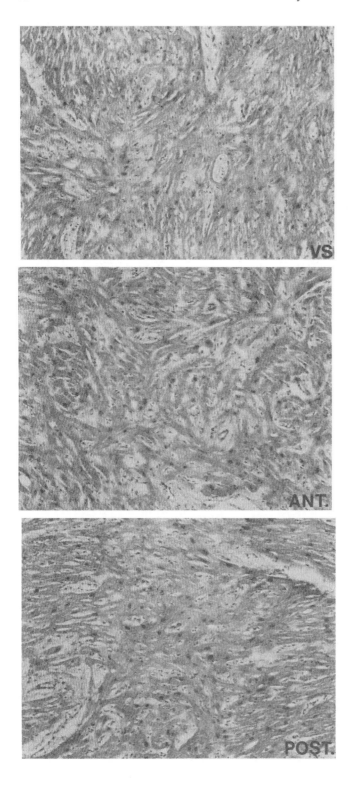

Cellular Disorganization in Hypertrophic Cardiomyopathy

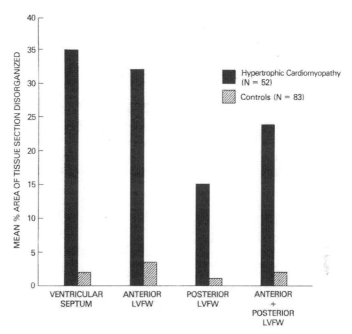

Fig. 10. Mean percent area of the tissue section occupied by disorganized cardiac muscle cells in 52 patients with hypertrophic cardiomyopathy and in 83 control patients. Shown separately for ventricular septum, anterior left ventricular free wall, posterior left ventricular free wall, and combined anterior and posterior left ventricular free wall. For each region of myocardium sampled, the percent disorganization in patients with hypertrophic cardiomyopathy significantly exceeded that in control patients ($P<0.001$). *LVFW*, left ventricular free wall

ent in the same patients (35±4%; $P<0.05$). As in the ventricular septum, type I (particularly I–A) was most commonly the predominant form of disorganization in the left ventricular free wall of patients with hypertrophic cardiomyopathy and controls.

The anterior left ventricular free wall section in patients with hypertrophic cardiomyopathy showed significantly more disorganization (32±4%) than the posterior free wall section (15±3%; $P<0.005$) (Fig. 10). The extent of disorganization in the anterior free wall did not differ significantly from that in the ventricular septum (35±4%); however, disorganization in the posterior free wall was significantly less than in the ventricular septum ($P<0.001$). In patients with hypertrophic cardiomyopathy, the overall left ventricular wall disorganization (combined ventricular septal and free wall tissue sections) (28±3%) significantly exceeded that in the control patients (2±0.5; $P<0.001$) (Fig. 11).

Fig. 9. Histologic sections of ventricular septum (*VS*) and anterior (*ANT*) and posterior (*POST*) left ventricular free wall from the patient with hypertrophic cardiomyopathy shown in Fig. 8. Note marked disorganization of cardiac muscle cells (type I) in each of the three tissue sections. Magnifications × 105 for each. Hematoxylin and eosin stain

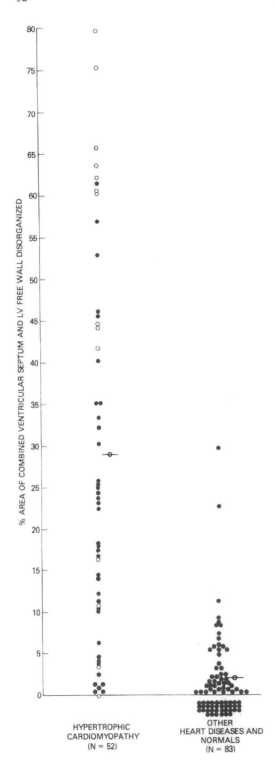

Fig. 11. Percent area of combined ventricular septal and left ventricular (*LV*) free wall tissue sections ("total left ventricular wall") occupied by disorganized cardiac muscle cells, in 52 patients with hypertrophic cardiomyopathy and in 83 control patients. Patients ($\leq$ 25 years of age) in whom sudden death was the initial manifestation of hypertrophic cardiomyopathy are indicated by open symbols. -⊖- = Mean values

Fig. 12. Histologic "maps" of the three sections of left ventricular wall from a subject with a structurally normal heart. Solid areas in anterior and posterior left ventricular free wall sections represent small foci of type I cellular disorganization. Striped areas represent normally arranged cardiac muscle cells that have been cut longitudinally. Clear areas contain cells cut transversely. Tissue sections are oriented with the left ventricular endocardium directed toward the bottom of the page. *LVFW*, left ventricular free wall

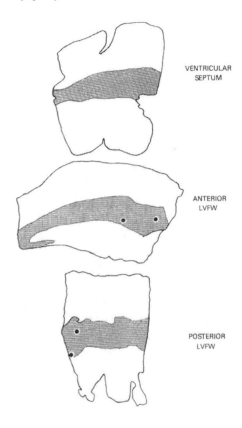

In contrast, left ventricular free wall disorganization was less common and less extensive in control patients than in patients with hypertrophic cardiomyopathy (Figs. 7, 11, and 12), although there was some overlap between the two groups. While 39 (47%) of the 83 controls showed some left ventricular free wall disorganization, only 16 (19%) of the patients with hypertrophic cardiomyopathy had areas of disorganization comprising 5% or more of the tissue section, and only one patient had 25% or more of the section involved (Fig. 7). The mean percent area of left ventricular free wall disorganized in control patients (2±0.5%) was also considerably less than in patients with hypertrophic cardiomyopathy (24±3%; $P < 0.001$). In the 83 control patients percent disorganization in the ventricular septum (2±1) or anterior (3±1) or posterior free wall (1.5±0.5) did differ significantly.

Correlation of Extent of Disorganization with Other Parameters

Clinical, hemodynamic, and anatomic parameters identified in the 52 patients with hypertrophic cardiomyopathy were analyzed to determine whether there was a correlation with the extent of left ventricular free wall or combined ventricular septal and free wall disorganization. There was no relation between the extent of disorganization and sex distribution, duration of symptoms, presence of atrial fibrillation,

Table 3. Correlation of extent of cellular disorganization with clinical parameters

Parameter	No. of patients	% area LVFW disorganized (mean±SEM)		% area of combined VS and LVFW disorganized (mean±SEM)	
1. *Age at death (years)*					
≦25	24	37±6	$P<0.001$	39±5	$P<0.001$
>25	28	13±3		17±3	
2. *Functional limitation (symptoms)*					
Absent	16[a]	41±6	$P<0.005$	43±6	$P<0.005$
Present	28[a]	19±4		24±3	
3. *Functional state and age*					
No functional limitation; ≦25 years	14[a]	43±7	$P<0.001$	45±7	$P<0.005$
Functional limitation; >25 years	19[a]	15±3		19±3	
4. *Obstruction to LV outflow*					
Absent[b] (basal and provoked)	5	22±10	NS	33±7	NS
Present[c] (basal)	24	18±5		21±4	

LV, left ventricular; LVFW, left ventricular free wall; VS, ventricular septum; NS, nonsignificant.
[a] Patients with associated coronary heart disease were excluded from these analyses.
[b] <30 mm Hg [c] ≧30 mm Hg

magnitude of left ventricular end-diastolic pressure, heart weight, ventricular septal thickness, or septal-free wall thickness ratio.

However, other parameters did show a statistically significant relation with the extent of disorganization. Disorganization in tissue sections from left ventricular free wall and combined ventricular septal and free wall was most marked in the younger patients and patients without functional limitation, particularly in the subgroup of 14 patients (≦ 25 years of age) without functional limitation, in whom sudden death was the initial manifestation of cardiac disease [20] (Table 3; Fig. 11). Nine of these 14 patients had more than 35% disorganization in each of the three regions of left ventricular wall sampled.

The extent of free wall and combined septal and free wall disorganization was also greater in five patients with nonobstructive hypertrophic cardiomyopathy (outflow gradient of <30 mmHg both at rest and with provocative maneuvers) than in 24 patients with obstruction to left ventricular outflow under basal conditions; however, this difference did not achieve statistical significance (Table 3).

Discussion

The results of this quantitative histologic study show that marked ventricular septal disorganization (involving at least 5% of the relevant areas of the tissue section) is both a highly sensitive (86%) and specific (92%) marker for hypertrophic cardiomyopathy [11–13]. In addition, in the large population of patients with hypertrophic cardiomyopathy studied, cellular disorganization commonly and extensively involved regions of the left ventricular free wall [14]. Ninety percent of the 52 patients had some disorganization present in the free wall sampled and in over 60% of the patients at least 5% of the free wall tissue sections was disorganized. In the patients with hypertrophic cardiomyopathy, the mean area of free wall tissue section disorganized was substantial ($24 \pm 3\%$), although less marked than that present in the septum ($35 \pm 4\%$). However, the extent of septal and free wall disorganization was similar in many patients. Of 45 patients with marked disorganization in the ventricular septum, 33 also had marked disorganization in the free wall.

Hence, these histologic data suggest that cardiac muscle cell disorganization may represent a diffuse cardiomyopathic process in many patients with hypertrophic cardiomyopathy. Furthermore, the preceeding two-dimensional echocardiographic analysis demonstrates that the gross distribution of left ventricular hypertrophy is diffuse in most patients with hypertrophic cardiomyopathy. The findings of these two studies substantiate our contention that the cardiomyopathic process in hypertrophic cardiomyopathy is not usually limited to the ventricular septum, but also typically involves other regions of the left ventricular wall.

Of note, left ventricular free wall disorganization was also common (i.e., 47%) in the 83 patients with normal hearts or cardiac diseases other than hypertrophic cardiomyopathy. However, foci of left ventricular free wall disorganization in these patients usually involved extremely small areas of myocardium (<5%), in contrast to the widespread disorganization present in most patients with hypertrophic cardiomyopathy. The specificity of marked left ventricular free wall disorganization (involving $\geq 5\%$ of the tissue section) in our necropsy population of 83 patients without hypertrophic cardiomyopathy was relatively high (i.e., 82%).

While the mechanism of sudden death in hypertrophic cardiomyopathy has not been definitively defined, high-grade ventricular arrhythmias have been indentified by 24-h ambulatory electrocardiograms in a substantial proportion of these patients [21]; furthermore, the occurrence of asymptomatic ventricular tachycardia may prospectively identify a subgroup of patients with hypertrophic cardiomyopathy who are at risk for subsequent sudden death [22, 23].

Therefore, of potential importance is the question of whether distribution and extent of cellular disorganization has any relation to clinical outcome in patients with hypertrophic cardiomyopathy. Our data demonstrated that left ventricular free wall and combined septal and free wall disorganization was most extensive in the younger (≤ 25 years of age) and least symptomatic patients studied, particularly those who had no functional limitation prior to their sudden and unexpected death. Hence, in those patients in whom cellular disorganization is extensive and distributed widely throughout the left ventricular wall, this pattern may represent a diffuse cardiomyopathic process and be a determinant of clinical outcome. The mechanism by which particularly marked and diffuse cardiac muscle cell disorganization may increase the likelihood of premature sudden death is unknown. However, it is possible that the disorganized arrangement of adjacent cardiac muscle cells in the ventricular walls of these patients may be inefficient in producing an orderly pattern of electrical depolarization or repolarization and, hence, could provide the substrate for malignant ventricular ectopy.

References

1. Maron BJ, Epstein SE (1979) Hypertrophic cardiomyopathy: A discussion of nomenclature. Am J Cardiol 43:1242
2. Menges H, Brandenburg RO, Brown AL (1961) The clinical, hemodynamic and pathologic diagnosis of muscular subvalvular aortic stenosis. Circulation 24:1126
3. Abbasi AS, MacAlpin RN, Eber LM, Pearce ML (1972) Echocardiographic diagnosis of idiopathic hypertrophic cardiomyopathy without outflow obstruction. Circulation 46:897
4. Henry WL, Clark CE, Epstein SE (1973) Asymmetric septal hypertrophy (ASH): Echocardiographic identification of the pathognomonic anatomic abnormality of IHSS. Circulation 47:225
5. Roberts WC (1973) Valvular, subvalvular and supravalvular aortic stenosis: morphologic features. Cardiovasc Clin 5:104
6. Maron BJ, Gottdiener JS, Epstein SE (1981) Patterns and significance of the distribution of left ventricular hypertrophy in hypertrophic cardiomyopathy: A wide-angle two-dimensional echocardiographic study of 125 patients. Am J Cardiol 48:418
7. Teare D (1958) Asymmetrical hypertrophy of the heart in young patients. Br Heart J 20:1
8. Van Noorden S, Olsen EG, Pearse AG (1971) Hypertrophic obstructive cardiomyopathy. A histological, histochemical and ultrastructural study of biopsy material. Cardiovasc Res 5:118
9. Ferrans VJ, Morrow AG, Roberts WC (1972) Myocardial ultrastructure in idiopathic hypertrophic subaortic stenosis: a study of operatively excised left ventricular outflow tract muscle in 14 patients. Circulation 45:769
10. Knieriem H-J, Stroobandt R, Meyer H, Bouregeois M (1975) Hypertrophic nonobstructive cardiomyopathy caused by disorder of the myofiber texture. Virchows Arch [Pathol Anat] 367:209
11. Maron BJ, Roberts WC (1979) Quantitative analysis of cardiac muscle cell disorganization in the ventricular septum of patients with hypertrophic cardiomyopathy. Circulation 59:689
12. Maron BJ, Sato N, Roberts WC, Edwards JE, Chandra RS (1979) Quantitative analysis of cardiac muscle cell disorganization in the ventricular septum: Comparison of fetuses and infants with and without congenital heart disease and patients with hypertrophic cardiomyopathy. Circulation 60:685
13. Maron BJ, Epstein SE (1980) Hypertrophic cardiomyopathy. Recent observations regarding the specificity of three hallmarks of the disease: asymmetric septal hypertrophy, septal disorganization and systolic anterior motion of the anterior mitral leaflet. Am J Cardiol 45:141
14. Wigle ED, Adelman AG, Silver MD (1971) Pathophysiological considerations in muscular subaortic stenosis. In: Wolstenholme GE, O'Connor M (eds) Hypertrophic Obstructive Cardiomyopathy. J & A Churchill, London, p 63
15. Maron BJ, Ferrans VJ, Henry WL, Clark CE, Redwood DR, Roberts WC, Morrow AG, Epstein SE (1974) Differences in distribution of myocardial abnormalities in patients with obstructive and nonobstructive asymmetric septal hypertrophy (ASH): light and electron microscopic findings. Circulation 50:436
16. Maron BJ, Edwards JE, Henry WL, Clark CE, Bingle CJ, Epstein SE (1974) Asymmetric septal hypertrophy (ASH) in infancy. Circulation 50:809
17. Maron BJ, Henry WL, Clark CE, Redwood DR, Roberts WC, Epstein SE (1976) Asymmetric septal hypertrophy in childhood. Circulation 53:9
18. Sutton MSJ, Lie JT, Anderson KR, O'Brien PC, Frye RL (1980) Histopathological specificity of hypertrophic obstructive cardiomyopathy. Myocardial fibre disarray and myocardial fibrosis. Brit Heart J 44:433

Cellular Disorganization in Hypertrophic Cardiomyopathy 57

19. Fujiwara H, Kawai C, Hamashima Y (1979) Myocardial fascicle and fiber disarray in 25 μ-thick sections. Circulation 59:1293
20. Maron BJ, Roberts WC, Edwards JE, McAllister HA, Foley DD, Epstein SE (1978) Sudden death in patients with hypertrophic cardiomyopathy: characterization of 26 patients without previous functional limitation. Am J Cardiol 41:803
21. Savage DD, Seides SF, Maron BJ, Meyers DJ, Epstein SE (1979) Prevalence of arrhythmias during 24-h electrocardiographic monitoring and exercise testing in patients with obstructive and nonobstructive hypertrophic cardiomyopathy. Circulation 59:866
22. Maron BJ, Savage DD, Wolfson JK, Epstein SE (1981) Prognostic significance of 24-hour ambulatory electrocardiographic monitoring in patients with hypertrophic cardiomyopathy: a prospective study. Am J Cardiol 48:252
23. McKenna WJ, England D, Oakley CM, Goodwin JF (1980) Detection of arrhythmia in hypertrophic cardiomyopathy: prospective study (Abstr). Circulation [Suppl III]:III-187

Left Ventricular Biopsy in Hypertrophic Cardiomyopathy: Light and Electron Microscopic Evaluations

B. Kunkel, M. Schneider, R. Hopf, G. Kober, K. Hübner, and M. Kaltenbach

The morphology of hypertrophic cardiomyopathy has been studied in myocardium excised surgically from the septum and in biopsy specimens from the right and left ventricle obtained during catheterization [1–3]. Characteristic changes in myocardial architecture, predominantly of the septal region, have been described by many authors [1, 2, 4, 5]. The reliability of endomyocardial biopsy in diagnosing hypertrophic cardiomyopathy remains controversial, however. The present study was carried out to evaluate the diagnostic implications of this method in patients with hypertrophic cardiomyopathy.

Patients and Methods

Left ventricular biopsies were performed in 24 patients with hypertrophic cardiomyopathy (HOCM). The diagnosis was established by echocardiography as well as right and left heart catheterization including coronary angiography and biplane ventriculography. All patients had intraventricular pressure gradients of more than 30 mmHg, consistent with classic hypertrophic obstructive cardiomyopathy.

The biopsy forceps (Olympus BF 5 B_2) was introduced into the left ventricle via the right brachial artery through a thin-walled guide catheter. In each patient, two specimens were excised from the left ventricular posterior wall, one for light and one for electron microscopy. Tissue samples for light microscopy were fixed in 4% formalin and embedded in paraffin. 5-μ-thick sections were routinely stained with Hematoxilin-Eosin and Goldner. Specimens for electron microscopy were fixed in 2.5% glutaraldehyde in phosphate buffer (pH 7.2), dehydrated with ether, and embedded in Vestopal. Ultrathin sections were examined with a Siemens Elmiscop 101.

The microscopic finding of the 24 patients with hypertrophic cardiomyopathy (HOCM) were compared with those obtained in 50 patients with advanced congestive cardiomyopathy (COCM) and 18 patients with aortic stenosis (AS).

For quantification of myocardial hypertrophy the fiber diameter was measured in at least 50 myocytes. The degree of hypertrophy was graded according to the mean cell diameter: below 16μ was considered normal, 16–20μ mild, 21–25μ moderate, and over 25μ severe hypertrophy.

The interstitial fibrous tissue was measured morphometrically by a point counting system according to the principles of Weibel [6]. The sections were divided into adjacent areas upon which a square grid consisting of 36 points was superimposed. According to the size of the specimen, 6–15 adjacent areas per section could be an-

Left Ventricular Biopsy in Hypertrophic Cardiomyopathy 59

alyzed. In this manner, 1080–1800 points per biopsy were counted. The connective tissue content was calculated using the following formula:

$$\frac{P_c}{P_t} \times 100 = \text{connective tissue volume \%}.$$

P_c = number of points following on connective tissue

P_t = total number of points

Ultrastructural analysis could be performed in 21 patients with HOCM, 18 patients with aortic valve disease, and 115 patients with advanced and suspected early COCM. Electron microscopic changes were graded by a previously described score system that allowed quantification of the various hypertrophic or degenerative changes [7]. Electron microscopy thus could be compared to clinical data.

Results

The results of light microscopy are summarized in Table 1. Myocardial hypertrophy was present in all patients with COCM and AS. In HOCM 19 of the 24 patients displayed some degree of hypertrophy in the posterior left ventricular wall; this change was not evident in the remaining five patients.

Degenerative cellular alterations with perinuclear vacuolization and reduction of the contractile material were observed much less often in HOCM (8%) than in COCM (24%). The highest incidence was found in AS (60%).

Two patients (2/24) with hypertrophic obstructive cardiomyopathy showed focal disarrangement of myofibers and stellated cells. This abnormality, however, was also seen in four patients (4/50) with COCM and in three patients (3/18) with AS.

Table 1. Histologic findings in patients with HOCM, COCM, and AS

	HOCM (n=24)		COCM (n=50)		AS (n=18)	
	n	%	n	%	n	%
Myocardial hypertrophy	19	79	50	100	18	100
Degenerative alterations of the cardiocytes	2	8	12	24	12	67
Irregular arrangement of cardiocytes	2	8	4	8	3	17
Interstitial fibrosis	8	32	39	78	18	100
Endocardial fibrosis	3	12	21	42	9	50
Smooth muscle cells within the endocardium	2	8	11	22	4	22
Inflammatory infiltrations	0	0	1	2	0	0
Increase in fibrocytes, fibroblasts, and histiocytes	1	4	10	20	2	11
Normal myocardium	1	4	0	0	0	0

HOCM, Hypertrophic obstructive cardiomyopathy; COCM, Congestive cardiomyopathy; AS, Aortic stenosis.

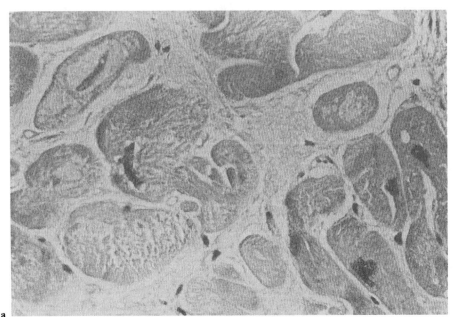
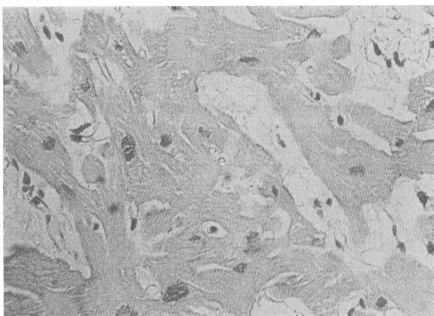

Fig. 1 a–d. The figures show typical examples of left ventricular biopsies of different myocardial diseases. **a** B. K. H. 41 years. HOCM. Intraventricular pressure gradient 64 mmHg. Myocardial biopsy: Normal arrangement of the markedly hypertrophied cardiac muscle cells (cell diameter 27.9 μm). **b** R. I. 24 yrs. HOCM. Intraventricular pressure gradient 30 mmHg. Myocardial biopsy: Small focus of cellular disorganization. Slight nuclear enlargement. Normal fiber diameter (15.4 μm). **c** G. R. 42 yrs. COCM. Ejection fraction 34%. Myocardial biopsy: Severe hypertrophy of the myocardial cells and marked diffuse interstitial fibrosis. (Fiber diameter 29.9 μ, interstitial fibrous tissue 26.2%). **d** D.G. 27 yrs. Aortic valve disease. Ejection fraction 32%. Myocardial biopsy: Severe myocardial hypertrophy with degenerative cellular changes. Marked diffuse interstitial fibrosis. (Fiber diameter 28.5 μm, interstitial fibrous tissue: 35%)

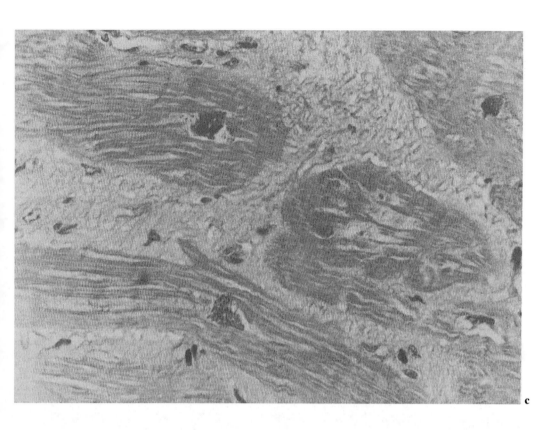

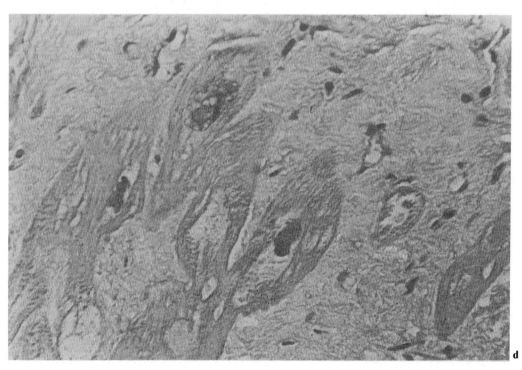

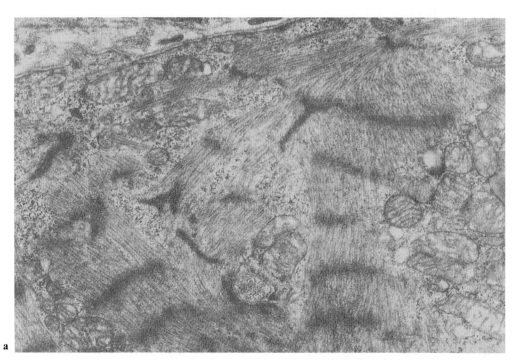
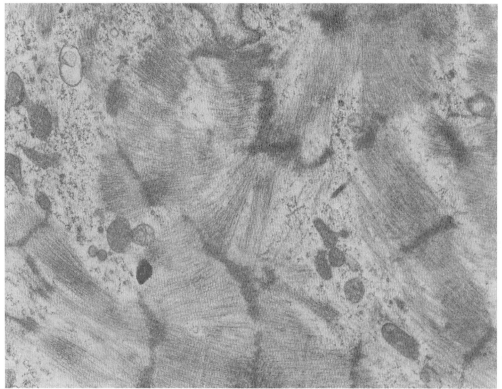

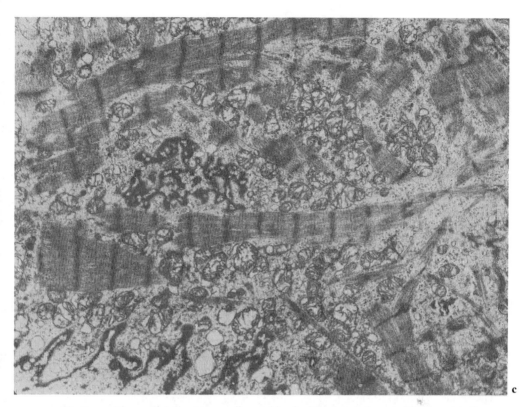

Fig. 2a–c. Myocardial disarray usually combined with z-band abnormalities is not pathognomonic for hypertrophic cardiomyopathy. It can be found in patients with myocardial hypertrophy regardless of its origin. **a** S. H. 54 yrs. HOCM. Intraventricular pressure gradient 80 mmHg. **b** G. R. 42 yrs. COCM left ventricular ejection fraction. 34% (same patient as Fig. 1c). **c** L. H. 52 yrs. aortic valve disease

Table 2. Quantification of myocardial hypertrophy according to muscle cell diameter

	HOCM n=24 n	HOCM %	COCM n=50 n	COCM %	AS n=18 n	AS %
Myocardial hypertrophy absent (< 16 μ)	5	21	0	0	0	0
mild (16 – 20 μ)	9	37	12	24	5	28
moderate (21 – 25 μ)	9	37	24	48	7	39
severe (< 25 μ)	1	4	14	28	6	33

Interstitial fibrosis of the left ventricular free wall occurred significantly more frequently in COCM (78%) and AS (100%) than in HOCM (32%). The same distribution was found for endocardial fibrosis with/without proliferation of smooth muscle cells. Inflammatory infiltrations were seen in only one COCM patient. An increase in fibrocytes, fibroblasts, and histiocytes in cardiac interstitium was observed considerably more often in COCM than in HOCM or AS.

Quantification of Myocardial Hypertrophy

The degree of myocardial hypertrophy was quantified according to the muscle cell diameter (Table 2). Absent or mild myocardial hypertrophy was more often present in hypertrophic cardiomyopathy than in both other groups. By contrast severe hypertrophy predominated in patients with aortic valve disease or congestive cardiomyopathy and occurred only sporadically in hypertrophy cardiomyopathy.

Quantification of Interstitial Fibrosis

Interstitial fibrosis was more frequent and more pronounced in the subendocardial layers of patients with COCM and AS than with HOCM (Table 3). Of HOCM patients, 12% had severe interstitial fibrosis, while 28% of advanced COCM and 33% of AS patients were found to have this change.

Electron Microscopy

The ultrastructural changes in hypertrophic cardiomyopathy and the other groups were due to myocardial hypertrophy or cellular degeneration. The most prominent elctron microscopic changes are compiled in Table 4.

Z-band abnormalities such as irregular widening and clumping of Z-band material or accumulation under the sacrolemmal membrane were common findings in hypertrophic cells of all three types of diseases. Myofibrillar disarray surprisingly occurred more frequently in biopsies of congestive cardiomyopathy and aortic valve disease than in hypertrophic cardiomyopathy. Myofibers with reduced contractile

Table 3. Quantification of interstitial fibrosis in patients with HOCM, COCM, and AS

Interstitial fibrosis	HOCM n = 24		COCM n = 50		AS n = 18	
	n	%	n	%	n	%
absent (< 5%)	15	62	11	22	0	0
mild (5 – 10%)	2	8	14	28	1	5,5
moderate (10 – 20%)	4	17	11	22	11	61
severe (> 20%)	3	12	14	28	6	33

Left Ventricular Biopsy in Hypertrophic Cardiomyopathy

Table 4. Ultrastructural findings in patients with HOCM, COCM, and AS

	HOCM n = 21		COCM n = 40		AS n = 18	
	n	%	n	%	n	%
Nuclear enlargement	18	85	40	100	18	100
Myofibrils						
Z-band abnormalities	11	52	27	68	8	44
Disarray	6	29	15	38	9	50
Lysis/loss	6	29	36	90	13	72
Mitochondria						
Increase in number	13	62	40	100	18	100
Reduction in number	1	4,8	25	63	12	67
Abnormal size/shape	8	38	33	83	12	67
Degeneration	9	43	30	75	8	44
Myelin figures	10	48	24	60	7	39
Lipid droplets	3	14	11	28	7	39
Lipofuscin granules	3	14	20	50	5	28
Hyperplasia/dilatation of the sarcoplasmatic reticulum	7	33	19	48	4	22
Hyperplasia/dilatation of the T system	11	52	21	53	15	83
Hypertrophic Golgi apparatus	13	62	19	48	10	56
Ergastoplasma	12	57	19	48	10	56

material were often found in patients with COCM and AS, whereas this alteration was seen only sporadically and to a mild degree in patients with hypertrophic cardiomyopathy. This is in accordance with the lower grade of hypertrophy and a usually normal left ventricular function in this group. Mitochondria showed numerous structural and quantitative abnormalities in all three groups. Cardiocytes with proliferation of mitochondria were found in all biopsies from congestive cardiomyopathy and aortic stenosis, whereas they were only seen in 62% of patients with HOCM. In COCM and AS, numerous other cells had a reduced number of mitochondria. This was rarely seen in hypertrophic cardiomyopathy. Mitochondrial degeneration and abnormal variations of size and shape were also more pronounced in the two other groups. Proliferation and dilatation of the T system was found significantly more frequently in the HOCM and AS groups than in HOCM. Myelin figures, lipid droplets, lipofuscin granules, and alterations of the sarcoplasmatic reticulum did not show major differences in the three groups.

Myocardial Biopsy and Ventricular Function

Left ventricular ejection fraction in relation to muscle cell diameter and ultrastructural alterations showed increasing myocardial hypertrophy and pronounced electronmicroscopic changes with decreasing ventricular pump function (Fig. 3). Patients with normal or slightly decreased ejection fraction usually had minor pathologic changes with mild hypertrophy and a low total electronmicroscopic score. Patients with reduced ejection fraction showed advanced myocardial hypertrophy and more extensive ultrastructural changes due to hypertrophy and cellular degeneration. This could be uniformly observed both in patients with congestive cardiomyopathy and aortic valve disease. Pathologic changes in HOCM were usually less severe according to the normal or hypercontractile patterns of the myocardium.

Severe myocardial scarring was found more often in patients with impaired ventricular function although there are enormous individual variations and the differences between the three functional groups are not significant.

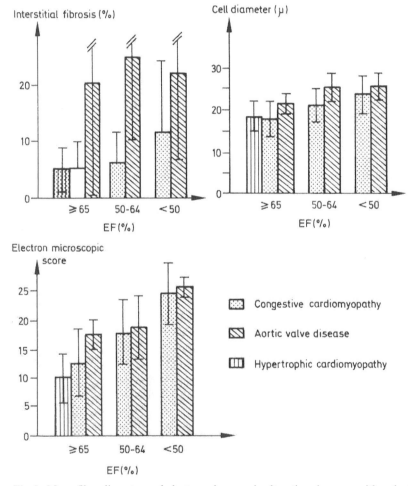

Fig. 3. Mean fiber diameter and electronmicroscopic alterations increase with reduction of the ejection fraction. HOCM shows minor pathologic changes similar to patients with aortic valve disease and suspected early COCM with normal EF. The interstitial fibrous tissue content varies markedly within the three groups

Discussion

The characteristic histologic appearance of hypertrophic cardiomyopathy consists of hypertrophied, abnormally shaped, irregular arranged muscle cells with abnormal arrangement of myofibrils and Z-band abnormalities [5,6]. The characteristic alterations were found by Ferrans [2] in operatively excised materials from the septal region in each of 15 patients. From right ventricular biopsies, Olsen [8] "confirmed" hypertrophic cardiomyopathy in six cases and "excluded" the diagnosis in 11 of 25. In eight cases "unhelpful" results were obtained. Davis [3] found the characteristic histologic appearance in biopsies from the left ventricular wall in only one of six cases. In our series, no fundamental structure differences were found between left ventricular biopsies of patients with hypertrophic cardiomyopathy, congestive cardiomyopathy, and aortic stenosis. Branching and abnormal arrangement of myocardial cells was seen in only two cases of hypertrophic cardiomyopathy but was also found in patients with congestive cardiomyopathy and aortic valve disease. Abnormal arrangement of singular myocardial cells evidently occurs to a certain degree in various kinds of myocardial hypertrophy. Ferrans [9] observed disarray of myocardial fibers in 10% of patients with congestive cardiomyopathy and in 18% of patients with congenital heart diseases associated with right ventricular hypertrophy and outflow tract obstruction. While a majority of myofibers in the ventricular septum of hypertrophic cardiomyopathy patients is affected, only very few myofibers show irregular arrangement in other diseases. Kawai and Matsumori [4] found various degrees of myofiber disarray in 60% of the biopsies from patients with congestive cardiomyopathy. From necropsy studies, he concluded that the probability of hitting the site of myocardial fiber disarray by right ventricular biopsy is not more than 33%. As pointed out by Maron et al., not the presence of cellular disarray but the number of myofibers involved in the intraventricular septum is characteristic for hypertrophic cardiomyopathy [10]. The specimens obtained by myocardial biopsy are usually too small to evaluate the extent of fiber disarray. Hence, hypertrophic cardiomyopathy cannot reliably be diagnosed from a few branched and irregularly arranged myocytes in the small biopsy specimen containing a very limited number of myocardial cells.

The most frequent findings observed in all three groups were myocardial hypertrophy and interstitial fibrosis. Both were considerably more pronounced in congestive cardiomyopathy and aortic valve disease than in hypertrophic cardiomyopathy. The latter showed no histologic evidence of hypertrophy in 21%, although all angiographic and echocardiographic characteristics of hypertrophic cardiomyopathy were present. This may be due to the fact that in aortic valve disease and congestive cardiomyopathy all regions of the heart are equally affected, whereas hypertrophic obstructive cardiomyopathy primarily represents a localized disorder of the myocardium. Hypertrophy of the free ventricular wall is possibly acquired during the course of disease [11]. Therefore, the severity of hypertrophy in the biopsy from the left ventricular free wall of patients with HOCM may provide information concerning the stage and progress of the disease as well as the response of the entire myocardium to the abnormal anatomic and functional conditions.

Electron microscopic analysis revealed the typical ultrastructural criteria of myocardial hypertrophy in all three groups. As in light microscopy, all changes were more pronounced in aortic valve disease and congestive cariomyopathy than in hypertrophic cardiomyopathy. Degenerative cellular changes as a consequence of myocardial hypertrophy – common findings in congestive cardiomyopathy and aortic valve disease [2, 12] – were rarely seen in HOCM. This finding is in accordance with the normal or hypercontractile status of the heart in HOCM. The degree of myocardial hypertrophy and resulting degenerative alterations increases with the impairment of ventricular function. Comparing histologic and functional parameters of patients with aortic valve disease and congestive cardiomyopathy, we were able to demonstrate that the degree of hypertrophy and the severity of cellular degeneration increase significantly as the ejection fraction decreases. Thus, the ultrastructural changes of the biopsies more probably reflect the degree of functional impairment of the myocardium than any specific disease entity.

Summary

Myocardial hypertrophy with or without degenerative alterations is the predominant finding in left ventricular biopsies from patients with hypertrophic and congestive cardiomyopathy and aortic valve disease. Small foci of cellular disorganization may occur in all three disease entities. Myofibrillar disarray was seen significantly more often in congestive cardiomyopathy and aortic valve disease than in hypertrophic cardiomyopathy. Hence, from the small myocardial biopsy, hypertrophic cardiomyopathy cannot be reliably diagnosed and differentiated from other diseases with myocardial hypertrophy. The degree of myocardial hypertrophy and consecutive cellular degeneration more probably reflects the functional patterns of the myocardium than any peculiar disease.

References

1. Van Norden S, Olsen EGJ, Pearce GE (1971) Hypertrophic obstructive cardiomyopathy. A biological histochemical and ultrastructural study of biopsy material. Cardiovasc Res 5:118–131
2. Ferrans VJ, Massumi RA, Shugoll GJ, Ali N, Roberts WC (1977) Ultrastructural studies of myocardial biopsies in 45 patients with obstructive or congestive cardiomyopathy. In: Bagust E, Rona S, Brink AJ (eds) Recent advances in cardiac structure and metabolism. Cardiomyopathies. University Park, Baltimore, pp 231–272
3. Davis MJ, Brooksby JAB, Jenkins S, Canvocic-Darracott S, Swanton RH, Coltard DJ, Webb-Peploe MM (1977) Left ventricular biopsy II: The value of light microscopy. Cath et Cardiovasc Diag 3:123–130
4. Kawai C, Matsumori A (1980) Myocardial biopsy. Am Rev Med 31:139–157
5. Maron BJ, Anan TJ, Roberts WC (1981) Quantitative analysis of the distribution of cardiac muscle cell disorganization in the left ventricular wall of patients with hypertrophic cardiomyopathy. Circulation 63:887–899
6. Weibel E, Kistler GS, Scherle WF (1966) Practical stereological methods for morphometric cytology. J Cell Biol 30:23–38

Left Ventricular Biopsy in Hypertrophic Cardiomyopathy

7. Kunkel B, Lapp H, Kober G, Kaltenbach M (1978) Correlation between clinical and morphologic findings and natural history in congestive cardiomyopathy. In: Kaltenbach M, Loogen F, Olsen ECJ (eds) Cardiomyopathy and myocardial biopsy. Springer, Berlin Heidelberg New York, pp 271–283
8. Olsen EGJ (1976) Pathologie der "primären" Kardiomyopathien. Muench Med Wochenschr 118:735–740
9. Ferrans VJ (1978) Myocardial ultrastructure in human cardiac hypertrophy. In: Kaltenbach M, Loogen F, Olsen EGJ (eds) Cardiomyopathy and myocardial biopsy. Springer, Berlin Heidelberg New York, pp 100–120
10. Maron BJ, Roberts WC (1979) Quantitative analysis of cardiac muscle cell disorganisation in the ventricular septum of patients with hypertrophic cardiomyopathy. Circulation 55:689
11. Roberts WC, Ferrans VJ, Buja LM (1974) Pathologic aspects of the idiopathic cardiomyopathies. Adv Cardiol 13:343–357
12. Maron BJ, Ferrans VJ, Roberts WC (1975) Myocardial ultrastructure in patients with chronic aortic valve disease. Am J Cardiol 35:725–739
13. Kunkel B (1981) Licht- und elektronenmikroskopische Untersuchung von Myokardbiopsien und ihre klinische Bedeutung. Habilitationsschrift, Universität Frankfurt am Main

Cardiomyopathy in Animals and Therapeutic Interventions

Synopsis

BARRY J. MARON

For those investigators interested in the clinical, pathophysiologic, and subcellular features of hypertrophic cardiomyopathy, availability of a spontaneously occurring or experimentally produced animal model of this disease suitable for controlled experimentation would be potentially useful. The three papers presented in this chapter describe some of the current data concerning available animal models and their potential use in experimental studies on hypertrophic cardiomyopathy.

In the first paper I present data characterizing a spontaneously occurring form of hypertrophic cardiomyopathy in cats and dogs that has been described at The Animal Medical Center (New York City) by Drs. Si-Kwang Liu and Lawrence Tilley. The cardiac structural abnormalities in these small animals with hypertrophic cardiomyopathy resemble (but are not identical to) that in patients having this disease. While cats and dogs with hypertrophic cardiomyopathy may prove to be useful in the study of human disease, it should be emphasized that these animals do not represent "identical models" of human disease and certain potentially important differences exist between the human and animal conditions. Also, the ability to practically utilize the feline and canine forms of hypertrophic cardiomyopathy experimentally would ultimately require the breeding of these animals in colonies, and this has not as yet been attempted.

The paper by Dr. Kaye formulates an interesting hypothesis that nerve-growth-factor may produce certain anatomical changes in puppies which resemble those of hypertrophic cardiomyopathy in patients. However, the author is properly cautious in avoiding any definitive conclusions regarding the equivalence of this model to human hypertrophic cardiomyopathy. Certainly, the ability to experimentally produce hypertrophic cardiomyopathy would provide an easily available source of subjects for laboratory investigation, as well as possibly providing insights into the basic mechanisms involved in the pathogenesis of hypertrophic cardiomyopathy.

The study of Dr. Lossnitzer demonstrates the way in which a spontaneously occurring cardiomyopathy in the Syrian golden hamster may be used to study the effects a pharmacologic agent such as verapamil has on myocardial morphology and metabolism. The cardiomyopathy in Syrian hamsters differs substantially (with regard to structural alterations) from hypertrophic cardiomyopathy in man and other animals. However, such spontaneously occurring animal diseases may still be useful for the study of certain selected alterations of the heart, e.g., disturbed myocardial calcium metabolism and the effects of a calcium-antagonistic drug on these abnormalities.

Spontaneously Occurring Hypertrophic Cardiomyopathy in Dogs and Cats: A Potential Animal Model of a Human Disease

BARRY J. MARON, SI-KWANG LIU, and LAWRENCE P. TILLEY

Summary

Cardiac morphologic features are described in 51 cats and ten dogs with spontaneously occurring hypertrophic cardiomyopathy. Each animal had a hypertrophied, but nondilated left ventricle in the absence of another cardiac or systemic disease capable of producing left ventricular hypertrophy. Death most commonly occurred suddenly and unexpectedly in dogs (occasionally in the absence of previous signs of cardiac disease), but was usually due to marked congestive heart failure in cats.

Disproportionate thickening of the ventricular septum with respect to the left ventricular free wall was present in eight (80%) of the ten dogs and 16 (31%) of the 51 cats. Marked ventricular septal disorganization (involving ≧ 5% of the tissue section), and similar in appearance to the characteristic lesion of patients with hypertrophic cardiomyopathy, was identified in two (20%) of the 10 dogs and 14 (27%) of the 51 cats. Therefore, cardiac muscle cell disorganization is not confined to the human variety of hypertrophic cardiomyopathy but appears to represent an anatomic linkage between different species in which this disease occurs.

Marked septal disorganization occurred only in those cats with disproportionate hypertrophy of the ventricular septum. Hence, about one-fourth of our cats with hypertrophic cardiomyopathy closely resembled the human form of this disease morphologically, with asymmetric left ventricular hypertrophy and marked disorganization of cardiac muscle cells in the ventricular septum.

Although not identical "models" of the human disease, feline and canine hypertrophic cardiomyopathy may prove useful in future investigations of the clinical, hemodynamic, and pathologic features of hypertrophic cardiomyopathy in man.

Hypertrophic cardiomyopathy is a disease of cardiac muscle in which the most characteristic anatomic feature is a hypertrophied, nondilated left ventricle [1] that is usually associated with a disproportionately thickened ventricular septum containing numerous disorganized cardiac muscle cells [2–13]. Since animal models of hypertrophic cardiomyopathy would be useful in the study of this condition, identification of a spontaneous cardiac disease in animals that is similar to hypertrophic cardiomyopathy in patients is of particular interest. Hence, the following report describes a primary cardiomyopathy in dogs [14] and cats [15, 16] that resembles hypertrophic cardiomyopathy in man.

Selection of Animals

The cardiovascular registry of the Animal Medical Center, 1975–1977, was reviewed. During that period 177 dogs and 243 cats with cardiac disease were examined at necropsy; 10 of the 177 dogs and 51 of the 243 cats were identified as having anatomic findings consistent with a primary hypertrophic cardiomyopathy. Ninety-five dogs and 65 cats with normal hearts (who died of noncardiac diseases) or acquired or congenital heart diseases other than hypertrophic cardiomyopathy were selected for study as controls (Table 1).

Table 1. Cardiac diseases in 160 control animals

Disease	No. of cats studied	No. of dogs studied
Dilated (congestive) cardiomyopathy [25]	16	19
Ventricular septal defect	5	2
Supravalvular aortic stenosis	2	0
Congenital malformation of mitral valve complex [25]	3	20
Congenital dysplasia of tricuspid valve [25]	3	13
Acquired mitral valvular disease	0	18
Discrete subaortic stenosis	0	4
Patent ductus arteriosus	0	6
Atrial septal defect	0	1
Tetralogy of Fallot	0	1
Normal	36	11
Total	65	95

Materials and Methods

Measurement of Ventricular Wall Thicknesses

Measurements of ventricular wall thicknesses were made in fixed specimens in the following two areas: (1) ventricular septum, at the point of maximum thickness, usually about one-half the distance between the base of the aortic valve and the apex of the left ventricle; and (2) the posterior left ventricular free wall, behind the mid-point of the posterior mitral leaflet, at a level corresponding to caudal margins of the mitral leaflets. In making measurements of ventricular wall thickness, care was taken to avoid including trabeculae, papillary muscles, or crista supraventricularis.

Preparation of Tissue

In each of the 116 cats studied (51 with hypertrophic cardiomyopathy and 65 controls), full wall thickness blocks of tissue were taken perpendicular to the long-axis of the left ventricle from: (1) ventricular septum at the point of maximal thickness; (2) posterior left ventricular wall about one-half the distance between the mitral valve anulus and left ventricular apex, and (3) anterior left ventricular wall about 1–2 cm lateral to the left anterior descending coronary artery. All tissue sections were embedded in paraffin, sectioned at a thickness of 6 μ, and stained with hematoxylin and eosin.

Quantitation of Cardiac Muscle Cell Arrangement

A technique previously described in detail [12] was used to quantitatively assess the extent of cardiac muscle cell disorganization in tissue sections of ventricular septum and left ventricular free wall. In brief, tissue sections in which cardiac muscle cell disorganization was judged to be present qualitatively were photographed and the images enlarged into 30×40 inch positive prints, resulting in an average magnification of about 1000–2000 times the original tissue section. A transparent cellulose overlay was then placed over the print, and the areas of myocardium occupied by disorganized cardiac muscle cells were outlined with a marking pen on the overlay. The transparent overlay was removed, photographed, and the image reproduced as a 5×7 inch print. Each area into which the tissue section had been divided was outlined separately with a fine point marking pen on ordinary tablet paper, and quantitated using a video planimetry system.

Results

Clinical Findings and Circumstances of Death

Dogs

Clinical findings in the 10 dogs with hypertrophic cardiomyopathy are summarized in Table 2. At death, ages ranged from 1 to 13 years (mean 6 years). Eight dogs were male and two were female.

Four of the ten dogs had evidence of congestive heart failure one week to one year prior to death. In two dogs cardiac decompensation was mild and was manifested by coughing, mild dyspnea, and radiographic evidence of pulmonary venous congestion. In two other dogs cardiac failure was marked, as evidenced by severe dyspnea, cardiomegaly, hepatomegaly, and pleural or pericardial effusions. Three of the four dogs with heart failure died unexpectedly while under anesthesia during operation (for repair of a skin laceration, pacemaker implantation, or pericardiocentesis); the remaining dog was put to death by request of the owner.

Six other dogs with hypertrophic cardiomyopathy had no evidence of cardiac disease prior to death. Three of these dogs died suddenly (one while being walked and two were found dead); two dogs died unexpectedly during operation for noncardiac abnormalities. The remaining dog died of causes apparently unrelated to heart disease, i.e., renal failure of undetermined etiology associated with disseminated intravascular coagulopathy.

Electrocardiographic recordings were obtained in five of the ten dogs with hypertrophic cardiomyopathy. Three dogs showed complete heart block, including one with a history of syncope (who died during implantation of a pacemaker). This latter dog and one other with complete heart block also showed evidence of bifascicular block (left axis deviation and right ventricular conduction delay) (Fig. 1).

Table 2. Clinical and necropsy findings in 10 dogs with hypertrophic cardiomyopathy

Age (yr)/Sex	Breed	Heart wt.		Ventricular wall thickness (mm)					VS dis-organi-zation[a]	Clinical history	Circumstances of death	Electro-cardiogram
		g	g/kg	VS	PW	AL	RV	VS/PW				
8/M	Doberman	311	9.5	21	14	23	7	1.5	0	No cardiac symptoms	1-week history renal failure[b]	–
4/M	German shepard	266	8.5	21	15	22	6	1.4	0	2-week his-tory mild CHF	During surgery for repair of skin lacera-tion; under anesthesia	–
9/F	Airedale	153	10.6	17	12	12	6	1.4	0	No cardiac symptoms	Sudden; found dead by owner	1° A–V block
7/M	German shepard	273	8.0	20	15	24	7	1.3	0	No cardiac symptoms	Sudden; while being walked	–
13/M	Poodle	98	10.8	13	10	11	4	1.3	12%	1-year history progressive CHF; syncope	Euthanasia	CHB; LAD, RVCD, possible RVH
6/F	German shepard	247	9.2	21	16	18	7	1.3	0	1-month his-tory mild CHF; syncope	During pacemaker implan-tation, under anesthesia	CHB; LAD, RVCD, possible RVH
1/M	Great Dane	385	10.4	22	19	21	6	1.2	0	No cardiac symptoms	Sudden; found dead by owner	–
3/M	Bulldog	193	10.1	19	16	15	7	1.2	14%	No cardiac symptoms	During surgery for ure-thral calculi; under anesthesia	CHB[c]

| 3/M | German shepard | 269 | 9.1 | 18 | 16 | 18 | 8 | 1.1 | 0 | No cardiac symptoms | During surgery for repair of fractured mandible; under anesthesia | – |
| 8/M | Boston terrier | 116 | 10.2 | 16 | 15 | 12 | 4 | 1.1 | 0 | 1-week history severe CHF; pericardial, pleural effusions, ascites | During pericardiocentesis | Normal |

VS, ventricular septum;   PW, posterior left ventricular free wall;   AL, anterolateral left ventricular free wall;   RV, right ventricular wall;   VS/PW, ventricular septal to posterior left ventricular free wall thickness ratio;   LVFW, left ventricular free wall;   0, absent;   –, data not available;   CHF, congestive heart failure;   1° A–V, first degree atrioventricular;   CHB, complete heart block;   LAD, left axis deviation;   RVCD, right ventricular conduction defect;   RVH, right ventricular hypertrophy.

[a] Expressed as the area of myocardium involved by disorganized cells relative to the area of myocardium containing longitudinally cut cardiac muscle cells [12].

[b] Disseminated intravascular coagulopathy at necropsy.

[c] Noted just prior to cardiac arrest on monitor; a complete scalar electrocardiogram was not obtained.

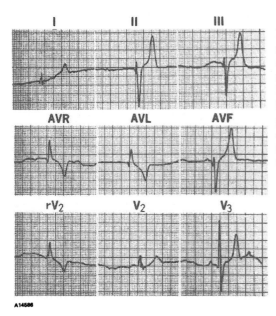

Fig. 1. Electrocardiogram recorded in a dog with hypertrophic cardiomyopathy 1 day prior to death. Note left anterior hemiblock and right ventricular conduction delay (QRS duration = 0.09 s; normal ≦ 0.06 s). T waves are peaked and upright in leads II, III, AVF, and V_3. rV_2 is obtained at right fifth interspace at chondrosternal junction

Of the two remaining dogs with electrocardiograms, one showed first degree atrioventricular block (PR interval = 0.15 s; normal ≦ 0.13 s) and the other was normal.

Cats

The 51 cats with hypertrophic cardiomyopathy ranged in age from 6 months to 16 years (mean 7 years); 39 were male and 12 were female. Cardiac failure was manifested by 22 (43%) of the cats and aortic thromboembolism was present in 21 (41%) of the animals. Eight (15%) cats died suddenly although each had manifested heart failure previously. The remaining 43 cats were euthanatized, 36 because of intractable heart failure and seven for reasons not related to cardiac disease such as pneumonia, anemia, osteosarcoma, urinary tract calculi, or traumatic injury.

Necropsy Data: Gross Anatomic Findings

Dogs

Fresh heart weights in the ten dogs with hypertrophic cardiomyopathy (9.6 ± 0.3 [SEM] g/kg) were significantly greater than in 11 dogs with normal hearts (6.6 ± 0.3 g/kg; $P<0.001$); heart weights in each of the ten dogs with hypertrophic cardiomyopathy were equal to or exceeded heart weights of each normal dog. However, heart weights in the dogs with hypertrophic cardiomyopathy (9.6 ± 0.3 g/kg) did not differ significantly from those in 84 dogs with aquired or congenital heart diseases (12.2 ± 0.5 g/kg).

In the ten dogs with hypertrophic cardiomyopathy, ventricular septal thickness ranged from 13 to 22 mm (mean 19) and posterior left ventricular free wall thickness ranged from 10 to 19 mm (mean 15). Disproportionate septal thickening (defined as a septal-free wall thickness ratio of >1.1)[1] was present in eight dogs (Figs, 2, 3); six had ratios ≧ 1.3, thereby meeting the diagnostic criterion for disproportionate septal thickening in patients with hypertrophic cardiomyopathy [7]. In none of the 95 control dogs (11 normals and 84 with acquired or congenital heart diseases) did the septal-free wall thickness ratio exceed 1.1 (Fig. 3). Mean septal-free wall thickness ratios in the ten dogs with hypertrophic cardiomyopathy (1.3 ± 0.04) was significantly greater than in dogs with normal hearts (1.0 ± 0.01; $P<0.001$) or in dogs with acquired or congenital heart disease (0.9 ± 0.01; $P<0.001$).

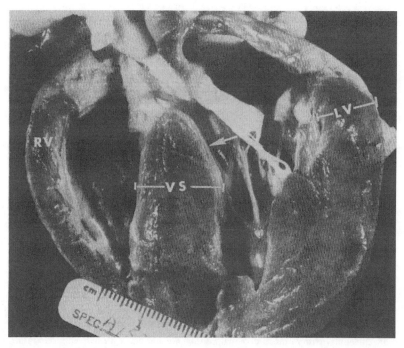

Fig. 2. Heart of a 9-year-old Airedale showing disproportionate thickening of the ventricular septum (*VS*) with respect to left ventricular free wall (*LV*). Fibrous plaque is evident on the left ventricular outflow tract (*arrow*); *RV*, right ventricular wall

In two of the ten dogs with hypertrophic cardiomyopathy, a fibrous endocardial plaque was present on the ventricular septum in the left ventricular outflow tract adjacent to the anterior mitral leaflet (Fig. 2). These endocardial plaques were similar in appearance to those in patients with hypertrophic cardiomyopathy [10]. In two other dogs a more diffuse fibrous tissue formation was present on the ventricular septum in the left ventricular outflow tract. In each of the ten dogs, the left ven-

---

[1] Our comparison of septal-free wall thickness ratios in animals with hypertrophic cardiomyopathy and control animals with normal hearts or other congenital or acquired heart diseases suggests that thickness ratios of >1.1 in dogs and ≧ 1.1 in cats are more appropriate diagnostic criteria for disproportionate septal thickening than the ≧ 1.3 "cut-off" that has been the conventional criterion employed in patients with hypertrophic cardiomyopathy [7].

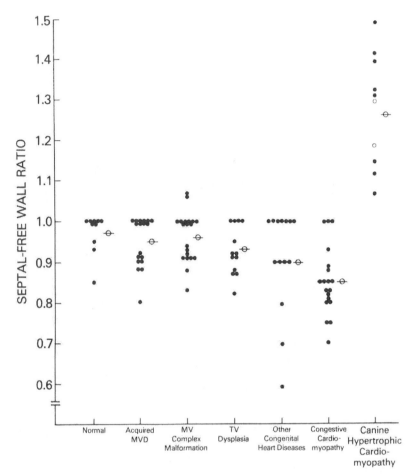

Fig. 3. Ventricular septal-left ventricular free wall thickness ratios in ten dogs with hypertrophic cardiomyopathy and 95 dogs with either normal hearts or with other acquired or congenital heart diseases. Subgroup of "other congenital heart diseases" includes four dogs with discrete subaortic stenosis, six with patent ductus arteriosus, two with ventricular septal defect, and one each with atrial septal defect and tetralogy of Fallot. Open symbols denote dogs with hypertrophic cardiomyopathy and marked septal disorganization

tricular cavity was moderately or markedly reduced in size; in two of these dogs the left atrium was moderately dilated. The cardiac valves appeared normal in each dog.

Cats

Heart weights in the 51 cats with hypertrophic cardiomyopathy (6.4±0.1 g/kg) were significantly greater than in 36 cats without cardiac disease (4.8±0.1 g/kg; $P<0.001$), but did not differ from the 29 cats with heart diseases other than hypertrophic cardiomyopathy (6.1±0.3 g/kg). Ventricular septal thicknesses in the 51 cats with hypertrophic cardiomyopathy ranged from 7 to 12 mm (mean 8); posterior free wall thicknesses ranged from 6 to 11 (mean 8).

Disproportionate thickening (defined as a ventricular septal to free wall thickness ratio of ≥ 1.1) was present in 16 (31%) of the 51 cats with hypertrophic cardiomyopathy, but in only three (4%) of the 65 control cats (Figs. 4, 5). Mean septal to posterior left ventricular wall ratios were significantly greater in the 51 cats with hypertrophic cardiomyopathy (1.0 ± 0.02) than in the 65 control cats (0.85 ± 0.01; $P < 0.001$).

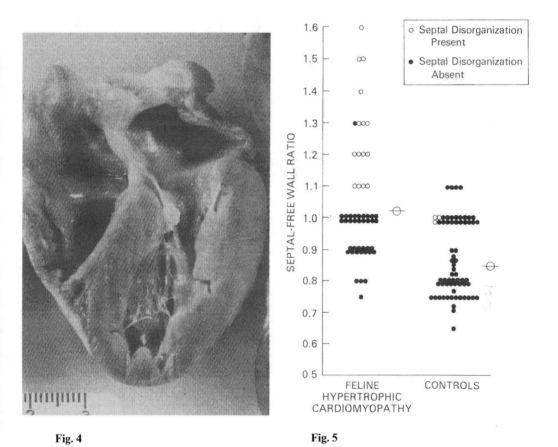

Fig. 4   Fig. 5

Fig. 4. Heart from a 2½-year-old male domestic cat showing disproportionate thickening of the cephalad portion of the ventricular septum with respect to the left ventricular free wall; septal to free wall thickness ratio is 1.3. At the point of maximum thickening, the septum bulges prominantly into the left ventricular outflow tract

Fig. 5. Ventricular septal-posterior free wall thickness ratios in 51 cats with hypertrophic cardiomyopathy and 65 control cats with normal hearts or with other acquired or congenital heart diseases. ⊖ = mean values

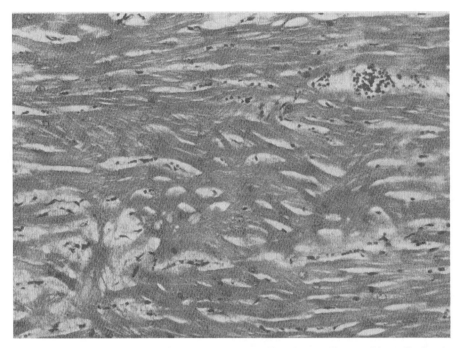

Fig. 6. Histologic section of ventricular septal myocardium from a 13-year-old poodle showing area of cardiac muscle cell disorganization in which adjacent cells are oriented obliquely and perpendicularly to each other. Magnification × 100. Hematoxylin and eosin stain

Necropsy Data: Quantitative Histologic Findings

Dogs

In eight of the ten dogs with hypertrophic cardiomyopathy and each of the 95 control animals studied, virtually all cardiac muscle cells in the ventricular septum were in normal parallel alignment. However, in the ventricular septum of two dogs with hypertrophic cardiomyopathy, a number of cardiac muscle cells were arranged perpendicularly or obliquely to each other (Figs. 6, 7). In quantitative terms, these areas

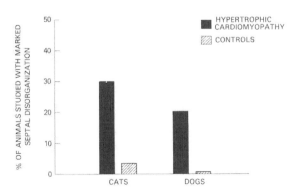

Fig. 7. Occurrence of marked ventricular septal disorganization ($\geq 5\%$) in dogs and cats with hypertrophic cardiomyopathy and comparison with control animals

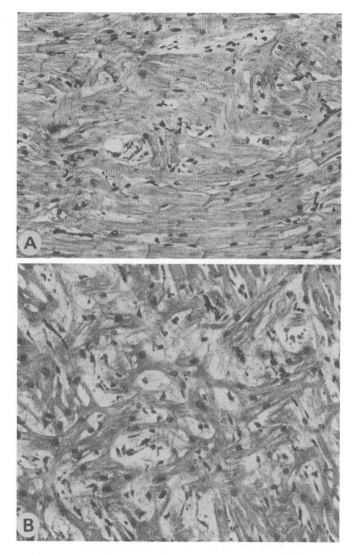

Fig. 8A, B. Histologic sections of ventricular septal myocardium from cats with hypertrophic cardiomyopathy showing cardiac muscle cell disorganization. (A) pattern in which small groups of cells are arranged at acute angles to other groups of cells (×220); (B) tangled arrangement of adjacent muscle cells (×200). Both sections stained with hematoxylin and eosin

of disorganized cardiac muscle cells were marked, i.e., occupied 14% and 12% of the tissue sections.

All cardiac muscle cells in the left ventricular free wall of nine of the ten dogs with hypertrophic cardiomyopathy were normally arranged. In the remaining dog, with a septal-free wall thickness ratio of 1.3, marked disorganization of cardiac muscle cells was present in the anterior and posterior left ventricular free walls (8% of the combined tissue sections).

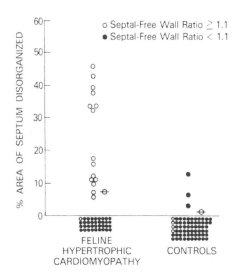

Fig. 9. Percent area of ventricular septum occupied by disorganized cardiac muscle cells in 51 cats with hypertrophic cardiomyopathy and in 65 control cats. ⊖ = mean values

Cats

Disorganized cardiac muscle cells were present in the ventricular septum of 15 (30%) of the 51 cats with hypertrophic cardiomyopathy (Figs. 7–9), and were absent in the remaining 36 cats. In 14 of the 15 cats disorganization was marked (involving 5% or more of the relevant areas of the tissue section; range, 6 to 46%), including seven cats in which >30% of the tissue section was involved (Figs. 7, 9). The remaining cat had septal disorganization involving 4% of the section. Septal disorganization was significantly more common in the cats with hypertrophic cardiomyopathy (15 of 51 or 30%) than in the controls (3 of 65 or 4%; $P<0.01$) (Figs. 7, 9); similarly, the extent of septal disorganization in the cats with hypertrophic cardiomyopathy (mean percent of section disorganized, $7\pm2\%$) was significantly greater than in the controls (mean percentage, $0.3\pm0.2\%$; $P<0.01$) (Figs. 7, 9).

Each of the 15 cats with septal disorganization had septal to free wall thickness ratios of ≥ 1.1, although one other cat with an abnormal thickness ratio had no disorganization (Figs. 5, 9).

Seven of the 15 cats with septal disorganization also had abnormally arranged cardiac muscle cells in the left ventricular free wall. Free wall disorganization ranged from 0.5% to 20% and involved >5% of the tissue section in four of the seven cats. The extent of free wall disorganization (mean $7\pm3\%$) was significantly less than that in the ventricular septum (mean $21\pm5\%$; $P<0.05$). Each of the seven cats with septal and free wall disorganization had abnormal septal to free wall ratios of ≥ 1.1 and four had marked ventricular septal thickening (10–12 mm).

Discussion

The present report describes the spontaneous occurrence of a primary hypertrophic cardiomyopathy in dogs and cats [14–16]. The clinical and pathologic findings in these animals are similar in many respects to that of hypertrophic cardiomyopathy in man. First, each of the dogs and cats showed marked cardiac hypertrophy. i.e., increased cardiac mass compared to animals with normal hearts. Second, the mean ventricular septal to left ventricular free wall thickness ratios in animals judged to have hypertrophic cardiomyopathy were significantly greater than in those animals with normal hearts or with other congenital or acquired heart diseases.

About one-fourth of the cats with hypertrophic cardiomyopathy showed marked disorganization of cardiac muscle cells in the ventricular septum (involving $\geq 5\%$ of the tissue section), similar in appearance and extent to the histologic hallmark of patients with hypertrophic cardiomyopathy [2, 5, 9, 12, 13]. Of note, each of the 15 cats with septal disorganization also had disproportionate thickening of the ventricular septum with respect to the left ventricular free wall (defined as a septal to free wall thickness ratio of ≥ 1.1 in cats). Hence, this study identified a subgroup of cats that resembled morphologically the form of hypertrophic cardiomyopathy which most commonly occurs in man, i.e., with asymmetric left ventricular hypertrophy and marked disorganization of cardiac muscle cells in the septum. However, the majority of cats studied (about 75%) showed a structural form of hypertrophic cardiomyopathy uncommonly observed in patients, i.e., characterized by symmetric (concentric) ventricular hypertrophy and normal arrangement of cardiac muscle cells in the septum [17]. At present, it is not clear whether these two morphologic forms of feline hypertrophic cardiomyopathy represent etiologically distinct diseases or are different phenotypic expressions of a single disease entity.

Septal disorganization was relatively uncommon (28%) in the overall population of 61 cats and dogs with hypertrophic cardiomyopathy. Hence, this histologic abnormality must be considered an insensitive marker of feline or canine hypertrophic cardiomyopathy. Nevertheless, when septal disorganization was present it was almost always marked; in 14 of the 15 cats and both dogs with disorganization, abnormally arranged cardiac muscle cells occupied >5% of the tissue section. On the other hand, marked septal disorganization was uncommon in cats and dogs with normal hearts or cardiac diseases other than hypertrophic cardiomyopathy (only 3 of the 160 controls); therefore, septal disorganization was a relatively specific finding (specificity = 98%) for feline and canine hypertrophic cardiomyopathy.

Disorganized architecture of the left ventricular free wall was infrequent in our population of cats and dogs with hypertrophic cardiomyopathy. Cardiac muscle cell disorganization was present in the free wall of only 7 of the 51 cats and only one of the ten dogs and was marked (> 5%) in just three animals. Of note, each of the seven cats with left ventricular free wall disorganization also had marked disorganization of cardiac muscle cells in the ventricular septum, as well as disproportionate septal thickening; four of these seven animals died suddenly and unexpectedly. Although we can not be definitive at this time, these findings do suggest that such cats have a more severe morphologic form of feline hypertrophic cardiomyopathy.

Of note, certain clinical features of dogs with hypertrophic cardiomyopathy are similar to those of many patients with this disease [18–22]. These points of similarity include predominance of the disease in males, the occurrence of sudden and unexpected death even without previous signs of cardiac disease, and the development of marked cardiac failure in some animals. However, one feature of hypertrophic cardiomyopathy in dogs that is distinctly uncommon in man is complete heart block [23]. Diffuse degenerative changes were present in the conduction system of two of our dogs with hypertrophic cardiomyopathy that may have been responsible for the complete heart block in these animals. However, such histopathologic abnormalities are not unique to dogs with hypertrophic cardiomyopathy and complete heart block; similar structural alterations have also been described in dogs with complete heart block that did not have a cardiomyopathy (unpublished observations) and in dogs without cardiac disease that died suddenly or were put to death by request of the owner [24].

In conclusion, it is evident from the data presented in this report that a primary myocardial disease, with certain pathologic features similar to those of hypertrophic cardiomyopathy in man, also occurs spontaneously in dogs and cats. The existence of this canine and feline disease may prove to be a valuable aid in the investigation of human cardiomyopathies.

References

1. Maron BJ, Epstein SE (1979) Hypertrophic cardiomyopathy: a discussion of nomenclature. Am J Cardiol 43:1242
2. Teare D (1958) Asymmetrical hypertrophy of the heart in young adults. Br Heart J 20:1
3. Menges H, Brandenburg RO, Brown AL (1972) The clinical, hemodynamic, and pathologic diagnosis of muscular subvalvular aortic stenosis. Circulation 24:1126
4. Abbasi AS, MacAlpin RN, Eber LM, Pearce ML (1972) Echocardiographic diagnosis of idiopathic hypertrophic cardiomyopathy without outflow obstruction. Circulation 46:897
5. Ferrans VJ, Morrow AG, Roberts WC (1972) Myocardial ultrastructure in idiopathic hypertrophic subaortic stenosis: A study of operatively excised left ventricular outflow tract muscle in 14 patients. Circulation 45:769
6. Abbasi AS, MacAlpin RN, Eber LM, Pearce ML (1973) Left ventricular hypertrophy diagnosed by echocardiography. N Engl J Med 289:118
7. Henry WL, Clark CE, Epstein SE (1973) Asymmetric septal hypertrophy: Echocardiographic identification of the pathognomonic anatomic abnormality of IHSS. Circulation 47:225
8. Maron BJ, Edwards JE, Henry WL, Clark CE, Bingle G, Epstein SE (1974) Asymmetric septal hypertrophy (ASH) in infancy. Circulation 50:809
9. Maron BJ, Ferrans VJ, Henry WL, Clark CE, Redwood DR, Roberts WC, Morrow AG, Epstein SE (1974) Differences in distribution of myocardial abnormalities in patients with obstructive and nonobstructive asymmetric septal hypertrophy (ASH): Light and electron microscopic findings. Circulation 50:436
10. Roberts WC, Ferrans VJ (1975) Pathological anatomy of the cardiomyopathies: Idiopathic dilated and hypertrophic types, infiltrative types, and endomyocardial disease with and without eosinophilia. Hum Pathol 6:287
11. Maron BJ, Henry WL, Clark CE, Redwood DR, Roberts WC, Epstein SE (1976) Asymmetric septal hypertrophy in childhood. Circulation 53:9
12. Maron BJ, Roberts WC (1979) Quantitative analysis of cardiac muscle cell disorganization in the ventricular septum of patients with hypertrophic cardiomyopathy. Circulation 59:689
13. Maron BJ, Sato N, Roberts WC, Edwards JE, Chandra RS (1979) Quantitative analysis of cardiac muscle cell disorganization in the ventricular septum. Comparison of fetuses and infants with and without congenital heart disease and patients with hypertrophic cardiomyopathy. Circulation 60:685

Spontaneously Occurring Hypertrophic Cardiomyopathy in Dogs and Cats 87

14. Liu S-K., Maron BJ, Tilley LP (1979) Hypertrophic cardiomyopathy in the dog. Am J Pathol 94:497
15. Tilley LP, Liu S-K, Gilbertson SR, Wagner BM, Lord PF (1977) Primary myocardial disease in the cat. Am J Pathol 86:493
16. Liu S-K, Maron BJ, Tilley LP (1981) Feline hypertrophic cardiomyopathy: Gross anatomic and quantitative histologic features. Am J Pathol 103:388
17. Maron BJ, Gottdiener JS, Roberts WC, Henry WL, Savage DD, Epstein SE (1977) Left ventricular outflow tract obstruction due to systolic anterior motion of the anterior mitral leaflet in patients with concentric left ventricular hypertrophy. Circulation 57:527
18. Frank S, Braunwald E (1968) Idiopathic hypertrophic subaortic stenosis: Clinical analysis of 126 patients with emphasis on the natural history. Circulation 137:759
19. Adelman AG, Wigle ED, Ranganathan N, Webb GD, Kidd BSL, Bigelow WG, Silver MD (1972) The clinical course in muscular subaortic stenosis: A retrospective and prospective study of 60 hemodynamically proven cases. Ann Intern Med 77:515
20. Shah PM, Adelman AG, Wigle ED, Gobel FL, Burchell HB, Hardarson T, Curiel R, De La Calzada C, Oakley CM, Goodwin JF (1973) The natural (and unnatural) history of hypertrophic obstructive cardiomyopathy: A multicenter study. Circ Res [Suppl II] 34, 35:179
21. Goodwin JF (1974) Prospects and predictions for the cardiomyopathies. Circulation 50:210
22. Maron BJ, Roberts WC, Edwards JE, McAllister HA, Foley DD, Epstein SE (1978) Sudden death in patients with hypertrophic cardiomyopathy: Characterization of 26 patients without previous functional limitation. Am J Cardiol 41:803
23. Spilkin S, Mitha AS, Matisonn RE, Chesler E (1977) Complete heart block in a case of idiopathic hypertrophic subaortic stenosis. Circulation 55:418
24. Meierhenry EF, Liu S-K (1978) Atrioventricular bundle degeneration associated with sudden death in the dog. J Am Vet Med Assoc 172:1418
25. Liu S-K (1977) Pathology of feline heart diseases. Vet Clin North Am 7:323

Cardiac Effects of Nerve Growth Factor in Dogs*

MICHAEL P. KAYE, DAVID J. WITZKE, DAVID J. WELLS, and VALENTIN FUSTER

Summary

Nerve growth factor, a protein necessary for the growth and maintenance of sympathetic nerves, was administered to newborn puppies and to pregnant bitches. Chemical analysis of the hearts of these animals at 3 months of age revealed a marked increase in myocardial norepinephrine. Gross and microscopic studies suggested myocardial hypertrophy. These changes occurring in the absence of systemic hypertension and caused by administration of nerve growth factor to dogs in the prenatal period raise questions concerning a potential role of nerve growth factor in the spontaneous development of myocardial abnormalities.

Introduction

Spontaneous elevation of circulating levels of catecholamines and the infusion of large doses of catecholamines have been shown to result in myocardial hypertrophy [1, 2] and the production of diffuse necrotic lesions in the myocardium [3, 4]. To demonstrate that ventricular hypertrophy could occur in the absence of a physiologically significant pressure overload, Laks et al. [5] showed that the chronic infusion of subhypertensive doses of norepinephrine resulted in the production of left ventricular hypertrophy. Summarizing the data obtained from their experiments, these investigators postulated that stress to the heart stimulates release of norepinephrine into the myocardium which then initiates the hypertrophy process.

On the basis of the evidence that norepinephrine induces myocardial hypertrophy either directly or by an increase in afterload, we investigated a technique of increasing endogenous myocardial catecholamine content to determine the possibility that this too might result in myocardial hypertrophy. Administration of nerve growth factor (NGF), a protein necessary for the growth and maintenance of sympathetic nerves [6], has been shown to cause an increase in myocardial catecholamine content in kittens [7] and puppies [8]. This manuscript reports data obtained from the chemical analysis of the myocardium of puppies treated with NGF in the prenatal or neonatal period together with the gross and microscopic changes occurring in the hearts of these animals.

---

* This investigation was supported in part by Research Grants HL–18123 and HL–20610 from the National Institutes of Health.

Methods

Fifty-six mongrel puppies from 15 litters were injected subcutaneously daily for the first 5 days of life with either 25000 units of 7S-NGF (Burroughs Wellcome) or 50000 units of β-NGF prepared in our laboratory by a modification of the technique of Mobley and associates [9]. Of the 56 treated puppies, 44 were killed at 3 months of age, 11 at 9 months and one at 1 year. An equal number of untreated littermates was used as controls. Additionally, two pregnant bitches were injected approximately one week before delivery with 25000 units per day of 7S-NGF for 5 days. A total of ten puppies from these litters survived and were killed for study at 3 months of age.

Myocardial Norepinephrine Content

For determination of myocardial catecholamine content, 13 untreated adult dogs and 12 of the 56 NGF-treated (3 months) and three untreated littermates were rapidly killed with intravenous barbiturate, their hearts were immediately excised, and samples were taken from eight segments: the right and left atria, right ventricular conus and sinus, left ventricular apex and base and high and low interventricular septum. These specimens were frozen in liquid nitrogen and stored on dry ice until they were analyzed. Norepinephrine concentration was measured in the eluate of the alumina column by the trihydroxyindole procedure as outlined by Valori et al. [10], which we have previously described.

Histologic and Ultrastructural Pathology

Myocardial fiber hypertrophy was quantitated in two groups of dogs: three NGF-treated and three untreated animals. In each group, two dogs were 3 months old at the time they were killed and one dog was 1 year old. In each heart, quantitative analysis of myocardial fiber diameter was performed from two myocardial specimens: one from the base of the septum and one from the base of the free left ventricular wall. In each heart tissue specimen, the myocardial fiber diameter was obtained by measuring from the photograph of the stained fiber longitudinal areas the diameter at the level of the nucleus of at least four myocardial fibers from each of four histologic preparations, and then taking the average results [11]. The fibers measured in each preparation are those considered to be most representative and easiest to measure.

Twenty-eight animals 3 months of age were anesthetized and subjected to in vivo retrograde cardiac perfusion-fixation with cold 2% glutaraldehyde at a rate of 12 ml/min for 20 minutes while the hearts were externally bathed in 2% cold glutaraldehyde. After the hearts were fixed, they were rapidly excised and placed in cold glutaraldehyde. Sections of each heart were made by "bread slicing" the ventricles perpendicular to the ventricular septum in equal thickness. Next, small samples of the myocardium (approximately 1-mm cubes) were removed from each of the preselected areas and placed in 3% cold glutaraldehyde in a 0.1 M phosphate buffer at pH 7.2 to 7.4 for 2 h at 4°C. The preselected areas examined included high and low sites in the ventricular septum, base and apex of the left and right ventricular free walls, and atria. The tissue samples were then rinsed twice in 0.1 M phosphate buffer and stored overnight at 4°C. Tissue samples for electron microscopy were posfixed in 1% osmium tetroxide in 0.1 M phosphate buffer for 1 h. They were then dehydrated with a graded series of ethanols to propylene oxide, starting with 60% alcohol for 5 min, 70% alcohol for 10 min, 80% alcohol for 10 min, 95% alcohol for 10 min, absolute alcohol for 10 min and then 5 min, propylene oxide for 10 min and then 5 min, 50:50 propylene oxide-Epon resin 812 overnight, and then pure Epon resin for at least 4 h. The sections were then embedded in Epon resin-812 Beem capsules and polymerized at 60° over a 48-h period. Next, 1-μm sections were cut by the use of glass knives on an ultramicrotome (Sorvall MT-2B) and stained with methylene blueazure 2 (50:50). These sections were examined by light microscopy for selection of areas for electron microscopic study. The final choice of areas for electron microscopy was limited only to those areas free of contraction bands and other tissue preparation artifacts. From the areas selected, thin sections of 600–700 Å were cut with diamond knives and mounted on 200-mesh, uncoated copper grids. The grids were stained with 7% uranyl acetate in methanol and lead citrate. All sections were examined on an electron microscope (Phillips 201).

Hemodynamic Data

Hemodynamic data were obtained from 30 treated and 20 control littermates studied while they were under either pentobarbital or α-chloralose anesthesia. From these studies, data suitable for detailed analysis and without evidence of catheter entrapment were obtained from 15 NGF-treated and eight control puppies. All left ventricular pressures were obtained with a Millar catheter-tip transducer, and aortic pressure was obtained with a 5F Rodriguez catheter and a P23dB Statham transducer. All hemodynamic data were recorded on a Brush Gould 200 recorder.

Results

Myocardial Norepinephrine Content

No statistically significant differences were noted in the hearts from the animals treated with 7S-NGF or β-NGF or from the hearts of puppies from the treated pregnant bitches. Table 1 summarizes the data obtained for myocardial norepinephrine content from the eight heart segments studied in control and NGF-treated littermates as well as in 13 adult untreated animals. It should be noted that not only did the NGF-treated puppies that were killed at 3 months of age have norepinephrine levels remarkably higher than those of their control littermates, but the norepinephrine levels were also considerably elevated over those of the adult controls.

Gross, Histologic, and Ultrastructural Pathology

At autopsy (3, 6, or 12 months of age), the absolute weights of the hearts of the dogs treated with NGF were greater than those of controls. For the entire group across

Table 1. Myocardial norepinephrine content (μg/g) ± SE

Region	Control littermates (n=3)	Nerve growth factor (n=12)	Adult controls (n=13)
Right atrium	1.08 ± 0.10	2.72 ± 0.24	1.95 ± 0.14
Left atrium	1.09 ± 0.05	2.89 ± 0.16	2.63 ± 0.21
Right ventricular conus	0.87 ± 0.06	1.35 ± 0.13	1.09 ± 0.08
Right ventricular sinus	0.80 ± 0.07	1.30 ± 0.12	0.79 ± 0.09
Left ventricular base	0.73 ± 0.07	1.43 ± 0.12	1.08 ± 0.09
Left ventricular apex	0.68 ± 0.06	1.18 ± 0.10	0.76 ± 0.09
High septum	0.64 ± 0.06	1.52 ± 0.12	1.06 ± 0.08
Low septum	0.61 ± 0.06	1.11 ± 0.15	0.80 ± 0.09

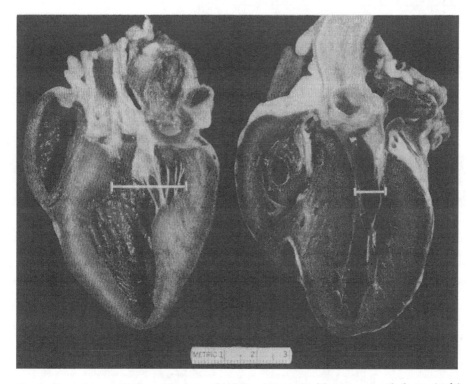

Fig. 1. Control heart (*left*) and hypertrophied heart treated with nerve growth factor (*right*) from puppies of same litter. Note decrease in size of left ventricular cavity and bulge of septum into left ventricle of treated dog. (Compare width of left ventricular outflow tracts as indicated by white lines.)

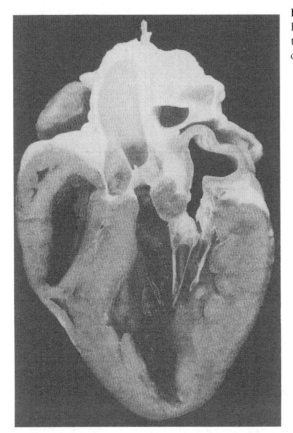

Fig. 2. Photograph of section of heart from nerve growth factor-treated puppy killed at 3 months of age

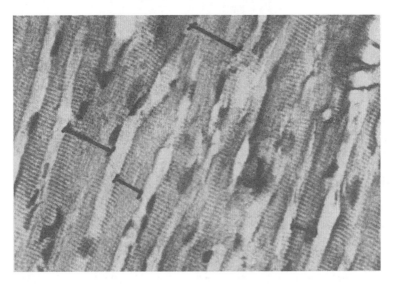

Fig. 3. Myocardial fibers from septum of control animal at 1 year of age ×1200

Cardiac Effects of Nerve Growth Factor

all ages, there was no significant difference in heart weight/body weight ratio. This result may be due to the variability in size of the mongrel litters. In the one litter in which ten puppies (five treated, five control) survived until they were killed at 3 months of age, the heart weight/body weight ratio of NGF-treated puppies was 0.675 ± 0.32 and that of the control littermates was 0.575 ± 0.28, values significantly different at the 0.04 level. The hearts excised from treated dogs had areas of hypertrophy that varied from asymmetric subaortic type (Fig. 1) to diffuse left ventricular hypertrophy with a severely compromised left ventricular cavity (Fig. 2).

Table 2. Myocardial fiber diameter

Dog no.	Septum (μm)	Free wall (μm)
Untreated		
1 [a]	6	–
2 [a]	6	5
3 [b]	9	11
Treated		
4 [a]	8	–
5 [a]	8	7
6 [b]	22	14

[a] Dog 3 months old.
[b] Dog 1 year old.

Right ventricular hypertrophy of varying degrees was seen in a majority of NGF-treated animals. The septal-free wall ratios of dogs treated with NGF varied from 1.2 to 3.2, with a mean of 1.9, whereas the ratios in controls were all 1.3 or less, with a mean of 1.2. None of the treated dogs had any gross left ventricular dilatation.

Nerve growth factor-treated dogs showed a myocardial fiber diameter of 13.0 μm (mean) in the septum and 10.0 μm (mean) in the free left ventricular wall, whereas untreated dogs showed a myocardial fiber diameter of 7.0 μm (mean) in the septum and 8.0 μm (mean) in the free left ventricular wall (Table 2) (Figs. 3, 4). The number of specimens studied did not permit meaningful statistical comparison.

On examination by electron microscopy, all treated dogs had some myocardial involvement, the most characteristic being the disorganization of myofilaments and myofibrils and the mitochondrial disruption. Myofibrillar disarray was the most characteristic abnormality noted; it varied in extent and severity but was a constant finding in all treated dogs (Figs. 5, 6). Mitochondrial alterations occurred in most of the hearts from the treated dogs (Fig. 7). The alterations consisted of swollen mitochondria with disrupted cristae and lamellar inclusion rings. The degree of mitochondrial involvement did not seem to be directly proportional to the amount of myofibrillar damage or disarray.

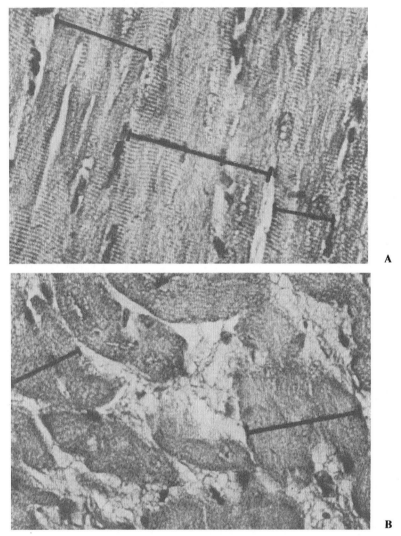

Fig. 4A, B. Myocardial fibers from septum of nerve growth factor-treated animal at 1 year of age. Observe significant myocardial fiber hypertrophy in longitudinal section (A) and in transverse section (B). × 1200

Fig. 5. Section from left ventricular base of untreated control dog, showing normal myofibrillar alignment and normally aligned mitochondria (*M*) with intact cristae and normal-appearing Z-bands (*Z*). × 10000

Fig. 6. Portion of right ventricular apex excised from treated dog, showing severe myofibrillar disarray with abnormal orientation of adjacent myofibrils (*arrows*) and pooling of mitochondria in areas of lesser contraction. × 7000

Cardiac Effects of Nerve Growth Factor

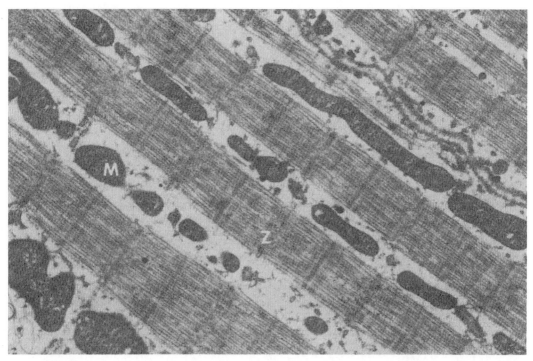

Fig. 5

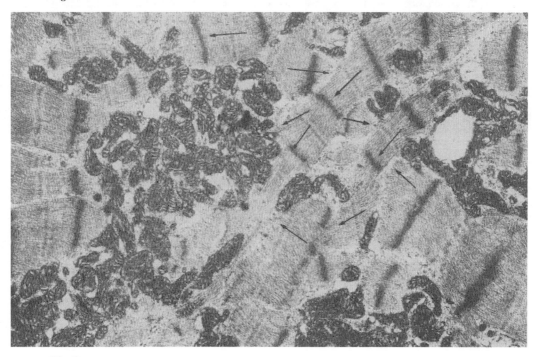

Fig. 6

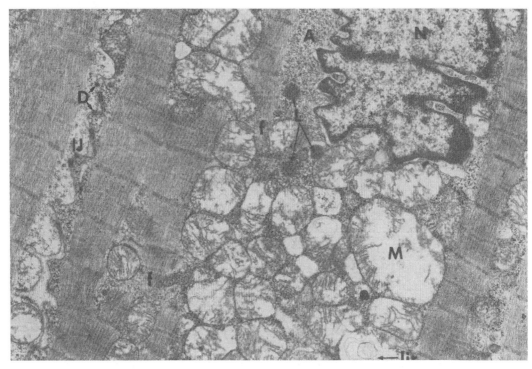

Fig. 7. Section of left ventricular base excised from offspring of treated bitch, showing fragmentation of myofibrils (*f*); loss of myofibrils with pooling of swollen mitochondria (*M*), many of which contain disrupted cristae and lamellar inclusion rings (*lir*); large nucleus (*N*) with irregularly contracted nuclear membrane; area of side-to-side intercellular junction (*IJ*) with small desmosomes (*D*); several lysosomes (*L*); and area of large accumulation of free ribosomes and glycogen particles (*A*). ×7000

The average aortic blood pressure in control animals was $173 \pm 33/124 \pm 31$ (SD) mmHg, whereas in NGF-treated animals aortic blood pressure was $167 \pm 52/126 \pm 43$ mmHg. Likewise, the left ventricular pressure did not differ significantly, being $178 \pm 34/7 \pm 4$ in controls and $180 \pm 58/7 \pm 3$ in NGF-treated animals. Four of the eight control dogs had a resting gradient across the left ventricular outflow tract, which averaged 10 mmHg. Upon stimulation with isoproterenol, three of these four dogs had an increase in this gradient, which averaged 20 mmHg. In the NGF-treated dogs, 10 of the 15 had a resting gradient averaging 20 mmHg. With isoproterenol stimulation, 9 of the 15 dogs had an average gradient of 56.7 mmHg. Because of the concern that the hypertrophy seen in our studies may be due to systemic hypertension, the data from current experiments were compared with those obtained from 40 adult untreated animals being studied for other purposes in our laboratory. In these animals aortic blood pressure averaged $155 \pm 34/124 \pm 29$ mmHg, which was not significantly different from that of either control or NGF-treated animals.

Discussion

The data obtained from our experiments in which NGF was administered to prenatal or neonatal puppies for 5 days indicate that such treatment results in an increase in myocardial catecholamine content. Moreover, although there was no significant difference in heart weight/body weight ratio between control and treated dogs, absolute weight of the hearts of treated dogs was greater than that of controls. The greater heart weight occurred in the absence of systemic hypertension. It is recognized that the data presented relative to myocardial hypertrophy are from preliminary observations and that a systematic study quantitating both gross and microscopic evidence of hypertrophy needs to be completed to verify the absolute validity of this model.

Other investigators have documented that myocardial catecholamine content directly reflects the degree of sympathetic innervation of a specific tissue [12, 13]. Our data imply, therefore, that administration of NGF results in an increase in sympathetic innervation of the heart. These results are consistent with the report by Nicolescu et al. [14], who demonstrated an increase in fluorescent-staining fibers in the hearts of kittens treated with NGF. The generally accepted action of NGF, that it enhances growth and development of the sympathetic nerve system, also lends support to the suggestion that the increased levels of myocardial catecholamines seen in the NGF-treated animals reflect an increased sympathetic innervation.

One might speculate that with the increase in endogenous myocardial catecholamines there is an increase in the release of this catecholamine. Increase in force of contraction consequent to norepinephrine release would result in hypertrophy. Since myofibrillar disarray prevails in embryonic hearts, abnormal stresses and therefore nonparallel force vectors set up in this way would tend to lead to an accentuation of the disarray. The data further indicate that the catecholamine content is higher at the base of the heart (right ventricular conus, high septum, left ventricular base) than at the apex and would be in keeping with the concept that a greater degree of hypertrophy may occur in these basal areas.

This study does again raise the question of a possible link between hypertrophic cardiomyopathies and abnormalities of the sympathetic nervous system. It further stimulates speculation on whether there is more than a fortuitous relationship between disorders of neural crest tissue – such as the Polani-Moynihan syndrome, pheochromocytoma, neurofibromatosis, and multiple lentiginosis – and hypertrophic cardiomyopathy.

Whether the hypertrophy induced by the administration of NGF to dogs is in any way related to human hypertrophic cardiomyopathies is not known. There are indeed some similarities, including the histologic disarray of muscle fibers, but these changes are not specific. Likewise, preponderance of septal hypertrophy is not specific and was not universal in our animals. It is well known that outflow-tract gradients can be demonstrated in so-called normal dogs by infusion of isoproterenol, and hence, the gradients seen in our experiments are not diagnostic of an anatomically abnormal state.

Nonetheless, it appears from both gross and microscopic studies that the administration of NGF to dogs in the perinatal period results in an increase in myocardial catecholamine content and myocardial hypertrophy, this in the absence of systemic hypertension. However, we are continuing to quantitate histologic specimens for further statistical evaluation of the magnitude of this hypertrophy.

References

1. Goodwin JF (1974) Prospects and predictions for the cardiomyopathies. Circulation 50:210–219
2. Gans JH, Cater MR (1970) Norepinephrine induced cardiac hypertrophy in dogs. Life Sci 9:731–740
3. Haft JL (1974) Cardiovascular injury induced by sympathetic catecholamines. Prog. Cardiovasc Dis 17:73–86
4. Ferrans VJ, Hibbs RG, Black WC, Weilbaecher DG (1964) Isoproterenol-induced myocardial necrosis: a histochemical and electron microscopic study. Am Heart J 68:71–90
5. Laks MM, Morady F, Swan HJC (1973) Myocardial hypertrophy produced by chronic infusion of subhypertensive doses of norepinephrine in the dog. Chest 64:75–78
6. Mobley WC, Server AC, Ishii DN, Riopelle RJ, Shooter EM (1977) Nerve growth factor. N Engl J Med 297:1096–1104; 1149–1158; 1211–1218
7. Zaimis E (1972) Nerve growth factor: The target cells. In: Zaimis E, Knight J (eds) Nerve growth factor and its antiserum. Athlone Press, London, pp 59–70
8. Witzke DJ, Kaye MP (1976) Hypertrophic cardiomyopathy induced by administration of nerve growth factor (Abstr). Circulation [Suppl 2] 54:88
9. Mobley WC, Schenken A, Shooter EM (1976) Characterization and isolation of proteolytically modified nerve growth factor. Biochemistry 15:5543–5551
10. Valori C, Brunori CA, Renzini V, Corea L (1970) Improved procedure for formation of epinephrine and norepinephrine fluorophors by the trihydroxyindole reaction. Anal Biochem 33:158–167
11. Fuster V, Danielson MA, Robb RA, Broadbent JC, Brown AL Jr, Elveback LR (1977) Quantitation of left ventricular myocardial fiber hypertrophy and interstitial tissue in human hearts with chronically increased volume and pressure overload. Circulation 55:504–508
12. Iversen LL, Glowinski JJ, Axelrod J (1966) The physiologic disposition and metabolism of norepinephrine in immunosympathectomized animals. J Pharmacol Exp Ther 151:273–284
13. Glowinski J, Axelrod J, Kopin IJ, Wurtman RJ (1964) Physiological disposition of H^3-norepinephrine in the developing rat. J Pharmacol Exp Ther 146:48–53
14. Nicolescu E, Kakari S, Zaimis E (1972) Studies of tissue monoamines by fluorescence microscopy. In: Zaimis E, Knight J (eds) Nerve growth factor and its antiserum. Athlone Press, London, pp 108–113

Prevention of Myocardial Cell Necrosis in the Syrian Hamster – Results of Long-Term Treatment

K. LOSSNITZER, A. KONRAD, D. ZEYER, and W. MOHR

Introduction

Several strains of Syrian hamsters afflicted with muscular dystrophy and cardiomyopathy were derived from inbred lines of *Mesocricetus auratus* through brother-sister-mating at the Bio-Research Institute in Cambridge from 1956 onward. In 1962 and 1966 Homburger et al. [1, 2] reported the first time that hereditary myopathy with heart muscle necroses may occur in breeds of Syrian golden hamsters. It is the great merit of Bajusz [3, 8] of having introduced between 1966 and 1969 the myopathic Syrian hamsters as reproducible disease model for cardiomyopathy into experimental cardiology. Since then many morphological, hemodynamic, biochemical, pharmacological as well as clinical studies have been performed in these hamsters. In 1968 Bajusz and Lossnitzer [9] as well as in 1975 Lossnitzer [10] presented the first thorough reviews about the features of this hereditary cardiomyopathy. It turned out that in several interrelated lines of this disease model the appearance of the cardiomyopathy differs. Contrary to the original strain BIO 14.6, in which the heart developed distinct hypertrophy besides necroses [5, 7, 11–13] the substrains BIO 8262 as well as UM-X 7.1 predominantly display cardiac myolysis, necrotization, scarring, and calcification [14–16]. Whereas in strains BIO 14.6 and UM-X 7.1 congestive heart failure develops in about 50% of the animals during the terminal stage of the disease, this feature can scarcely be observed in strain BIO 8262.

As our working group is mainly interested in the pathogenesis of myocardial necrosis, we decided to investigate strain BIO 8262 and labeled its cardiomyopathy "dystrophic" according to skeletal muscular dystrophy with which the hamsters are additionally afflicted.

Our studies performed between 1968 and 1978 demonstrated that there exists a disturbance of myocardial calcium metabolism in these hamsters [4, 17–22]. This metabolic aberration is concealed prior to the onset of myocardial necrotization and calcification, which generally begins in these hamsters about the 40th day of their life. However, it can already be evidenced by pharmacological means in so-called prenecrotic 30-day-old animals [22, 23]. Fleckenstein and his group [24–30] demonstrated myocardial calcium overload as the determinant factor in the pathogenetical chain leading to cardiac necrotization in isoproterenol-treated rats. Therefore, the latent disturbance of myocardial calcium metabolism in the genetically cardiomyopathic hamsters became of great importance to us.

On the basis of numerous experiments, Fleckenstein and his working group [30–32] ascribed cardioprotective properties to several substances interfering with the calcium dependent process of excitation-contraction coupling in myocardial cells. They named these substances calcium antagonists. A direct and competitive blockade of calcium conductivity via the slow inward channel was unequivocally shown for verapamil [33, 34], which is one of these substances. However, the calcium antagonistic potency of other substances was indirectly proven by radio-calcium uptake studies [24–32].

Thus, the administration of calcium antagonists to hamsters with spontaneously occurring cardiomyopathy appeared as a challenging enticement, not only to derive more insight into the pathogenesis of the hamster cardiomyopathy, but also to establish the concept of myocardial calcium overload and calcium antagonism as a more common pathogenetical principle and therapeutic regimen. If long-term treatment was initiated during the prenecrotic stage of the cardiomyopathy and continued into the necrotizing phase, the as yet latent cardiomyopathic hearts ought to be protected from obvious degeneration; i.e., necrotization as well as calcification. Since Angelakos et al. [35, 36] assume increased sympathetic activity as the pathogenetic cause of the hamster cardiomyopathy, long-term treatment with β-adrenoceptor blocking substances should be as efficient. The well-known enhancing effect of β-adrenergic catecholamines on myocardial calcium metabolism [31, 34, 37–44] provides a fairly logical basis for the above reasoning. However, recently there was also a report by Späh and Fleckenstein [45] about reciprocal effects of β-adrenergic catecholamines on inward fluxes across the myocardial sarcolemma membrane of calcium and magnesium ions. As magnesium salts are known to be cardioprotective agents in the electrolyte-steroid cardiopathy [46, 47], as well as in the isoproterenol cardiopathy [25, 31, 48, 49], it made sense to also apply a magnesium salt for cardioprotection in the dystrophic cardiomyopathy of the hamster.

Material and Methods

582 genetically cardiomyopathic (BIO 8262 inbred strain) and 26 healthy (CLAC inbred strain) hamsters of both sexes were used in the experiments. They were housed under identical conditions in air-conditioned rooms with artificial light in a 12-h day and night cycle. Normal laboratory diet (Ssniff-H-hamster chow) and tap water were offered ad libitum.

Spontaneous Course of Calcification and Necrotization

In order to demonstrate grossly the parallelism of myocardial necrotization and calcification 90 cardiomyopathic hamsters between the age of 27 and 78 days were divided into eight age groups (Fig. 1) and killed under ether anesthesia. Thereafter their hearts were excised. Left ventricular myocardium with intracellular septum was assayed for its calcium content by atomic absorption spectrophotometry as described elsewhere [19, 21, 50]. The same procedure was applied to 26 genetically healthy hamsters aged 27–82 days.

66 cardiomyopathic hamsters again between the age of 27 and 78 days were grouped and killed as previously (Fig. 1); however, their hearts were histologically

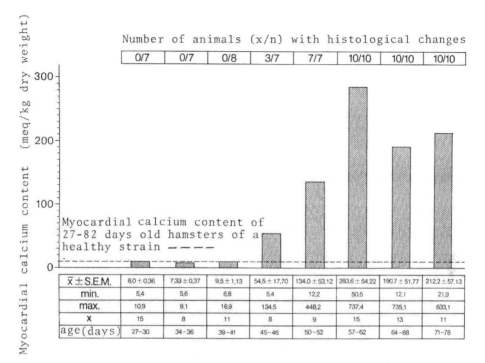

Fig. 1. Time course survey of histological changes and calcium content in myocardium of cardiomyopathic hamsters (strain BIO 8262). Transition from prenecrotic into necrotizing stage of myocardium occurs between the 40th and 50th day of life, while the myocardial calcium content is progressively increasing. There is a continuous rise of the latter until about the 60th day of life. Prior to the onset of overt myocardial degeneration (until the 41th day of life) myocardial calcium content of the cardiomyopathic hamsters resembles that of animals from a healthy strain

examined. Only one section was made through the middle of both ventricles in a plane vertical to the heart axis. The method for preparation and staining of the slices is described elsewhere [14, 22]. Gross histological evaluation was performed looking for fresh necroses and resorptive changes.

Long-Term Treatment

Biochemical Studies

Action of Verapamil on Spontaneous Myocardial Calcification

For this experiment 50 cardiomyopathic hamsters 30 days of age were used. 37 animals were divided into four groups and injected s.c. with 1, 3, 5, and 10 mg verapamil/kg b.wt. b.i.d. for 30 days. Verpamil (Knoll AG, Ludwigshafen) was dissolved in saline solution (0.9%) to obtain the appropriate amount of drug in a suitable volume. At the commencement of the experiments the animals were weighed; subsequently the weighing procedure was repeated four times at weekly intervals. 13 hamsters remained untreated serving as controls. On the 60th day of life the animals were killed and their hearts excised. Left ventricular myocardium and septum were analyzed for myocardial calcium content.

Action of Various β-Adrenoceptor Blocking Substances on Spontaneous Myocardial Calcification

For these experiments 276 cardiomyopathic hamsters between 28 and 31 days of age were used. 95 animals remained untreated, while 181 hamsters were injected s.c. with various β-adrenoceptor blocking substances for 30 days. The β-adrenoceptor blocking substances (propranolol, atenolol, practolol (ICI-Pharma, Plankstadt), alprenolol (Astra-Chemicals, Wedel), and pindolol (Sandoz AG, Nürnberg)) were dissolved in 0.9% saline solution in suitable amounts in order to obtain an appropriate injection volume adjusted to body weight and dose. The hamsters were killed on the 58th day and on the 61th day the hearts were excised and prepared for calcium analysis.

Propranolol was injected s.c. in doses of 1, 3, 10, and 30 mg/kg b.wt. b.i.d., alprenolol in doses of 2, 6, and 20 mg/kg b.wt. b.i.d., pindolol in doses of 2, 6, 20, and 60 mg/kg b.wt. b.i.d., atenolol in doses of 10, 30, 100, and 300 mg/kg b.wt. b.i.d. and practolol in doses of 10, 30, 100, and 300 mg/kg b.wt. b.i.d.

Action of Mg-aspartate · HCl on Spontaneous Myocardial Calcification

29 hamsters 30 days of age were divided into three groups and injected through a stomach tube p.o. with 8, 23, and 46 meq Mg-aspartate · HCl/kg b.wt. b.i.d. for 30 days. Mg-aspartate · HCl (Verla-Pharm, Tutzing) as powder was dissolved in suitable amounts with aqua demineralisata in order to adjust the injection volume to the required dose and to the body weight.

Histological Studies

The histological studies are considered as supplementary part for demonstration of the interrelationship between pharmacological suppression of myocardial calcium accumulation and prevention of myocardial degeneration.

For these studies 60 cardiomyopathic hamsters from several offsprings 30 days of age were used. Three series of ten hamsters each were chronically treated for 30 days with verapamil, propranolol, or Mg-aspartate · HCl, whereas three series of ten untreated siblings remained as controls. On the 60th day of life the animals were killed and their hearts prepared for histological evaluation as already described elsewhere [22]. For these experiments the highest doses of verapamil, propranolol, and Mg-aspartate · HCl as already applied in the biochemical studies were administered by the same route since they had proven to be effective in preventing myocardial calcium accumulation.

Results

Spontaneous Course of Calcification and Necrotization

In Fig. 1 the biochemical and histological results are summarized. Whereas the myocardial calcium content of the healthy hamsters does not differ within the age

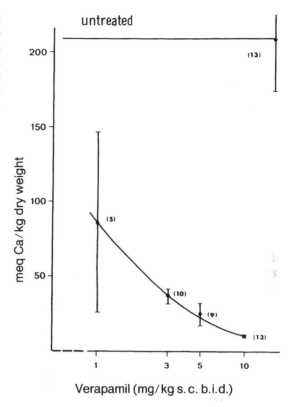

Fig. 2. Myocardial calcium content of 60-day-old cardiomyopathic hamsters after chronic treatment with various doses of verapamil and of untreated animals of the same age. With increasing dosage of the drug calcium content decreases concomitantly. Values represent the mean±SEM. The numbers of animals are given in parentheses

range between 27 and 82 days (amounting to 8.38±1.47 meq/kg dry weight), its behavior in the cardiomyopathic hamsters is quite different. Up to the 36th day no significant alteration occurs, and up to the 41st day only a slight increase from 8.0±0.36 and 7.33±0.37 to 9.5±1.13 meq/kg dry weight becomes evident. However, hamsters of 45 and 46 days of age do partly exhibit a tremendous augmentation of their myocardial calcium content, which reaches 134.5 meq/kg dry weight at maximum. The average myocardial calcium content, however, is 54.5±17.70 meq/kg dry weight in this age group. With increasing age up to the 62nd day of life it continuously and tremendously rises up to individual values, which are about 100 times as high as in the youngest cardiomyopathic or in the normal hamsters. The mean value of the myocardial calcium content in 57–62 day old animals is 283.6±54.22 meq/kg dry weight. Later on, up to the 78th day there is no further increment.

The histological examination does not reveal morphological changes in myocardium of 27–41 day old cardiomyopathic hamsters. In three out of seven 45–46 day old animals fresh necrotic foci become evident, and in the subsequent age groups no heart examined is free of fresh necroses as well as of resorptive and calcific changes.

Long-Term Treatment

Myocardial Calcium Content

In Fig. 2 the behavior of the myocardial calcium content of chronically treated cardiomyopathic hamsters is demonstrated under influence of various doses of verapamil. As small an amount as 1 mg/kg b.i.d. is able to avoid full calcification as it occurs in untreated controls. The myocardial calcium content amounts only to 85.8 ± 136.6 meq/kg dry weight, whereas that of the untreated animals is 209.1 ± 130.8 meq/kg dry weight. With increasing doses of verapamil myocardial calcification is further depressed. Thus, 10 mg/kg b.i.d. of verapamil almost completely prevents calcification; myocardial calcium content amounts to 9.8 ± 2.2 meq/kg dry weight, which is nearly identical with that of healthy hamsters (their myocardial calcium content is 8.38 ± 1.47 meq/kg dry weight; Fig. 1).

Figure 3 reflects the behavior of calcification in the cardiomyopathic hearts under chronic influence of various β-adrenergic blocking agents. Propranolol, alprenolol, and pindolol suppress myocardial calcification in a dose-dependent manner. Propranolol 30 mg/kg b.i.d. unequivocally prevents calcification, as

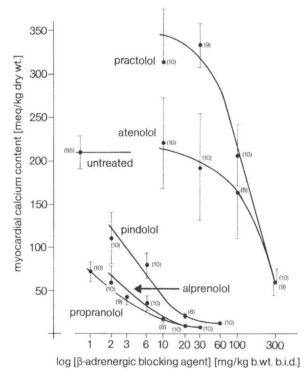

Fig. 3. Myocardial calcium content of 58–61 day old cardiomyopathic hamsters after chronic treatment with various doses of several β-adrenoceptor blocking substances and of untreated animals of the same age. Whereas the lower doses of practolol seem to increase myocardial calcium content, propranolol, alprenolol, pindolol, and atenolol do not so, at least in the doses used. With increasing dosage they only diminish the myocardial calcium content. Values represent the mean ± SEM. The numbers of animals are given in parentheses

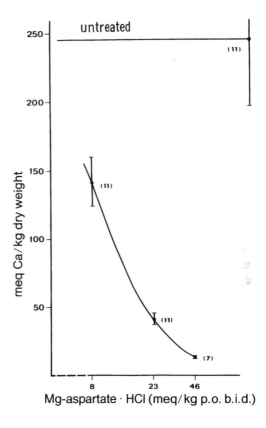

Fig. 4. Myocardial calcium content of 60-day-old cardiomyopathic hamsters after chronic treatment with various doses of Mg-aspartate. HCl and of untreated animals of the same age. With increasing dosage of the drug, calcium content abates. Values represent the mean ± SEM. The numbers of animals are given in parentheses

myocardial calcium content is 8.35 ± 0.75 meq/kg dry weight. Alprenolol 20 mg/kg b.i.d. and pindolol 60 mg/kg b.i.d. are almost as effective, myocardial calcium content being 10.39 ± 0.75 and 12.98 ± 3.97 meq/kg dry weight, respectively. However, even very high doses of atenolol and practolol (up to 300 mg/kg b.i.d.) are unable to totally prevent calcification, although a certain dose-dependent decrease is evident. Furthermore, it is noteworthy that the initial doses of 10 and 30 mg/kg b.i.d. of practolol seem to augment calcification. While the myocardial calcium content of untreated hamsters is 208.57 ± 183.88 meq/kg dry weight, that of animals treated with 10 and 30 mg/kg b.i.d. practolol amounts to 314.88 ± 188.31 and 334.02 ± 73.81 meq/kg dry weight, respectively.

The influence of chronic oral administration of Mg-aspartate · HCl on spontaneous calcification of the cardiomyopathic hearts is demonstrated in Fig. 4. The myocardial calcium content of the untreated control group of hamsters is 245.3 ± 161.1 meq/kg dry weight. Even 8 meq/kg b.i.d. partly suppresses myocardial calcification, although 142.5 ± 58.6 meq calcium/kg dry weight is still far above that calcium level of healthy hamsters. However, augmentation of the dose of the magnesium salt runs in parallel with an increase of its anticalcific activity. Thus, 46 meq Mg-aspartate · HCl/kg b.i.d. prevents at least gross myocardial calcification. The myocardial calcium content is 13.2 ± 1.9 meq/kg dry weight under this dose and only slightly differs from that of healthy hamsters (8.38 ± 1.47 meq/kg dry weight).

Histological Studies

The findings derived from the chronic verapamil-treated hamsters are summarized in Table 1. All untreated hamsters are afflicted with myocardial scar formation and calcification, the latter mainly appearing within giant cells. In six of these animals older necroses with resorptive changes and calcification can be detected. However, fresh myolytic foci or necrotic lesions without calcification but with mononuclear round cell infiltration are only discernible in four animals. Myolytic foci are not found in any of the treated hamsters, and only two animals manifest resorptive changes with as well as without calcification. Scar formation and calcification can also be detected in only two of the treated hamsters.

By a more sensitive examination (counting the number of slices containing the specified lesions) an even better impression of the beneficial therapeutic effect is evident. Whereas fresh myolytic foci can be seen in 7 out of the 40 heart slices from the untreated hamsters, these lesions are not seen in any of the 40 slices from the treatment group. There is also a clear-cut reduction of resorptive changes. A still better evaluation of the advantageous influence of the magnesium salt is possible comparing the fibrotic foci between the treated and the untreated group: In 35 slices from the untreated and only in four from the treated hearts can fibrotic lesions be discovered.

The clearest difference between the untreated and treated group, however, is evident when each single focus appearing within the 40 slices examined is counted. A total number of 9 myolytic foci, 17 resorptive lesions without and 60 with calcification, and 104 fibrotic lesions is present in the untreated group; no myolytic focus, only four resorptive foci with and three without calcification, and only eight fibrotic foci are detectable in the treated group.

In Table 2 the results obtained from the chronic propranolol-treatment are depicted. As in the verapamil group all hearts of the untreated hamsters are afflicted with fibrotic and calcific lesions, whereas only two of the ten treated animals disclose such lesions. Differences in resorptive changes are also observed (Table 2). A myolytic focus appears in only one untreated hamster and in none of the treated animals.

Table 1. Histological results in 60-day-old cardiomyopathic hamsters after 30-day long-term treatment with 10 mg s.c. verapamil/kg b.wt. b.i.d.

	Number of animals with lesions		Number of slices with lesions		Total number of discovered foci	
	Un-treated	Vera-pamil	Un-treated	Vera-pamil	Un-treated	Vera-pamil
Myolysis	4/10	0/10	7/40	0/40	9	0
Resorptive changes without calcification	4/10	2/10	9/40	3/40	17	4
Resorptive changes with calcification	6/10	2/10	17/40	3/40	60	3
Fibrosis with calcification	10/10	2/10	35/40	4/40	104	8

Prevention of Myocardial Cell Necrosis in the Syrian Hamster

Table 2. Histological results in 58–61 day old cardiomyopathic hamsters after 30-day long-term treatment with 30 mg s.c. propranolol/kg b.wt. b.i.d.

	Number of animals with lesions		Number of slices with lesions		Total number of discovered foci	
	Un-treated	Propran-olol	Un-treated	Propran-olol	Un-treated	Propran-olol
Myolysis	1/10	0/10	1/40	0/40	1	0
Resorptive changes without calcification	3/10	2/10	5/40	2/40	6	2
Resorptive changes with calcification	6/10	3/10	13/40	4/40	35	4
Fibrosis with calcification	10/10	2/10	36/40	3/40	106	6

Table 3. Histological results in 60-day-old cardiomyopathic hamsters after 30-day long-term treatment with 46 meq p.o. Mg-aspartate · HCl/kg b.wt. b.i.d.

	Number of animals with lesions		Number of slices with lesions		Total number of discovered foci	
	Un-treated	Mg-asp. HCl	Un-treated	Mg-asp. HCl	Un-treated	Mg-asp. HCl
Myolysis	3/10	0/10	5/40	0/40	5	0
Resorptive changes without calcification	5/10	4/10	9/40	4/40	20	6
Resorptive changes with calcification	8/10	2/10	18/40	4/40	62	6
Fibrosis with calcification	10/10	3/10	30/40	4/40	73	4

The therapeutic effect of propranolol is better evidenced by counting the slices exhibiting the various kinds of alterations. In only three slices scar formation as well as resorptive changes with calcification is present, whereas these structural changes are seen in 36 and 13 slices, respectively, of the untreated control group. Mere resorptive changes as well as myolysis are also less commonly observed in the treated hearts.

As in the verapamil experiments, the clearest survey is obtained by counting each single focus. Far fewer lesions are present in the treatment group (Table 2).

Table 3 demonstrates the results of the chronic treatment with Mg-aspartate · HCl. With each method of assessment an improvement in outcome is evident in the treatment group.

Discussion

The time course survey studying the transition from the prenecrotic to the necrotizing phase of the cardiomyopathy of the hamsters demonstrates an unequivocal interrelationship between cardiac necrotization and calcification, which appears to be quantitative in nature. Thus, the amount of myocardial calcium content might be taken as at least a semiquantitative measure of the degree of cardiac degeneration, and myocardial calcification in the cardiomyopathic hamsters could be considered as the biochemical marker of the onset and of the intensity of the disease. As disturbance of myocardial calcium metabolism has been proven the determinant pathogenetical – although not etiological – factor for myocardial necrotization of this cardiomyopathy [18, 20, 22, 51–54], the above-stated proposal seems to be fairly reasonable.

If long-term treatment with a drug suppresses myocardial calcification, dose-dependent diminution of calcium accumulation should reflect cardioprotection. Hence, dose-effect curves with respect to cardioprotection can be established. Keeping myocardial calcium content on about that observed in genetically healthy hamsters would necessarily indicate full cardioprotection, i.e., prevention of myocardial cell necrosis. This influence is supported by the results of the histological experiments, in which it was observed that verapamil, propranolol, and Mg-aspartate · HCl could almost completely suppress myocardial calcification. Moreover, the dose-effect relationship that occurred provides a pharmacological basis of correlating the cardioprotective potencies of various substances.

Verapamil has been shown to block competitively transsarcolemmal calcium conductivity of myocardial fibers and interfere with excitation contraction coupling [28, 33, 34]. Thus its beneficial effect on spontaneous calcium accumulation, as well as on necrotization, is compatible with the previous assumption of myocardial calcium overload being the determinant factor for the development of irreversible and progressive myocellular decay in the cardiomyopathic hamsters [18, 20, 22, 54]. This finding occurring in a hereditary spontaneous disease model strongly supports the postulation of Fleckenstein, who considers myocardial calcium overload as the fundamental and decisive principle in myocardial necrotization [24–32]. However, his ideas were based only on findings in the parmacological disease model of the isoproterenol-treated rat.

Interlinking the electrophysiological property of verapamil with its salutary effect on the hamster heart muscle might provide more insight into the course of the disease process. Besides a genetically induced defect in the myofibrillar apparatus (reflected by a disturbance of myofibril formation in hearts of embryonic [55] and newborn [12, 13, 56, 57] hamsters of the related strain BIO 14.6), an additional functional defect of the sarcolemma provoking myocardial calcium overload can be assumed. Rona et al. [58] were able to demonstrate sarcolemmal permeability alterations as the first manifestation of early cardiac muscle cell injury induced by various catecholamines in the rat. Both defective sarcolemma as well as disturbed myofibril formation might be taken as an early prenecrotic consequence of the genetical aberration in the cardiomyopathic hamsters. During the prenecrotic phase of the hamster disease, a very limited and as yet concealed flooding of myocardial cells with calcium is conceivable, leading only to ultrastructural changes reported as

Prevention of Myocardial Cell Necrosis in the Syrian Hamster

focal myolysis and fraying of myofilaments [12, 13, 57, 59]. The delayed onset of gross myocardial necrotization at about the 40th day of life of the hamsters points to a progressive sarcolemmal defect.

The cause of this progression, however, remains a matter of question. The primarily defective myofibrillar formation could possibly induce augmentation of myocardial sympathetic tone as a feed-back mechanism to compensate for reduced contractility. This reasoning is supported by the findings of Angelakos et al. [35, 36], who found increased cardiac sympathetic nerve activity with increased norepinephrine turnover prior to the development of myocardial lesions. The interrelationship between increased transmembrane calcium influx, cardiac contractility, and catecholamine stimulus is a well-established concept [28, 34, 38–44]. Therefore, long-term treatment with β-adrenoceptor blocking substances, commencing during the prenecrotic stage of the cardiomyopathy, was thought to prevent the development of myocardial necrosis.

This assumption was based on findings of Nayler [41] and of Bloom and Davis [37], who reported increased myocardial calcium accumulation by epinephrine and by isoproterenol, respectively, which could be prevented by pretreatment with propranolol. Our findings, however, disagree in part with the above conclusion. Whereas only those β-adrenoceptor blocking agents that also possess membrane stabilizing properties exerted full cardioprotection, in the order of their known nonspecific membrane efficacy [60, 61], neither of the two exclusive β-adrenoceptor blocking substances, i.e., atenolol and practolol, were able to completely suppress myocardial calcium accumulation.

In addition, the magnitude of the applied dosages that counteracted calcium accumulation seems to be far above the level providing total β-adrenoceptor blockade. These results suggest no influence of endogenously stimulated adrenergic activity on the development of the detrimental cell membrane defect. Nevertheless, practolol, possessing intrinsic sympathetic activity [61], did enhance myocardial calcium accumulation in lower doses. Interestingly, minor adrenergic stimulation turned out to be more harmful, i.e., calcium promoting, to prenecrotic cardiomyopathic than to normal myocardium, which has been shown by earlier comparative experiments in young hamsters [22, 23].

Not only direct β-adrenoceptor stimulation, but also ischemia (especially after reperfusion) will lead to enhanced myocardial calcium accumulation. Mitochondria are mainly afflicted [62, 63], but gross myocardial damage also occurs [41, 42]. Pretreatment before coronary occlusion not only with propranolol [62–66], but also with practolol [67] and the calcium antagonistic substances verapamil and nifedipine [66] exerted protective effects on myocardium. The protective effects of practolol as well as failure of d-propranolol to exert any protection [68] indicate that myocardial ischemic injury can be reduced by β-adrenergic blockade. However, our results applying β-adrenoceptor blocking substances with and without nonspecific membrane properties suggest that at least in the cardiomyopathy of the Syrian hamsters, augmented adrenergic influence does not seem to contribute to the onset of gross cardiac degeneration.

The cardioprotective effect of various Mg salts has been reported by several authors [46, 47, 49, 69, 70]. Janke et al. [48] postulate that if myocardial cells are damaged, high doses of Mg salts which elevate extracellular Mg-level will prevent progressive efflux of Mg-ions from the intracellular site. This latter process is interlinked with enhanced calcium influx. Späh and Fleckenstein [45] were able to demonstrate a preferential Mg-carrying transport system in the excited myocardial sarcolemma. This transport system can be blocked by catecholamines, while that carrying calcium ions is stimulated. It is hypothesized that high doses of Mg ions counterbalance intracellular calcium overload, which coincides with energy-consuming calcium sequestration in mitochondria [71]. Moreover, magnesium was shown to cause a marked decrease in the initial rates of respiration-supported calcium uptake by isolated heart mitochondria [72]. Hence, mitochondrial calcification will be avoided by prevention of cellular magnesium loss and vital mitochondrial phosphorylating ability of high energy phosphates retained. In addition, Jasmin et al. [52, 53] suggest that mitochondria of the diseased hamsters might be afflicted with abnormal respiratory function. These mitochondria are also higher in their cholesterol content. Biochemical [73] and recent electron microscopic studies [74] on myocardium of cardiomyopathic hamsters reveal calcification that begins in the mitochondria as also observed in damaged cardiomyocytes of Mg-deficient rats [75]. Earlier experiments performed in the cardiomyopathic hamsters of strain BIO 14.6 also showed intracellular magnesium deficiency in prenecrotic hearts [4]. These results led to our trial of chronic administration of a Mg salt into the hamsters.

The successful results obtained by the long-term experiments with Mg-aspartate · HCl in suppressing myocardial calcium accumulation as well as in protecting the cardiomyopathic hearts from gross degeneration confirm the above developed concepts. Compared with verapamil, magnesium seems to act as a weak intracellular calcium antagonist, not only in several pharmacological disease models, but also in spontaneously cardiomyopathic hamsters.

In conclusion, the cardiomyopathy of the Syrian hamster, representing a spontaneous disease model, offers a unique opportunity to evaluate the mechanism and potency of cardioprotective drugs. Although it is impossible to clarify the trigger mechanism inducing myocardial calcium overload in the cardiomyopathic hamster its crucial role for myocardial necrotization was emphasized by evaluating and correlating the effect of several cardioprotective drugs. i.e., verapamil, Mg-aspartate · HCl, and β-adrenoceptor blockers with respect to myocardial calcium accumulation and to morphological changes. It turned out thereby that stimulated adrenergic activity is not likely to provoke myocardial calcium overload in this hereditary disease.

References

1. Homburger F, Baker JR, Nixon CW, Wilgram G (1962) New hereditary disease of Syrian hamster. Primary generalized polymyopathy and cardiac necrosis. Arch Intern Med 110:660–662
2. Homburger F, Nixon CW, Eppenberger M, Baker JR (1966) Hereditary myopathy in the Syrian hamsters: Studies on pathogenesis. Ann NY Acad Sci 138:14–27
3. Bajusz E, Homburger F, Baker JR, Opie LH (1966) The heart muscle in muscular dystrophy with special reference to involvement of the cardiovascular system in the hereditary myopathy of the hamster. Ann NY Acad Sci 138:213–229

Prevention of Myocardial Cell Necrosis in the Syrian Hamster 111

4. Bajusz E, Lossnitzer K (1968) A new disease model of chronic congestive heart failure: studies on its pathogenesis. Trans NY Acad Sci 30:939–948
5. Bajusz E (1969) Hereditary cardiomyopathy: A new disease model. Am Heart J 77:686–696
6. Bajusz E, Baker JR, Nixon CW, Homburger F (1969) Spontaneous hereditary myocardial degeneration and congestive heart failure in a strain of Syrian hamster. Ann NY Acad Sci 156:105–129
7. Bajusz E, Büchner F, Onishi S, Rickers K (1969) Hypertrophie des Herzmuskels bei erbbedingter Myopathie. Naturwiss. 56:568–569
8. Bajusz E, Homburger F, Baker JR, Bogdanoff P (1969) Dissociation of factors influencing myocardial degeneration and general cardiovascular failure. Ann NY Acad Sci 156:396–420
9. Bajusz E, Lossnitzer K (1968) Ein neues Krankheitsmodell: Erbliche nichtvaskuläre Myokarddegeneration mit Herzinsuffizienz. Muench Med Wochenschr 110:1756–1768
10. Lossnitzer K (1975) Genetic induction of a cardiomyopathy. In: Schmier J, Eichler O (eds) Heart and circulation. Springer, Berlin Heidelberg New York. Handbook of Experimental Pharmacology, vol XVI/3, pp 309–344
11. Alousi A, Beards JA (1972) Catecholamine, protein, and RNA content in advanced congestive heart failure in the Syrian hamster. Recent Adv Stud Cardiac Struct Metab I:279–288
12. Büchner F, Onishi S (1970) Herzhypertrophie und Herzinsuffizienz in der Sicht der Elektronenmikroskopie. Urban & Schwarzenberg, Munich Berlin Vienna
13. Büchner F (1971) Qualitative morphology of heart failure. Methods Achiev Exp Pathol 5:60–120
14. Mohr W, Lossnitzer K (1974) Morphologische Untersuchungen an Hamstern des Stammes BIO 8262 mit erblicher Myopathie und Kardiomyopathie. Beitr Pathol 153:178–193
15. Mohr W, Lossnitzer K, Schwarz J (1978) The cardiomyopathy of the Syrian hamster (strain BIO 8262) – hypertrophic or dystrophic? Basic Res Cardiol 73:34–46
16. Jasmin G, Eu HY (1979) Cardiomyopathy in hamster dystrophy. Ann NY Acad Sci 317:46–58
17. Lossnitzer K, Bajusz E (1971) Myokardiale Elektrolytveränderungen bei einer erblichen Kardiomyopathie am Krankheitsmodell des syrischen Goldhamsters. Verh Dtsch Ges Inn Med 77:910–914
18. Lossnitzer K, Mohr W (1973) Prevention of myocardial necroses in myopathic hamsters. J Int Res Comm Syst 1:14
19. Lossnitzer K, Bajusz E (1974) Water and electrolyte alterations during the life course of the BIO 14.6 Syrian golden hamster. A disease model of a hereditary cardiomyopathy. J Mol Cell Cardiol 6:163–177
20. Lossnitzer K, Janke J, Hein B, Stauch M, Fleckenstein A (1975) Disturbed myocardial calcium metabolism – A possible pathogenetic factor in the hereditary cardiomyopathy of the Syrian hamster. Recent Adv Stud Cardiac Struct Metab 6:283–290
21. Lossnitzer K, Steinhardt B, Grewe N, Stauch M (1975) Charakteristische Elektrolytveränderungen bei der erblichen Myopathie und Kardiomyopathie des syrischen Goldhamsters (Stamm BIO 8262). Basic Res Cardiol 70:508–520
22. Lossnitzer K, Mohr W, Konrad A, Guggenmoos R (1978) The hereditary cardiomyopathy in the Syrian golden hamster – Influence of verapamil as calcium antagonist. In: Kaltenbach M, Loogen F, Olsen EGJ (eds) Cardiomyopathy and myocardial biopsy. Springer, Berlin Heidelberg New York, pp 27–37
23. Bajusz E, Baker JR, Nixon CW (1966) Effects of catecholamines upon cardiac and skeletal muscles of dystrophic hamsters. Fed Proc 25:475
24. Fleckenstein A (1968) Myokardstoffwechsel und Nekrose. In: VI Symposium Dtsch Ges für Fortschr auf dem Geb d Inn Med. Georg Thieme, Stuttgart, pp 94–109

25. Fleckenstein A, Janke J, Döring H-J, Leder O (1971) Die intrazelluläre Überladung mit Kalzium als entscheidender Kausalfaktor bei der Entstehung nicht-coronarogener Myokard-Nekrosen. Verh Dtsch Ges Kreislaufforsch 37:345–353
26. Fleckenstein A, Janke J, Döring H-J, Pachinger O (1973) Ca overload as the determinant factor in the production of catecholamine-induced myocardial lesions. Recent Adv Stud Cardiac Struct Metab 2:455–466
27. Fleckenstein A, Janke J, Döring H-J, Leder O (1974) Myocardial fiber necrosis due to intracellular Ca overload – A new principle in cardiac pathophysiology. Recent Adv Stud Cardiac Struct Metab 4:563–580
28. Fleckenstein A, Döring H-J, Janke J, Byon YK (1975) Basic actions of ions and drugs on myocardial high-energy phosphate metabolism and contractility. In: Schmier J, Eichler O (eds) Heart and Circulation. Springer, Berlin Heidelberg New York. Handbook of experimental pharmacology, vol XVI/3, pp 345–405
29. Fleckenstein A, Janke J, Döring H-J, Leder O (1975) Key role of Ca in the production of non-coronarogenic myocardial necroses. Recent Adv Stud Cardiac Struct Metab 6:21–32
30. Fleckenstein A (1980) Steuerung der myokardialen Kontraktilität, ATP-Spaltung, Atmungsintensität und Schrittmacherfunktion durch Calcium-ionen – Wirkungsmechanismus der Calcium-antagonisten. In: Fleckenstein A, Roskamm H (eds) Calcium-Antagonismus. Springer, Berlin Heidelberg New York, pp 1–28
31. Fleckenstein A (1971) Specific inhibitors and promotors of calcium action in the excitation-contraction coupling of heart muscle and their role in the prevention or production of myocardial lesions. In: Harris P, Opie L (eds) Calcium and the heart. Academic Press, London New York, pp 135–188
32. Fleckenstein A (1975) Fundamentale Herz- und Gefäßwirkungen Ca-antagonistischer Koronartherapeutika. Med Klin 70:1665–1674
33. Kohlhardt M, Bauer B, Krause H, Fleckenstein A (1972) Differentiation of the transmembrane Na and Ca channels in mammalian cardiac fibres by the use of specific inhibitors. Pflügers Arch 335:309–322
34. Thyrum PT (1974) Inotropic stimuli and systolic transmembrane calcium flow in depolarized guinea-pig atria. J Pharmacol Exp Ther 188:166–179
35. Angelakos ET, Carballo LC, Daniels JB, King MB, Bajusz E (1972) Adrenergic neurohumors in the heart of hamsters with hereditary myopathy during cardiac hypertrophy and failure. Recent Adv Stud Cardiac Struct Metab 1:262–278
36. Angelakos ET, King MD, Carballo LC (1973) Cardiac adrenergic innervation in hamsters with hereditary myocardiopathy: chemical and histochemical studies. Recent Adv Cardiac Struct Metab 2:519–531
37. Bloom S, Davis D (1974) Isoproterenol myocytolysis and myocardial calcium. Recent Adv Stud Cardiac Struct Metab 4:581–590
38. Entman ML (1970) Calcium and cardiac contractility. Am J Med Sci 259:164–167
39. Katz AM, Repke DI (1973) Calcium-membrane interactions in the myocardium: effects of ouabain, epinephrine and 3′,5′-cyclic adenosine monophosphate. Am J Cardiol 31:193–201
40. Morgenstern M, Noack E, Köhler E (1972) The effects of isoprenaline and thyramine on the calcium uptake, the total calcium content and the contraction force of isolated guinea-pig atria in dependence of different extracellular hydrogen ion concentrations. Naunyn Schmiedebergs Arch Pharmacol 274:125–137
41. Nayler WG (1967) Some factors involved in the maintenance and regulation of cardiac contractility. Circ Res [Suppl III] 20, 21:213–220
42. Pappano AJ (1970) Calcium dependent action potentials produced by catecholamines in guinea-pig atrial muscle fibers depolarized by potassium. Circ Res 27:379–390
43. Reuter H (1965) Über die Wirkung von Adrenalin auf den cellulären Ca-Umsatz des Meerschweinchenvorhofs. Naunyn Schmiedebergs Arch Pharmacol 251:401–412

Prevention of Myocardial Cell Necrosis in the Syrian Hamster

44. Shigenobu K, Sperelakis N (1972) Calcium current channels induced by catecholamines in chick embryonic hearts whose fast sodium channels are blocked by tetrodotoxin or elevated potassium. Circ Res 31:932–952
45. Späh F, Fleckenstein A (1979) Evidence of a new, preferentially Mg-carrying, transport system besides the fast Na and the slow Ca channels in the excited myocardial sarcolemma membrane. J Mol Cell Cardiol 11:1109–1127
46. Bajusz E (1963) Conditioning factors for cardiac necroses. Karger, Basel New York
47. Selye H (1961) The pluricausal cardiopathies. Thomas, Springfield
48. Janke J, Fleckenstein A, Hein B, Leder O, Sigel H (1975) Prevention of myocardial Ca-overload and necrotization by Mg and K salts or acidosis. Recent Adv Stud Cardiac Struct Metab 6:33–42
49. Lehr D, Cahu R, Kaplan J (1972) Prevention of experimental myocardial necrosis by electrolyte solutions. Recent Adv Stud Cardiac Struct Metab 1:684–698
50. Lossnitzer K (1973) Zur quantitativen Bestimmung von K, Na, Mg, Ca im Herzmuskelgewebe. In: Horatz K, Rittmeyer O (eds) Kalium-Magnesium-Aspartat. Medicus, Berlin, pp 33–40
51. Jasmin G, Bajusz E (1975) Prevention of myocardial degeneration in hamsters with hereditary cardiomyopathy. Recent Adv Stud Cardiac Struct Metab 6:219–229
52. Jasmin G, Solymoss B, Proschek L (1979) Therapeutic trials in hamster dystrophy. Ann NY Acad Sci 317:338–348
53. Jasmin G, Proschek L (1980) Prevention of myocardial degeneration in hamsters with hereditary cardiomyopathy. In: Fleckenstein A, Roskamm H (eds) Calcium-Antagonismus. Springer, Berlin Heidelberg New York, pp 144–150
54. Lossnitzer K, Konrad A, Jakob M (1980) Kardioprotektion durch Kalziumantagonisten bei erblich kardiomyopathischen Hamstern. In: Fleckenstein A, Roskamm H (eds) Calcium-Antagonismus. Springer, Berlin Heidelberg New York, pp 151–171
55. Wada A, Fushimi H, Takemura K, Imu Y, Onishi S (1977) Cardiomyocytes in the embryonal stage of Syrian hamsters with a hereditary cardiomyopathy. J Mol Cell Cardiol 9:799–805
56. Bester AJ, Gevers W (1975) The synthesis of myofibrillar and soluble proteins in cell-free systems and in intact cultured muscle cells from newborn polymyopathic hamsters. J Mol Cell Cardiol 7:325–344
57. Büchner F, Onishi S, Wada A (1978) Cardiomyopathy associated with systemic myopathy. Genetic defect of actomyosin influencing muscular structure and function. Urban & Schwarzenberg, Baltimore Munich
58. Rona G, Boutet M, Hüttner I (1975) Membrane permeability alterations as manifestation of early cardiac muscle cell injury. Recent Adv Stud Cardiac Struc Metab 6:439–451
59. Paterson RA, Layberry RA, Nadkarni BB (1972) Cardiac failure in the hamster. A biochemical and electron microscopic study. Lab Invest 26:755–766
60. Hellenbrecht D, Lemmer B, Wiethold G, Grobecker H (1973) Measurement of hydrophobicity, surface activity, local anaesthesia, and myocardial conduction velocity as quantitative parameters of the non-specific membrane affinity of nine β-adrenergic blocking agents. Naunyn Schmiedebergs Arch Pharmacol 277:211–226
61. Saameli K (1972) Die pharmakologische Charakterisierung β-sympathikolytischer Substanzen. In: Dengler HJ (ed) Die therapeutische Anwendung β-sympathikolytischer Stoffe. Schattauer, Stuttgart New York, pp 3–30
62. Maroko PR, Kjekshus JK, Sobel BE, Watanabe T, Covell JW, Ross J Jr, Braunwald E (1971) Factors influencing infarct size following experimental coronary artery occlusions. Circulation 43:67–62
63. Reimer KA, Rasmussen MM, Jennings RB (1973) Reduction by propranolol of myocardial necrosis following temporary coronary artery occlusion in dogs. Circ Res 33:353–363

64. Ergin MA, Dastgir G, Butt KMH, Stuckey JH (1976) Prolonged epicardial mapping of myocardial infarction: The effects of propranolol and intra-aortic balloon pumping following coronary artery occlusion. J Thorac and Cardiovasc Surg 72:892–899
65. Hillis LD, Askenazi J, Braunwald E, Radvani P, Muller JE, Fishbein MC, Maroko PR (1976) Use of changes in the epicardial QRS complex to assess interventions which modify the extent of myocardial necrosis following coronary artery occlusion. Circulation 54:591–598
66. Nayler WG, Ferrari R, Williams A (1980) Protective effect of pretreatment with verapamil, nifedipine and propranolol on mitochondrial function in the ischemic and reperfused myocardium. Am J Cardiol 46:242–248
67. Libby P, Maroko PR, Covell JW, Malloch CI, Ross J Jr, Braunwald E (1973) Effect of practolol on the extent of myocardial ischaemic injury after experimental coronary occlusion and its effects on ventricular function in the normal and ischaemic heart. Cardiovasc Res 7:167–173
68. Reimer KA, Rasmussen MM, Jennings RB (1976) On the nature of protection by propranolol against myocardial necrosis after temporary coronary occlusion in dogs. Am J Cardiol 37:520–527
69. Fedelesova M, Ziegelhöffer A, Luknarova O, Kostolansky S (1975) Prevention by K^+, Mg^{2+}-aspartate of isoproterenol-induced metabolic changes in the myocardium. Recent Adv Stud Cardiac Struct Metab 4:59–73
70. Slezak J, Tribulova N (1975) Morphological changes after combined administration of isoproterenol and K^+, Mg^{2+}-aspartate as a physiological Ca^{2+} antagonist. Recent Adv Stud Cardiac Struct Metab 6:75–84
71. Lehninger AL (1970) Mitochondria and calcium ion transport. The fifth jubilee lecture. Biochem J 119:129–138
72. Sordahl LA, Silver BB (1975) Pathological accumulation of calcium by mitochondria: modulation by magnesium. Recent Adv Stud Cardiac Struct Metab 6:85–93
73. Wrogemann K, Blanchear MC, Thakar JH, Mezon BJ (1975) On the role of mitochondria in the hereditary cardiomyopathy of the Syrian hamster. Recent Adv Stud Cardiac Struct Metab 6:231–241
74. Galle J, Mohr W, Lossnitzer K, Haferkamp O (1981) Development of necrosis and its sequelae in the myocardium of polymyopathic hamsters (BIO 8262). An electron microscopic study. Virchow Arch [Cell Pathol] 36:87–100
75. Heggtveit HA, Herman L, Mishra RK (1964) Cardiac necrosis and calcification in experimental magnesium deficiency. A light and electron microscopic study. Am J Pathol 45:757–782
76. Nadkarni BB, Hunt B, Heggtveit HA (1972) Early ultrastructural and biochemical changes in the myopathic hamster heart. Recent Adv Stud Cardiac Struct Metab I:251–261
77. Shen AC, Jennings RB (1972) Myocardial calcium and magnesium in acute ischemic injury. Am J Pathol 67:417–440
78. Shen AC, Jennings RB (1972) Kinetics of calcium accumulation in acute myocardial ischemic injury. Am J Pathol 67:441–452

Prevention by Verapamil of Isoproterenol-Induced Hypertrophic Cardiomyopathy in Rats

A. FLECKENSTEIN, M. FREY, and J. KEIDEL

It is a well-known fact that hypertrophy of both ventricles as well as disseminated or confluent myocardial necroses can be experimentally produced in rats by overdoses of the β-adrenergic stimulant isoproterenol. Thus not only cardiomyopathic Syrian hamsters [1, 2], but also isoproterenol-treated hypertrophic rat hearts are valuable disease models for pathophysiological studies on hypertrophic cardiomyopathy.

Significance of Intracellular Calcium Overload in the Pathogenesis of Myocardial Necrotization: Cardioprotection by Calcium Antagonists

Heart muscle fibers undergo severe functional and structural alterations resulting in necrotization, as soon as extracellular Ca ions penetrate excessively into the sarcoplasm, so that the capacities of the processes that extrude or sequester Ca are overpowered (see Fig. 1). Previous work with ^{45}Ca has shown that a number of non-coronarogenic cardiomyopathies result from an overload with intracellular Ca [3, 9]. This applies particularly to cardiac lesions caused by large doses of sympathomimetic amines, especially isoproterenol, since extreme stimulation of β-receptors increases the transmembrane Ca influx enormously. For instance, in rats with a single subcutaneous dose of 30 mg isoproterenol/kg, the myocardial Ca content is increased by a factor of 4 for several hours followed by development of disseminated myocardial necroses. A deleterious augmentation of Ca uptake in rat hearts is also brought about by overdoses of vitamin D_3 or dihydrotachysterol or by feeding the animals with a K- or Mg-deficient diet. This Ca overload produces (a) excessive activation of Ca-dependent intracellular ATPases and (b) swelling and functional deterioration of mitochondria, so that a massive deficiency of the cardiac high-energy phosphates occurs leading to structural damage as in anoxia or ischemia. Factors which sensitize the myocardium to catecholamine-induced necrotization act by potentiation of intracellular Ca uptake [4, 7]. Conversely, as we first described in 1968, the hearts can be protected against deleterious Ca overload by suitable doses of Ca-antagonistic substances such as prenylamine, verapamil, or D 600, which are capable of reducing transmembrane Ca uptake almost to normal (Figs. 2, 3). The Ca antagonists nifedipine and fendiline also counteract iso-proterenol-induced Ca overload [5]. Thereby the Ca antagonists prevent ATP and creatine phosphate exhaustion as well as myocardial necrotization [3, 9]. In comparison with β-blockers that only neutralize the catecholamine effects on Ca uptake, the Ca antagonists possess a broader scale of action since they interfere with

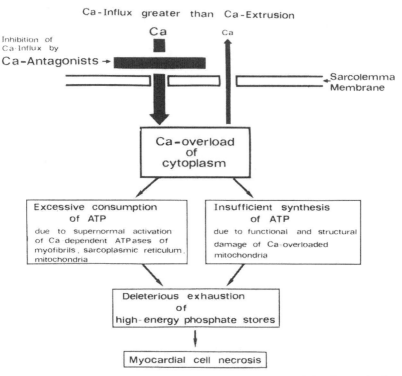

Fig. 1. Scheme of myocardial necrotization produced by intracellular Ca overload

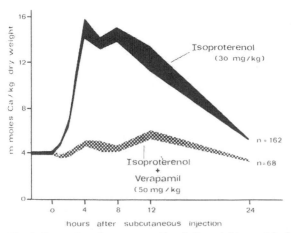

Fig. 2. Protection by verapamil of the right ventricular myocardium of rats against isoproterenol-induced Ca overload during an observation period of 24 h. Administration of 30 mg/kg isoproterenol with and without verapamil (50 mg/kg) at separate subcutaneous injection sites [5]

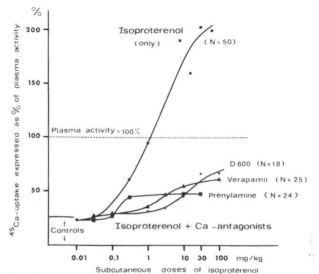

Fig. 3. Prevention of excessive isoproterenol-induced uptake of labeled Ca into the right ventricular myocardium of rats by three Ca-antagonistic compounds: Log dose-response curves of the isoproterenol-induced radiocalcium incorporation obtained with or without simultaneous administration of D 600 (10 mg/kg), verapamil (17 mg/kg), or prenylamine (250 mg/kg). All measurements were made 6 h after subcutaneous injection of the drugs [4]

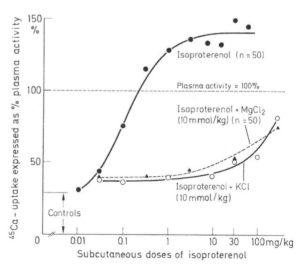

Fig. 4. Prevention of excessive isoproterenol-induced ^{45}Ca uptake into the inner layer of the left ventricular myocardium of rats by a single oral standard dose of KCl (10 mmol/kg) or MgCl$_2$ (10 mmol/kg). The log dose-response curves were obtained 6 h after simultaneous injection of 10 μCi ^{45}Ca/kg (intraperitoneally) and of the different amounts of isoproterenol (subcutaneously), with and without KCl or MgCl$_2$. The salt solutions were always given with a stomach tube just before the isoproterenol and ^{45}Ca administration [4]

practically all types of Ca overload irrespective of the particular origin. Ca overload and myocardial fiber damage are also inhibited by increasing the plasma concentration of natural Ca-antagonistic cations (K, Mg, or H) in order to counterbalance Ca according to the ratio:

$$\frac{Ca}{Mg, K, H}$$

The cardioprotective effects of oral doses of KCl or $MgCl_2$ are shown in Fig. 4. On the other hand, if Mg, K, or H ion concentrations are too low, Ca uptake, high-energy phosphate breakdown, and necrotization are facilitated.

Influence of Verapamil and Calcium-Antagonistic K and Mg Salts on Isoproterenol-Induced Cardiomegaly

Whereas isoproterenol-induced myocardial necrotization develops within a few hours following a high acute dose of the drug, cardiomegaly results from chronic subcutaneous administration of smaller amounts of isoproterenol (1 mg/kg daily for 7 days). This dosage roughly doubles the myocardial Ca concentration. For instance, in 157 experiments of the latter type, the ratio of ventricular weight (expressed in mg) over body weight (expressed in g) rose from 0.56 to 0.8 (right ventricle) and from 2.02 to 2.65 (left ventricle). In addition, after 7 days, scarce

Table 1. Inhibition of both isoproterenol-induced cardiac hypertrophy and isoproterenol-induced increase in apical hydroxyproline content of rats by simultaneous prophylactic administration of verapamil, or of verapamil in combination with KCl or $MgCl_2$

All rats received a daily subcutaneous dose of 1 mg isoproterenol per kg body weight for 7 consecutive days

Simultaneous cardioprotective treatment	Inhibition % of isoproterenol-induced ventricular hypertrophy		Inhibition % of isoproterenol-induced increase in hydroxy-proline content (apex)
	Right	Left	
With verapamil	34.5 (± 4.3)	65.7 (±3.2)	79.8 (±12.1)
With verapamil + KCl	58.5 (±14.2)	106.5 (±9.0)	110 (±23.5)
With verapamil + $MgCl_2$	88.6 (± 8.6)	118.6 (±9.9)	82.6 (± 8.6)

The figures indicate the degree of inhibition expressed in percent by which the isoproterenol effects could be reduced with the help of verapamil and the Ca-antagonistic salts.
Verapamil was administered in the form of daily subcutaneous doses of 15 mg/kg body weight for a period of 7 days simultaneously with isoproterenol, at different injection sites. However, KCl (twice daily 5 mmol/kg) and $MgCl_2$ (twice daily 12.5 mmol/kg) were administered during the 7-day period with a stomach tube [11].

disseminated necroses in the stage of healing were discernible in the apical region of the left ventricle. This was accompanied by an increase in the hydroxyproline content of the apical tissue, an observation which is indicative of a proliferation of connective tissue that replaces necrotic cardiac fibers (hydroxyproline represents 13% of the collagen mass).

However, the most important finding was that the same Ca-antagonistic treatment which prevented acute isoproterenol-induced myocardial necrotization, i.e., administration of verapamil, KCl, or $MgCl_2$, also inhibited isoproterenol-induced cardiac hypertrophy. Table 1 represents a quantitative evaluation of our results. The figures represent the degree of inhibition (expressed in percent) of the isoproterenol effects on ventricular weight (in relation to body weight) and on the apical hydroxyproline content. As can be easily seen from these data, verapamil alone (daily doses of 15 mg/kg subcutaneously administered for 7 days) inhibited the isoproterenol-induced growth of the relative ventricular mass by 65.7% ($\pm 3,2\%$), and the concomitant increase in the hydroxyproline content by 79.8% ($\pm 12.1\%$). However, the most efficient treatment consisted of combining the subcutaneous administration of verapamil with oral doses of KCl or $MgCl_2$ twice daily for 7 days. With this regimen, the isoproterenol-induced left ventricular hypertrophy and the rise in hydroxyproline could be completely prevented in most cases. The inhibition of left ventricular hypertrophy by 118.6% ($\pm 9.9\%$) (!) which was observed in the isoproterenol-treated rats under the therapy with verapamil $+ MgCl_2$ means that in this series, the relative ventricular weights were found to be even smaller than those of the control animals without any drug application. The right ventricles too responded favorably to the Ca-antagonistic therapy although its efficacy did not reach the 100% mark.

Discussion

The experiments indicate that both disseminated cardiac necroses and ventricular hypertrophy produced by isoproterenol are different consequences of the same myocardial alteration, which basically consists of intracellular Ca overload: Thus moderate chronic increases in myocardial Ca content, following application of relatively small doses of isoproterenol, seem to initiate ventricular hypertrophy, whereas higher degrees of acute Ca overload will produce necrotization. In keeping with this, isoproterenol-induced hypertrophy *and* myocardial lesions can be prevented, at least in part, by verapamil, KCl, or $MgCl_2$ because these agents counteract excessive myocardial Ca uptake. However, most effective is a combined application of verapamil together with these salts. This might also be an important hint for practical therapy.

Cardioprotection with verapamil is a phenomenon that must be explained on a cellular level. Accordingly, verapamil operates as an antidote against the necrotizing effects of overdoses of β-adrenergic stimulants even in tissue cultures of human heart muscle cells [10]. These observations clearly demonstrate that the cardioprotective actions of verapamil are not connected with certain hemodynamic effects that might be beneficial to the heart in situ such as an improvement of oxygen supply, reduction of preload or afterload, decrease in heart rate, etc. Our findings extend the classic work by Rona and his associates [12] on isoproterenol with respect to cardiac hypertrophy and simultaneously demonstrate again its high informative value.

References

1. Lossnitzer K, Janke J, Hein B, Stauch M, Fleckenstein A (1975) Disturbed myocardial calcium metabolism: A possible pathogenetic factor in the hereditary cardiomyopathy of the Syrian hamster. In: Fleckenstein A, Rona G (eds) Pathophysiology and morphology of myocardial cell alterations. Recent Adv Stud Cardiac Struct Metab, vol 6. University Park Press, Baltimore London Tokyo, pp 207–217
2. Lossnitzer K, Konrad A, Jakob M (1980) Kardioprotektion durch Kalzium-Antagonisten bei erblich kardiomyopathischen Hamstern. In: Fleckenstein A, Roskamm H (eds) Calcium-Antagonismus. Springer, Berlin Heidelberg New York, pp 159–171
3. Fleckenstein A, (1968) Myokardstoffwechsel und Nekrose. In: Heilmeyer L, Holtmeier H-J (eds) Herzinfarkt und Schock. Thieme, Stuttgart, pp 94–109
4. Fleckenstein A (1971) Specific inhibitors and promoters of calcium action in the excitation-contraction coupling of heart muscle and their role in the prevention or production of myocardial lesions. Proc meeting internat study group for research in cardiac metabolism, London 1970. In: Harris P, Opie L (eds) Calcium and the Heart. Academic Press, London New York, pp 135–188
5. Fleckenstein A (1980) Steuerung der myocardialen Kontraktilität, ATP-Spaltung, Atmungsintensität und Schrittmacher-Funktion durch Calcium-Ionen – Wirkungsmechanismus der Calcium-Antagonisten. In: Fleckenstein A, Roskamm H (eds) Calcium-Antagonismus. Springer, Berlin Heidelberg New York, pp 1–28
6. Fleckenstein A, Döring HJ, Janke J, Byon YK (1975) Basic actions of ions and drugs on myocardial high-energy phosphate metabolism and contractility. In: Schmier J, Eichler O (eds) Heart and circulation. Springer, Berlin Heidelberg New York (Handbook of experimental pharmacology, vol 16, part 3, pp 345–405)
7. Fleckenstein A, Janke J, Döring HJ, Leder O (1971) Die intracelluläre Überladung mit Kalzium als entscheidender Kausalfaktor bei der Entstehung nicht-coronarogener Myokard-Nekrosen. Verh Dtsch Ges Kreislaufforsch 37:345–353
8. Fleckenstein A, Janke J, Döring HJ, Leder O (1975) Key role of Ca in the production of noncoronarogenic myocardial necroses. In: Fleckenstein A, Rona G (eds) Pathophysiology and morphology of myocardial cell alterations. Recent Adv Stud Cardiac Struct Metab, vol 6. University Park Press, Baltimore London Tokyo, pp 21–32
9. Fleckenstein A, Janke J, Döring HJ, Pachinger O (1973) Ca overload as the determinant factor in the production of catecholamine-induced myocardial lesions. In: Bajusz E, Rona G (eds) Cardiomyopathies. Recent Adv Stud Cardiac Struct Metab, vol 2. University Park Press, Baltimore London Tokyo, pp 455–466
10. Hofmann W, Schleich A, Schroeter D, Weidinger H, Wiest W (1977) Der Einfluß von β-Sympathomimetika und sog. Ca^{++}-antagonistischer Hemmstoffe auf den menschlichen Herzmuskel in vitro. Virchows Arch [Pathol Anat] 373:85–95
11. Janke J, Fleckenstein A, Frey (1978) Schutzeffekt von Ca^{++}-Antagonisten bei der Isoproterenol-induzierten hypertrophischen Cardiomyopathie der Ratte. Verh Dtsch Ges Kreislaufforsch 44:206–207
12. Rona G, Kahn DS, Chappel CI (1963) Studies on infarct-like myocardial necrosis produced by isoproterenol: A review. Rev canad Biol 22:241–255

Effects of Acute Administration of Verapamil in Patients with Hypertrophic Cardiomyopathy

Synopsis

S. E. EPSTEIN

In Chap. 3, the groups from Bethesda, Frankfurt, and Hamburg present data that provide considerable insights into the mechanisms of action of verapamil and other calcium antagonist drugs, as well as into the pathophysiologic mechanisms that may contribute importantly to the natural history of the disease. Thus, it is clear that verapamil diminishes the left ventricular outflow tract gradient present in those patients with the obstructive form of HCM. It does this, at least in the large majority of patients, without causing serious elevation of left ventricular filling pressures. Reduction of gradient, with resultant decrease in intraventricular pressures, undoubtedly plays a role in the beneficial therapeutic effects of this drug in patients with HCM. That this is not the only mechanism responsible for its salutary clinical effects is suggested by the fact that there is no close correlation between reduction in gradient and improvement in exercise capacity, and that patients without obstruction also improve symptomatically.

In this regard, renewed interest has focused on the diastolic abnormalities that have long been known to be present in patients with this disease. With the use of echocardiographic and radionuclide techniques, it has become clear that a large proportion of patients with HCM have impaired left ventricular filling, independent of the presence or absence of left ventricular outflow tract obstruction. It is therefore intriguing to note the preliminary evidence that verapamil has a profound effect on such abnormalities, leading either to normal or considerably improved filling patterns.

The hemodynamic and myocardial contractile effects of the various calcium antagonists are extremely complicated, depending not only on dose, but also on route of administration. Rapid intravenous injection of these drugs will likely cause hypotension, with resulting baroreceptor-mediated reflexes causing alterations in the degree of sympathetic and parasympathetic cardiac stimulation. These reflex alterations can mask the primary effects of calcium antagonist drugs on the sinus and AV nodes, as well as on the myocardium itself. Reflex alterations in autonomic tone to the heart are not as marked after oral administration of the drugs, and are absent when the drugs are given directly into the coronary arteries. Once these considerations are taken into account, it is clear that verapamil depresses sinus note automaticity and conduction velocity of the AV node, actions that nifedipine lacks. Thus, patients have a lower sinus rate during exercise when on verapamil therapy than when taking nifedipine. Moreover, in patients with atrial fibrillation the ventricular response usually can be adequately controlled by verapamil alone. While these characteristics of verapamil may have therapeutic advantages in certain circumstances, they also can (albeit rarely) lead to difficulties. Excessive sinus node

Synopsis

slowing, and even sinus arrest can occur as well as high degrees of AV block, including complete heart block.

Evidence also indicates that calcium antagonists have negative inotropic effects in several experimental preparations. However, how important these negative inotropic actions are to the mechanisms responsible for the drugs' therapeutic efficacy, or to their potential for deleterious clinical effects, is uncertain.

Acute Hemodynamic Effects of Verapamil in Hypertrophic Cardiomyopathy*

DOUGLAS R. ROSING, KENNETH M. KENT, ROBERT O. BONOW, and STEPHEN E. EPSTEIN

For many years propranolol has been the primary pharmacologic therapeutic agent for symptomatic patients with hypertrophic cardiomyopathy [1–3]. The salutary hemodynamic and symptomatic effects produced by propranolol derive from its inhibition of sympathetic stimulation to the heart [4, 5]. However, there is no evidence that the drug alters the primary cardiomyopathic process. In addition, many patients remain or return to their severely symptomatic states, and some die, despite its administration [2, 3].

If propranolol therapy fails to control symptoms in patients with obstruction to left ventricular outflow, an operation such as septal myotomy-myectomy must be considered. As discussed by Dr. Maron (see this symposium p. 238 ff), this operation provides marked symptomatic benefit to the vast majority of patients with obstruction to left ventricular outflow, but the operative risks are between 5 and 10% [6, 7]. Moreover, operation is not a viable option for patients without obstruction. It is therefore clear that new approaches to the nonoperative treatment of this disease are necessary.

Dr. Epstein described the hypercontractile state of the left ventricle in patients with hypertrophic cardiomyopathy (see this symposium p. 14). One concept proposed to explain this hypercontractility is that there are increased amounts of norepinephrine in the left ventricle of patients with hypertrophic cardiomyopathy [8]. However, this hypothesis has never been confirmed and at present we have no explanation for the hypercontractile state in this disorder.

Since increases in myocardial cell calcium content increase myocardial contractility [9], we were intrigued by the studies of the hereditary cardiomyopathy of Syrian hamsters which were just discussed by Dr. Lossnitzer (see this symposium p. 99, [10, 11]). These studies demonstrated that myocardial calcium uptake and content are increased and that the metabolic and anatomic abnormalities can be prevented by the administration of verapamil, an agent which blocks inward calcium transport across cell membranes.

No evidence exists suggesting that the cardiomyopathy of the Syrian hamster is the same disease as hypertrophic cardiomyopathy in man. However, the finding of a hyperdynamic left ventricle in hypertrophic cardiomyopathy in man at least raises the possibility that myocardial calcium overload might, as in the Syrian hamster, account for some of the cardiac abnormalities leading to symptoms and death [12]. A report by Kaltenbach and associates [13], indicating that the administration of verapamil to patients with hypertrophic cardiomyopathy reduces symptoms, and the anecdotal report by Goodwin [14] proposing that drugs like verapamil, which

---

* Part of this paper has previously been published in Circulation 60: 1201–1208, 1979

Acute Hemodynamic Effects of Verapamil in Hypertrophic Cardiomyopathy 125

inhibit inward calcium transport through the so-called slow channel, might be beneficial in patients with hypertrophic cardiomyopathy, suggested that this was a hypothesis worthy of further exploration. We therefore performed the following study designed to examine the hemodynamic effects of verapamil in a group of patients with hypertrophic cardiomyopathy [15].

Methods

Subjects

Twenty-seven patients, 16 men and 11 women, ranging in age from 21 to 68 (mean age ± SEM, 44 ± 3) years, displayed echocardiographic evidence of myocardial hypertrophy of a nondilated left ventricle in the absence of other types of acquired or congenital heart disease which might produce left ventricular hypertrophy. All agreed to participate in the study according to a protocol approved by the Clinical Research Subpanel of the National Heart, Lung, and Blood Institute. The criterion for the obstructive form of hypertrophic cardiomyopathy was the presence of at least a 30 mmHg subaortic peak systolic pressure gradient in the basal state or with provocation with Valsalva maneuver, amyl nitrite inhalation, or intravenous isoproterenol infusion. The criterion for the nonobstructive form of hypertrophic cardiomyopathy was the absence of such a gradient. Twenty-six patients fulfilled the criteria for obstructive hypertrophic cardiomyopathy. The one patient without obstruction at the time of study had had a previous septal myotomy-myectomy.

Twenty-one patients underwent hemodynamic study because of clinically important dyspnea, angina, presyncope, or syncope, despite an adequate trial of propranolol. Propranolol had been administered in doses ranging from 80 to 480 mg per day, median dose 320 mg. Two other patients exhibited the same severe symptomatology, but were not able to tolerate propranolol. The remaining four patients were in a stable condition and underwent catheterization for diagnostic purposes only. Cardiac medications were discontinued at least five drug half-lifes prior to catheterization. Each patient received intramuscular pentobarbital 1 hour prior to study, and nothing was taken by mouth for at least 8 h. Informed consent for all procedures was obtained from each patient.

Hemodynamic Measurements

Left ventricular pressure was obtained through a pigtail catheter (end hole only, no side holes) placed in the apex of the left ventricle by the retrograde femoral technique. Catheter entrapment [16] was excluded by the guidelines proposed by Wigle et al. [17]. Pulmonary artery wedge pressure was obtained through a Cournand catheter placed by the antegrade femoral technique. Cardiac output was determined from indocyanine green dye dilution curves.

All patients were in normal sinus rhythm when hemodynamic measurements were made. Measurements were initially recorded in the control state and then 10–20 min after the initiation of each dose of verapamil. In all patients who had basal left ventricular outflow tract gradients less than 70 mmHg and in an occasional patient with a gradient between 70 and 90 mmHg, Valsalva maneuver, amyl nitrite inhalation, and intravenous isoproterenol infusion were performed after basal measurements were obtained. When possible, left ventricular outflow gradients obtained before and during verapamil infusion were compared at similar heart rates (± 10 beats/min) and systolic blood pressures (± 15 mmHg). Although verapamil administration sometimes lowered systemic systolic blood pressure by more than 15 mmHg compared to the control state, systolic pressure was never more than 15 mmHg above that of the control state.

Verpamil Infusions

Verapamil was infused into a peripheral vein in three dosages: 0.007, 0.014, and 0.021 mg/kg/min. Each infusion was preceded by a 0.1 mg/kg bolus of verapamil administered over 2 min. In the first ten patients studied, only 0.007 mg/kg/min was utilized and hemodynamic measurements were made at 10 and 20 min. When multiple dosages were administered, measurements were made after 10 min of infusion whereupon the next increment in drug dosage was begun preceded by a repeat bolus administration.

Left Ventricular Function

Gated Tc-99m radionuclide angiography was performed in six of these patients in order to assess left ventricular systolic and diastolic function at rest, and to determine the effects of oral verapamil administration on left ventricular function. High-temporal resolution time-activity curves were analyzed to determine left ventricular ejection fraction, peak left ventricular ejection, and filling rate (expressed in end-diastolic volumes per second), and time to peak filling rate (measured from end systole). The techniques employed in these studies have been described previously (Bonow RO, Bacharach SL, Green MV, Kent KM, Rosing DR, Lipson LC, Leon MB, Epstein SE (1981). Impaired left ventricular diastolic filling in patients with coronary artery disease: Assessment with radionuclide cineangiography, circulation 64:315–323). The radionuclide determinations were made with patients on no medications and again when they had been on oral verapamil treatment for approximately 5 days.

Statistics

Data were analyzed statistically using the two-tailed Student t test for paired data.

Results

Basal Hemodynamics

The two higher verapamil dosages produced a small increase in heart rate while systolic blood pressure decreased significantly at all three dose levels (Table 1, Figs. 1, 2). Mean pulmonary artery wedge pressure for the overall group did not change significantly with increasing verapamil dosages (Table 1, Fig. 3). However, in

Acute Hemodynamic Effects of Verapamil in Hypertrophic Cardiomyopathy

Table 1. Hemodynamic effects of verapamil

	No. of patients	Control	Verapamil infusion (mg/kg/min)		
			0.007	0.014	0.021
Heart rate	27	76 ± 3	77 ± 3		
(beats/min)	17	72 ± 3	76 ± 3^c	83 ± 3^d	
	11	72 ± 3	74 ± 3	80 ± 4^b	81 ± 6
Systolic blood pressure	27	116 ± 4	107 ± 3^c		
(mmHg)	17	118 ± 6	113 ± 4	107 ± 4^c	
	11	118 ± 8	112 ± 6	107 ± 5^a	99 ± 5^c
Mean pulmonary artery	25	14 ± 1	13 ± 1		
wedge pressure (mmHg)	17	14 ± 2	15 ± 1	15 ± 1	
	11	15 ± 3	15 ± 2	15 ± 2	15 ± 1
Left ventricular end-	25	16 ± 2	16 ± 1		
diastolic pressure (mmHg)	16	16 ± 2	16 ± 1	15 ± 1	
	10	17 ± 3	17 ± 2	16 ± 1	15 ± 1
Cardiac index	24	2.6 ± 0.1	2.7 ± 0.2		
(liters/min/M²)	15	2.6 ± 0.2	3.0 ± 0.3	3.0 ± 0.3	
	11	2.5 ± 0.2	2.7 ± 0.2^b	2.9 ± 0.3	2.8 ± 0.2^a

mean values $\pm$ SEM.
[a] $P<0.05$ compared to control.
[b] $P<0.01$ compared to control.
[c] $P<0.005$ compared to control.
[d] $P<0.001$ compared to control.

five of seven patients a high control wedge pressure fell by 4 to 12 mmHg. Only four of 19 patients with normal control wedge pressure developed an abnormal mean pulmonary artery wedge pressure (>15 mmHg) during verapamil infusion (Fig. 3). Left ventricular end-diastolic pressure for the group did not change significantly (Table 1, Fig. 4). However, left ventricular end-diastolic pressure fell (ten patients) or was unchanged (two patients) in 12 of the 15 patients who had abnormal pressures in the control state. The decrease in pressure ranged from 1 to 14 mmHg (Fig. 4). Five of ten patients with normal control end-diastolic pressures developed abnormal pressures (>12 mmHg) during verapamil infusion. Cardiac index was maintained during verapamil infusion and showed a significant increase at the highest dose of verapamil when there was a mild rise from a control value of 2.5 ± 0.2 to 2.8 ± 0.2 liters/min/M² ($P<0.05$; Table 1, Fig. 5).

In the 14 patients with a basal left ventricular outflow tract gradient of at least 30 mmHg, the mean basal gradient decreased with increasing verapamil infusions (Table 2, Fig. 6). Three patients had their basal gradients reduced to less than 30 mmHg by the drug infusions. The only patient who showed a marked increase in gradient with verapamil administration (35–80 mmHg) had a simultaneous fall in systolic blood pressure from 160–105 mmHg.

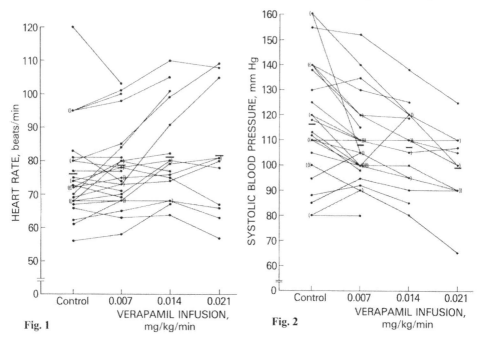

Fig. 1. Effect of increasing doses of verapamil on heart rate. *Horizontal bars* indicate mean values [15]

Fig. 2. Effect of increasing doses of verapamil on systolic blood pressure. *Horizontal bars* indicate mean values [15]

Table 2. Effect of verapamil on left ventricular outflow tract gradients (mmHg)

	No. of patients	Control	Verapamil infusion (mg/kg/min)		
			0.007	0.014	0.021
Basal gradient	14	86± 7	64± 8[a]		
	7	93±10	63±12[a]	51±12[b]	
	5	94±14	71±13	60±14[a]	49±14
Valsalva induced	12	90± 8	74± 9		
	5	81± 6	78± 7	63± 9	
	3	76± 5	88± 2	76± 5	63±13
Amyl nitrite induced	10	80±10	56±11[b]		
	8	72±10	44±13[a]	37±11[a]	
	5	69±15	56±11	49±14	39±13
Isoproterenol induced	9	107±15	79±14[c]		
	8	106±18	81±18[a]	66±14[c]	
	5	108±29	86±26	77±20[a]	70±21[b]

Mean values ± SEM.
[a] $P<0.05$ compared to control.
[b] $P<0.01$ compared to control.
[c] $P<0.005$ compared to control.

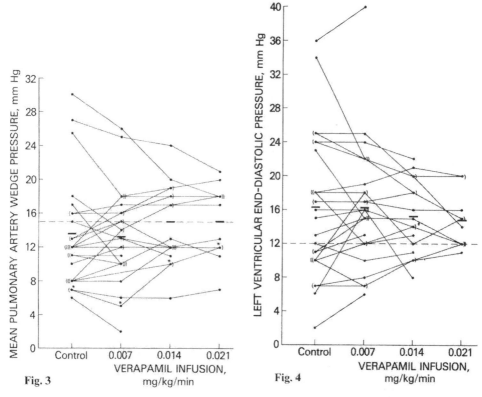

Fig. 3. Effect of increasing doses of verapamil on mean pulmonary artery wedge pressure. *Horizontal bars* indicate mean values. *Broken line* indicates upper limit of normal pressure. *Asterisk* (*) indicates direct left atrial measurements obtained when the catheter crossed a patent foramen ovale [15]

Fig. 4. Effect of increasing doses of verapamil on left ventricular end-diastolic pressure. *Horizontal bars* indicate mean values. *Broken line* indicates upper limit of normal pressure [15]

Provocable Gradients

In the control state, 12 of 15 patients who performed a Valsalva maneuver developed a left ventricular outflow tract gradient of at least 30 mmHg. In eight of these 12 patients, a 25% or greater decrease in the Valsalva induced gradient occurred during the verapamil infusion (Table 2, Fig. 7). Two of the four non-responders had a markedly lower systolic blood pressure with the Valsalva maneuver during verapamil infusion (Fig. 7).

Amyl nitrite inhalation produced a gradient of at least 30 mmHg in the control situation in 11 of 12 patients to whom it was administered. Verapamil reduced the amyl nitrite induced gradient more than 25% in nine of these 11 patients (Table 2, Fig. 7). Both patients in whom verapamil had no effect on the gradient induced by amyl nitrite had a systolic blood pressure more than 30 mmHg lower than in the control state at the time of the peak gradient measurement (Fig. 7). One of these patients received only the lowest dose of verapamil.

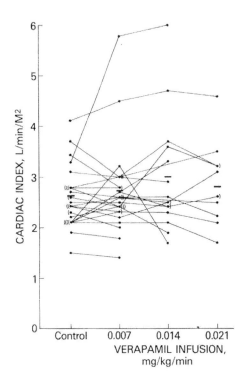

Fig. 5. Effect of increasing doses of verapamil on cardiac output. *Horizontal bars* indicate mean values [15]

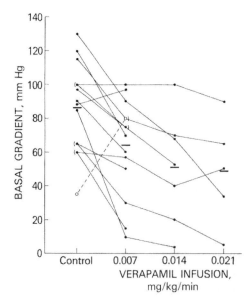

Fig. 6. Effect of increasing doses of verapamil on basal left ventricular outflow tract gradient. *Broken line with open circles* depicts patient whose systolic blood pressure decreased 15 mmHg during verapamil administration. *Horizontal bars* indicate mean values [15]

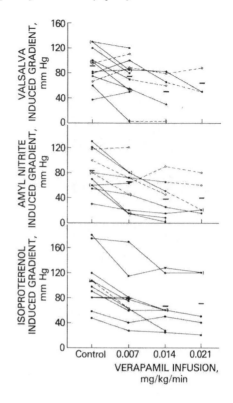

Fig. 7. Effect of increasing doses of verapamil on left ventricular outflow tract gradients produced by Valsalva maneuver (*top*), amyl nitrite inhalation (*middle*), and isoproterenol infusion (*bottom*). Broken lines with *open circles* depict times when systolic blood pressure was more than 15 mmHg below control value. *Horizontal bars* indicate mean values [15]

All ten patients who received an isoproterenol infusion developed a gradient of at least 30 mmHg in the control state. Verapamil decreased the isoproterenol evoked gradient at least 25% in all 10 patients (Table 2, Fig. 7).

Left Ventricular Function

Examples of time-activity curves generated during radionuclide angiography in a normal individual and one with hypertrophic cardiomyopathy are illustrated in Fig. 8. Patients with hypertrophic cardiomyopathy had normal or supranormal left ventricular ejection fractions. Most patients had either a diminished peak filling rate or a prolonged time to peak filling rate, or both abnormalities, compared with normal subjects [18]. When the studies were repeated with patients on short-term verapamil therapy, the abnormalities in diastolic filling improved or normalized (Fig. 9). Three patients both increased peak filling rate and decreased time to peak filling, while the other three improved one of the two indices of diastolic function. There was no consistent change, however, in left ventricular systolic function, as measured by ejection fraction and peak ejection rate.

Adverse Effects

In two patients systolic blood pressure decreased to less than 90 mmHg and for this reason they did not receive the highest dose of verapamil. P-R prolongation occurred

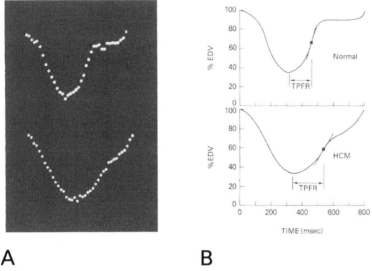

Fig. 8A. Unretouched time-activity curves obtained from a 22-year-old normal volunteer and a 16-year-old patient with hypertrophic cardiomyopathy (HCM). **B** Schematic representations of the two curves. The patient with HCM had similar heart rate (74 vs 78 beats/min), ejection fraction (67 vs 65%) and ejection time (340 vs 320 ms) compared to the normal individual. However, in the patient with HCM, peak filling rate was diminished (2.2 vs 3.6 EDV/s) and time to peak filling rate (TPFR) is prolonged (198 vs 155 ms). [18]

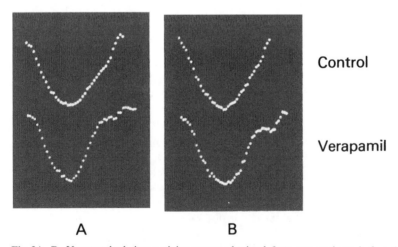

Fig. 9A, B. Unretouched time-activity curves obtained from two patients before (control) and during verapamil therapy. Verapamil results in increased peak filling rate (1.9 to 3.4 EDV/s in patient **A**, and 2.4 to 3.4 EDV/s in patient **B**) and reduced time to peak filling rate (165 to 150 ms in patient **A**, and 380 to 218 ms in patient **B**) [18]

in all patients with the longest P-R interval attained being 380 ms (from a control of 200 ms). The mean P-R interval in the control state was 177 ± 6 ms and increased to 199 ± 6 ($P<0.001$), 218 ± 10 ($P<0.001$), and 244 ± 17 ($P<0.005$) ms with increasing doses of verapamil. Two patients had occasional nonconducted sinus beats at the highest dose. No other abnormalities in cardiac conduction or adverse effects were noted.

Discussion

The present study demonstrates that the intravenous administration of verapamil to patients with hypertrophic cardiomyopathy diminished basal and provoked left ventricular outflow tract gradients in a dose-related manner (Table 2, Figs. 6, 7), while cardiac output either remained the same or slightly increased (Table 1, Fig. 5). The observation that cardiac output was maintained at a time when the left ventricular outflow gradient was reduced indicates that the fall in gradient resulted from an actual increase in the effective orifice size of the left ventricular outflow tract.

In addition to having no detrimental effect on cardiac output, verapamil administration produced no clinically important increase in mean pulmonary artery wedge or left ventricular end-diastolic pressures. Although left-sided filling pressures rose following verapamil in a number of patients, these increases occurred mainly in patients who had normal pressures in the control state, and in no patient did either pressure rise above 20 mmHg. Wedge and end-diastolic pressures decreased or did not change in most patients who began the study with abnormal left-sided filling pressures (Figs. 3, 4). An additional beneficial effect obtained from the oral administration of verapamil was the enhanced early left ventricular filling manifested by an increase in peak filling rate and a decrease in time to peak filling. We observed no drug effect on left ventricular systolic function.

Despite these beneficial hemodynamic effects of verapamil, several considerations must be kept in mind. First, only 11 of our 27 patients received the highest (0.021 mg/kg/min) dose of verapamil used in this study. It is possible that clinically important increases in left heart filling pressures might have been observed if more patients had received the higher doses. Second, reductions in ventricular afterload (systemic resistance) may increase left ventricular outflow obstruction in patients with obstructive hypertrophic cardiomyopathy [19]. Several patients in this study in whom systemic systolic blood pressure dropped more than 15 mmHg had no decrease in left ventricular outflow tract gradient, and one patient actually had a marked increase in gradient. Hence, it is possible that left ventricular outflow obstruction might be increased and the clinical situation worsened in a patient who responds to the drug with an appreciable decrease in systemic arterial pressure. Finally, we know that verapamil blood levels obtained with the two highest intravenous doses used in this study are usually higher than those obtained with the presently recommended oral doses of the drug. As with other drugs that have a high hepatic extraction from the portal blood before reaching the systemic circulation, there will probably be great individual variation in the blood levels and consequently in the hemodynamic effect of a given dosage. Thus, our results should not be construed as indicating that verapamil, when administered as a therapeutic agent, can usually be expected to be effective and totally safe. Although oral administration in clinically indicated dosages did not compromise left ventricular systolic function and improved diastolic filling events, patients receiving this medication must still be watched closely for signs of congestive heart failure. In addition, they must be watched for signs of depression of the sinus node and of conduction in the atrioventricular tissue, and blood pressure must be frequently monitored in both the supine and upright positions to insure that there is no tendency for an excessive decrease in peripheral vascular resistance.

The basic pharmacologic mechanisms by which verapamil exerts its diverse effects are presently unclear. Although earlier studies suggested verapamil had β-adrenergic receptor blocking activity [20], subsequent investigations have refuted this concept [21]. More recently, verapamil has been shown to inhibit transmembrane fluxes of calcium [22]. It appears that the drug specifically interferes with calcium transport occurring through the so-called slow channel [23]. Although there is some evidence that verapamil blocks other ion fluxes through the slow channel [24], it is unclear whether such ionic transport actually occurs normally, and, if so, what effect verapamil has on this transport.

Regardless of its precise biochemical effects, verapamil's major cardiovascular actions are to diminish the rate of conduction through atrioventricular tissue [25] and relax vascular smooth muscle [26, 27] as well as other smooth muscle throughout the body [28]. Potential adverse effects of the drug accrue from its ability to depress sinus node function [29] to produce atrioventricular block [29], and to cause severe hypotension secondary to its vasodilatory activity. The drug has been shown to be capable of decreasing myocardial contractility in vitro at high concentration [30]. Although depression in contractility also occurs experimentally in vivo [29] other studies have failed to demonstrate this finding [32–34]. These conflicting results may be a consequence of the different drug doses used, the different experimental models, and the relative contributions of the direct and indirect actions of verapamil in the various studies. Findings from our laboratory that oral verapamil administered to patients with coronary artery disease tends to decrease left ventricular ejection fraction while ejection fractions are unchanged in patients with hypertrophic cardiomyopathy demonstrate the variable effect of the drug on left ventricular systolic function. However, the tendency for verapamil to improve diastolic events has been a more consistent finding [18, 35].

The mechanisms responsible for the beneficial hemodynamic effects of verapamil in patients with hypertrophic cardiomyopathy probably derive, as do its adverse effects, from inhibition of calcium movement into the myocardial cell. Any agent producing a decrease in the contractile state of the heart should, nonspecifically, diminish the degree of left ventricular outflow obstruction present in patients with hypertrophic cardiomyopathy [4]. This is believed to be the major mechanism by which propranolol reduces the outflow gradient in such patients. Although our results indicate that verapamil does not reduce left ventricular

---

1 Bonow RO, Bacharach SL, Green MV, Kent KM, Rosing DR, Lipson LC, Leon MB, Epstein SE (1981) Impaired left ventricular diastolic filling in patients with coronary artery disease: Assessment with radionuclide cineangiography, Circulation 64:315–323

contractility as measured by global left ventricular ejection fraction, it is possible that other indices of left ventricular systolic function or regional function is affected in a manner which would explain the reduction in left ventricular outflow obstruction. However, we have demonstrated that verapamil enhances early diastolic filling in these patients [18]. If this improvement in myocardial relaxation increases left ventricular diastolic volume, it is possible that this result could decrease left ventricular obstruction by increasing the size of the left ventricular outflow tract. Furthermore, an improvement in relaxation should reduce left ventricular diastolic pressure for a given volume, and this effect should not only enhance myocardial perfusion but should also reduce elevated pulmonary venous pressures, a finding in some patients in this study. Further investigation will have to determine whether or not any of these considerations do occur, and what effect they have in patients with hypertrophic cardiomyopathy.

Regardless of whether the beneficial hemodynamic effects exerted by verapamil are due to an as yet unmeasured effect of the drug on myocardial contractile state, or because verapamil improves left ventricular diastolic function, our results suggest that verapamil may offer the physician a new alternative to propranolol and operation in the treatment of this disorder. Moreover, if results of further studies suggest a *specific* role of calcium antagonists in the treatment of hypertrophic cardiomyopathy, it is possible that a much broader application of verapamil to the therapy of this disease may be indicated.

Acknowledgment. We thank Knoll Pharmaceutical Company of Whippany, New Jersey for supplying us with verapamil. Sincere appreciation is also extended to Mary Denise Ochsenschlager, R. N., and Nancy P. Condit, R. N. for their technical assistance.

References

1. Cohen LS, Braunwald E (1967) Amelioration of angina pectoris in idiopathic hypertrophic subaortic stenosis with β-adrenergic blockade. Circulation 35:847
2. Swan DA, Bell B, Oakley CM, Goodwin J (1971) Analysis of symptomatic course and prognosis and treatment of hypertrophic obstructive cardiomyopathy. Br Heart J 33:671
3. Adelman AG, Wigle ED, Ranganathan N, Webb GD, Kidd BSL, Bigelow WG, Silver MD (1972) The clinical course in muscular subaortic stenosis: A retrospective and prospective study of 60 hemodynamically proved cases. Ann Intern Med 77:515
4. Harrison DC, Braunwald E, Glick G, Mason DT, Chidsey CA, Ross J Jr (1964) Effects of β-adrenergic blockade on the circulation with particular reference to observations in patients with hypertrophic subaortic stenosis. Circulation 29:84
5. Epstein SE, Henry WL, Clark CE, Roberts WC, Maron BJ, Ferrans VJ, Redwood DR, Morrow AG (1974) Asymmetric septal hypertrophy. Ann Intern Med 81:650
6. Morrow AG, Reitz BA, Epstein SE, Henry WL, Conkle DM, Itscoitz SB, Redwood DR (1975) Operative treatment in hypertrophic subaortic stenosis: Techniques and the results of pre- and postoperative assessments in 83 patients. Circulation 52:88
7. Maron BJ, Merrill WH, Freier PA, Kent KM, Epstein SE, Morrow AG (1978) Long-term clinical course and symptomatic status of patients after operation for hypertrophic subaortic stenosis. Circulation 57:1205
8. Pearse AGE (1964) Cardiomyopathies. In: Ciba foundation symposium. Churchill, London, pp 132–164

9. Nayler WG (1967) Calcium exchange in cardiac muscle. A basic mechanism of drug action. Am Heart J 73:379
10. Bajusz E, Lossnitzer K (1968) Ein neues Krankheitsmodell: Erbliche nichtvaskuläre Myokarddegeneration mit Herzinsuffizienz. Muench Med Wochenschr 110:1756
11. Lossnitzer K, Janke J, Hein B, Stauch M, Fleckenstein A (1975) Disturbed myocardial calcium metabolism: A possible pathogenetic factor in the hereditary cardiomyopathy of the Syrian hamster. Recent Adv Stud Cardiac Struct Metab 6:207–217
12. Dhalla NS (1976) Involvement of membrane systems in heart failure due to intracellular calcium overload and deficiency. J Mol Cell Cardiol 8:661
13. Kaltenbach M, Hopf R, Keller M (1976) Calciumantagonistische Therapie bei hypertroph-obstruktiver Kardiomyopathie. Dtsch Med Wochenschr 101:1284
14. Goodwin JF, Krikler DM (1976) Arrhythmia as a cause of sudden death in hypertrophic cardiomyopathy. Lancet 2:937
15. Rosing DR, Kent KM, Borer JS, Seides SF, Maron BJ, Epstein SE (1979) Verapamil therapy: A new approach to the pharmacologic treatment of hypertrophic cardiomyopathy. I. Hemodynamic effects. Circulation 60:1201–1207
16. White RI Jr, Criley JM, Lewis KB, Ross RS (1967) Experimental production of intracavitary pressure differences: Possible significance in the interpretation of human hemodynamic studies. Am J Cardiol 19:806
17. Wigle ED, Marquis Y, Auger P (1967) Muscular subaortic stenosis: Initial left ventricular inflow tract pressure in the assessment of intraventricular pressure differences in man. Circulation 35:1100
18. Bonow RO, Rosing DR, Bacharach SL, Green MV, Kent KM, Lipson LC, Maron BJ, Leon MB, Epstein SE (1981) Effects of verapamil on left ventricular systolic function and diastolic filling in patients with hypertrophic cardiomyopathy: assessment with radionuclide cineangiography. Circulation 64:181–196
19. Wigle ED, David PR, Labrosse CJ, McMeekan J (1965) Muscular subaortic stenosis. The interrelation of wall tension, outflow tract "distending pressure" and orifice radius. Am J Cardiol 15:761
20. Melville KI, Benfey BC (1965) Coronary vasodilatory and cardiac adrenergic blocking effects of iproveratril. Can J Physiol Pharmacol 43:339
21. Nayler WG, McInnes I, Swann JB, Price JM, Carson V, Race D, Lowe TE (1968) Some effects of iproveratril (isoptin) on the cardiovascular system. J Pharmacol Exp Ther 161:247
22. Kohlhardt M, Bauer B, Krause H, Fleckenstein A (1972) New selective inhibitors of the transmembrane Ca conductivity in mammalian myocardial fibers. Studies with the voltage clamp technique. Experientia 28:288
23. Cranefield PF, Aronson RS, Wit AL (1974) Effect of verapamil on the normal action potential and on a calcium-dependent slow response of canine cardiac Purkinje fibers. Circ Res 34:204
24. Shigenobu K, Schneider JA, Sperelakis N (1974) Verapamil blockade of slow Na^+ and Ca^{++} responses in myocardial cells. J Pharmacol Exp Ther 190:280
25. Heng MK, Singh BN, Roche AHG, Norris RM, Mercer CJ (1975) Effects of intravenous verapamil on cardiac arrhythmias and on the electrocardiogram. Am Heart J 90:487
26. Ross G, Jorgensen CR (1967) Cardiovascular actions of iproveratril. J Pharmacol Exp Ther 158:504
27. Singh BN, Roche AHG (1977) Effects of intravenous verapamil on hemodynamics in patients with heart disease. Am Heart J 94:593
28. Golenhofen K, Lammel E (1972) Selective suppresson of some components of spontaneous activity in various types of smooth muscle by iproveratril (verapamil). Pflugers Arch 331:233

Acute Hemodynamic Effects of Verapamil in Hypertrophic Cardiomyopathy 137

29. Singh BN, Ellrodt G, Peter CT (1978) Verapamil: A review of its pharmacological properties and therapeutic use. Drugs 15:169
30. Nayler WG, Szeto J (1972) Effect of verapamil on contractility, oxygen utilization, and calcium exchangeability in mammalian heart muscle. Cardiovasc Res 6:120
31. Newman RK, Bishop VS, Peterson DF, Leroux EJ, Horwitz LD (1977) Effect of verapamil on left ventricular performance in conscious dogs. J Pharmacol Exp Ther 201:723
32. Atterhög JH, Ekelund LG (1975) Haemodynamic effects of intravenous verapamil at rest and during exercise in subjectively healthy middle-aged men. Eur J Clin Pharmacol 8:317
33. Seabra-Gomes R, Richards A, Sutton R (1976) Hemodynamic effects of verapamil and practalol in man. Eur J Cardiol 4:79
34. Smith HJ, Goldstein RA, Griffith JM, Kent KM, Epstein SE (1976) Regional contractility: Selective depression of ischemic myocardium by verapamil. Circulation 54:629
35. Hanrath P, Mathey DG, Kremer P, Sonntag F, Bleifeld W (1980) Effect of verapamil on left ventricular isovolumic relaxation time and regional left ventricular filling in hypertrophic cardiomyopathy. Am J Cardiol 45:1258

Hemodynamics and Contractility After Oral, Intravenous, and Intracoronary Application of Calcium Antagonists

WULF-DIRK BUSSMANN, RÜDIGER HOPF, ALEXANDER TROMPLER, and MARTIN KALTENBACH

Summary

Nifedipine and verapamil are widely used in many cardiac diseases. However, the influence on left ventricular contractility is not entirely clear. This study was designed to verify a possible negative inotropic effect of both drugs. Isovolumic and auxotonic contractility were measured following oral application, intravenous infusion, intravenous bolus injection, and intracoronary administration.

Given orally, *nifedipine* has no cardiodepressive effect. Stroke volume increased indicating improvement of auxotonic contractility due to marked arterial vasodilatation. However, intracoronary injection unmasks the negative inotropic effect of nifedipine which is, however, of short duration.

After oral application, slow intravenous infusion as well as intracoronary injection of verapamil a negative inotropic effect is demonstrated. Following intravenous bolus injection, however, left ventricular contractility remains unaltered presumably due to increased sympathetic activity.

The therapeutic effect of verapamil in patients with hypertrophic cardiomyopathy thus may include influences on systolic as well as on diastolic left ventricular function.

Introduction

For a long time the treatment of hypertrophic obstructive cardiomyopathy has been a domain of beta-blocking agents. Since the report of Kaltenbach et al. showed a favorable influence of verapamil therapy on this disease [1], multiple efforts were undertaken to illuminate the effects of calcium antagonists [2–8].

From animal experiments it is known that calcium antagonists in larger doses have a negative inotropic effect on the heart muscle [9]. Clinically, however, marked cardiac depression has not been observed. Calcium antagonists are widely used in coronary artery disease because they have good antianginal activity. They have also been applied to preserve ischemic myocardium. Nowadays beneficial effects have been shown in hypertrophic obstructive cardiomyopathy via a mechanism which probably modifies the calcium-mediated hypertrophic process directly.

This study was designed to determine whether nifedipine and verapamil exert negative inotropic effects in clinical circumstances. Answering this question definitively is not easy because the agents have multiple actions. For example, heart rate may be affected directly or reflexly, a reduction in afterload may induce better contraction, and direct relaxation of coronary arteries could improve coronary perfusion.

Nifedipine

Methods

22 patients with acute myocardial infarction were studied. They were subdivided into two groups: group I with a left ventricular filling pressure below and group II above 20 mmHg. On the 3rd or 4th day after myocardial infarction both groups received 20 mg nifedipine orally, after 60 min an additional 40 mg. Arterial blood pressure, diastolic pulmonary artery pressure (left ventricular filling pressure), heart rate, and cardiac output (thermodilution) were monitored.

Results

Following 20 mg nifedipine, a decrease in arterial blood pressure was observed, both in patients with left ventricular filling pressures below and above 20 mmHg.

Left ventricular filling pressure remained unchanged. There was a significant increase in cardiac output in both groups. Heart rate did not change significantly (Fig. 1).

After repeated medication with 40 mg, following 1 h after the first dose, heart rate was still unchanged, whereas arterial blood pressure decreased further. At the same time, cardiac output increased. Left ventricular filling pressure remained unchanged (Fig. 2).

Discussion

Following the intracoronary injection of nifedipine, Serruys and coworkers found a direct negative inotropic effect [6, 7]. Reifart and Kober investigated the time course of this cardiodepressive effect. Several minutes following injection of 0.1 mg nifedipine, decreased contractility returned toward baseline (unpublished data).

Our results, however, obtained after acute myocardial infarction, indicate that any negative inotropic potential of nifedipine seems to play a major role clinically: the direct action on the heart is overridden by marked vasodilatation and decrease in systematic vascular resistance. Thus, the effect of nifedipine can be understood as typical vasodilatation: reduced afterload causes an increase in cardiac output. It is also possible that the increase in cardiac output may be partly due to the effect of nifedipine on coronary arterial diameter and the influence on myocardial ischemia.

In summary, despite an intrinsic negative inotropic effect of nifedipine, no cardiac depression has been observed unter clinical conditions. Due to arterial vasodilatation cardiac output even increased.

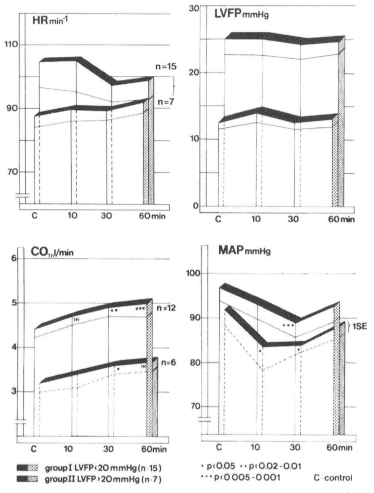

Fig. 1. Hemodynamic effects of 20 mg nifedipine orally in patients with acute myocardial infarction. In both groups with and without left ventricular failure (group II and I) heart rate (*HR*) and left ventricular filling pressure (*LVFP*) were unchanged. Cardiac output (*CO*) significantly increased and mean arterial pressure (*MAP*) decreased. Systemic vascular resistance was markedly reduced (not shown)

Verapamil

Methods

Thirty patients with acute myocardial infarction received a continued infusion of verapamil at a rate of 10 mg/h. A control group (n = 15) received no specific therapy. Pulmonary pressures and cardiac output were monitored by Swan-Ganz-Catheter. In addition, in seven of the patients radionuclide ejection fraction was determined after a 5-mg bolus injection of verapamil.

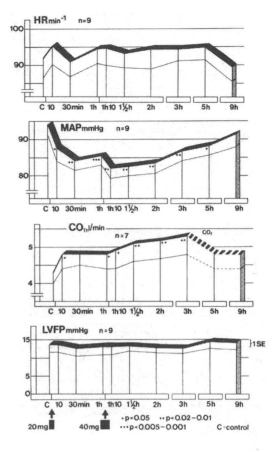

Fig. 2. Hemodynamic effects of oral nifedipine after an initial dose of 20 mg and repeated medication of 40 mg after 1 h. Observation time: 9 h. Significant decrease of mean arterial pressure (*MAP*) along with a marked increase in cardiac output (*CO*). No effect on heart rate (*HR*) and left ventricular filling pressure (*LVFP*)

Patients with a confirmed diagnosis of hypertrophic obstructive cardiomyopathy underwent the following trial: 11 patients were studied following 10 mg i.v. bolus injection of verapamil at rest and during exercise (100 Watt) using a catheter tip manometer in the left ventricle. 13 patients received 160 mg orally and measurements were taken using a fluid filled catheter system 60 min later.

In seven cases with coronary heart disease verapamil was infused over 3–5 min selectively in the left or right coronary artery. Max. dP/dt and pressures were assessed conventionally; in only a few cases a catheter tip manometer was used.

Results

10 mg verapamil per hour by continuous intravenous infusion in patients with recent myocardial infarction did not change heart rate and/or pulmonary artery pressure. There was no change in cardiac output in contrast to nifedipine (Fig. 3). Arterial blood pressure decreased significantly (minus 12 mmHg). Coronary perfusion pressure also decreased. Despite the decrease of arterial pressure, systemic vascular resistance decreased only slightly (Fig. 4).

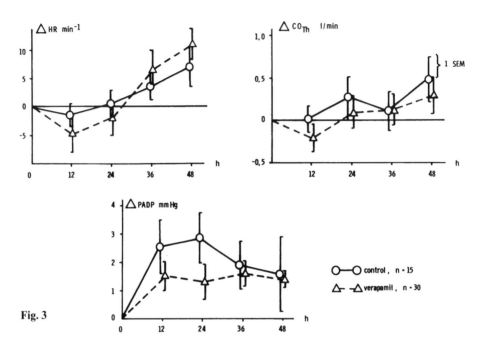

Fig. 3

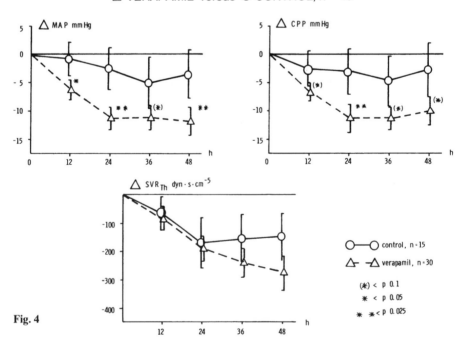

Fig. 4

Fig. 5. Intravenous injection of verapamil, 5 mg in seven patients with coronary artery disease (*CAD*) and recent myocardial infarction. Ejection fraction decreased initially in four but increased in three patients. Mean values slightly decreased and returned toward control 15 min later

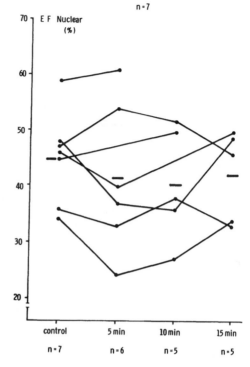

Radionuclide left ventricular ejection fraction showed no consistent changes following i.v. bolus injection of verapamil. In four patients ejection fraction decreased, in three ejection fraction increased. The mean value of ejection fraction tended to decrease but values returned to control 15 min later (Fig. 5).

Following a 10-mg bolus injection of verapamil in patients with hypertrophic obstructive cardiomyopathy, isovolumic contractility did not change. At rest and during exercise max dP/dt remained unchanged before and after verapamil (Fig. 6). Heart rate increased.

The oral medication with 160 mg verapamil resulted in decreased isovolumic contractility. Heart rate and left ventricular end-diastolic pressure were unchanged and left ventricular systolic pressure decreased (Fig. 7).

Following intracoronary infusion of 1.8 mg verapamil left ventricular isovolumic contractility was markedly reduced. This was obvious despite the decrease in heart

Fig. 3. Intravenous infusion of verapamil in a dose of 10 mg/h for 48 h in 30 patients with acute myocardial infarction compared to 15 controls. No significant changes in heart rate (*delta HR*), cardiac output (*delta CO*), and diastolic pulmonary artery pressure (*delta PADP*)

Fig. 4. Intravenous infusion of verapamil in a dose of 10 mg/h for 48 h in 30 patients with acute myocardial infarction compared to 15 controls. Mean arterial pressure (*delta MAP*) and coronary perfusion pressure (*delta CPP*) were significantly reduced during verapamil treatment compared to controls. Slight decrease in systemic vascular resistance (*delta SVR*) at 36 and 48 h

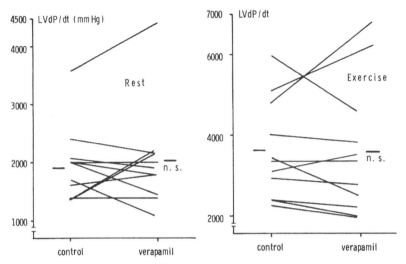

Fig. 6. Ten minutes following intravenous injection of verapamil, 10 mg in patients with hypertrophic obstructive cardiomyopathy (*HOCM*) left ventricular isovolumic contractility (*LV dP/dt*) was unchanged at rest and during exercise. Heart rate, however, increased (not shown in the figure)

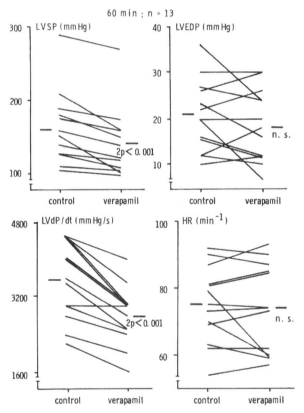

Fig. 7. Left ventricular function following oral application of 160 mg verapamil in patients with hypertrophic obstructive cardiomyopathy (*HOCM*). Left ventricular max dP/dt decreased significantly. Left ventricular systolic pressure (*LVSP*) decreased slightly. No major changes in left ventricular end-diastolic pressure (*LVEDP*) and heart rate (*HR*)

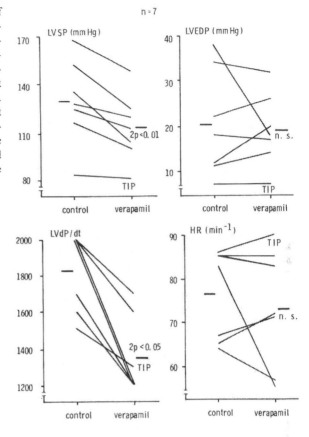

Fig. 8. Intracoronary infusion of 1.8 mg verapamil in seven patients with coronary artery disease. Marked decrease of isovolumic left ventricular contractility (*LVdP/dt*) and systolic left ventricular pressure (*LVSP*). No significant changes in left ventricular end-diastolic pressure (*LVEDP*) and heart rate (*HR*). *Tip:* values obtained with a tip manometer in one patient

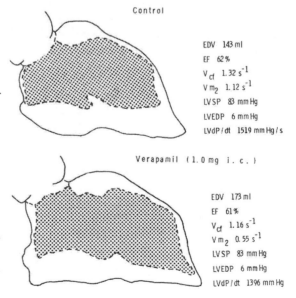

Fig. 9. Influence of intracoronary verapamil on isovolumic and auxotonic contractility parameters. Infusion of 1.0 mg verapamil into the left coronary artery. Increase of end-diastolic volume (*EDV*) without major change in the ejection fraction (*EF*). Decrease of the velocity of mean circumferential fiber shortening (*VCF*) and the velocity of the middle anterior hemiaxis (*Vm$_2$*). Regional wall motion deteriorated in the anterior and apical wall. No change in systolic and end-diastolic left ventricular pressure (*LVSP, LVEDP*). Marked decrease in left ventricular max dP/dt

rate in three patients. Again a drop in systolic ventricular pressure was observed (Fig. 8). Verapamil blood levels determined in several patients following intracoronary injection were found too low to cause any systemic effects.

Using an angiographic catheter with a manometer at the tip simultaneous measurements of isovolumic and auxotonic contractility indices were obtained. An example is shown in Fig. 9.

Selective injection of 1.0 mg verapamil into the left anterior descending branch induced a decrease of isovolumic and auxotonic contractility. Max dP/dt declined from 1519 to 1396 mmHg/s without major changes in systolic or diastolic left ventricular pressure. Enddiastolic and endsystolic volume increased and ejection fraction decreased slightly. Regional function was impaired in the perfusion area of the LAD.

Discussion

The influence of verapamil on hemodynamics and contractility was observed in different groups of patients. This may lead to difficulties in interpretation. However, generally the calcium antagonistic action of verapamil on the myocardium itself should be similar both in patients with coronary artery disease or in patients with hypertrophic obstructive cardiomyopathy.

The route of application: orally, intravenous infusion, intravenous bolus injection, and intracoronary infusion have major importance for interpretation of the results. The bolus injection induces acute changes in the circulatory system and reflex discharge becomes apparent. Intravenous infusion of verapamil or oral application of the drug results in slow changes in hemodynamics and less or absent sympathetic discharge. Intracoronary infusion of the drug acts directly on the myocardium and the intrinsic effects become apparent.

Slow verapamil infusion in patients with acute myocardial infarction had no effect on cardiac output or stroke volume despite a marked decrease of arterial blood pressure. Left ventricular isovolumic contractility or auxotonic ejection fraction were not directly measured. However, unchanged cardiac output and stroke volume in the presence of decreased arterial blood pressure can be taken as the consequence of intrinsic negative inotropism during the continuous 2-day drug infusion.

Like intravenous infusion oral application of verapamil does not induce sudden circulatory changes or eliminated excessive sympathetic discharge. Again arterial pressure decreased. The maximal rate of left ventricular pressure rose, max dP/dt significantly decreased. This indicates a definite negative inotropic effect. The decrease in arterial pressure may also be due to the cardio-depressive effect of the drug, since systemic vascular resistance did not change markedly.

Following intravenous bolus injection of verapamil the hemodynamic profile is different. It is important to follow the time course following injection for several minutes. Ejection fraction measured every 5 min tended to decrease but values returned to control 10–15 min later. Heart rate increased at the same time. Similar results were obtained regarding left ventricular isovolumic contractility in HOCM: no change in contractility but increased heart rate. Sympathetic discharge to the heart apparently increased. Usually an incrasee in heart rate is followed by an increase in max dP/dt. The fact that this increase in contractility was not observed suggests that the intrinsic negative inotropic effect of verapamil was only counterbalanced by increased sympathetic tone. Thus following rapid intravenous administration of the drug left ventricular contractility is largely unchanged. Apparently increased sympathetic discharge is responsible for this.

To further clarify verapamil's intrinsic negative inotropic effect, the drug was applied via the intracoronary route. Isovolumic and auxotonic contractility markedly decreased. Cardiac depression led to a decrease in arterial pressure since peripheral effects were absent indicated by very low blood concentrations. These results are in accordance with those of Serruys et al. [8].

In conclusion slow intravenous infusion or oral administration verapamil decreased left ventricular contractility. Intravenous bolus injection of verapamil had less effects on contractility since by a reflex mechanism the negative inotropic influence is reduced.

The beneficial effects of verapamil in patients with hypertrophic obstructive cardiomyopathy may go along with a mild decrease in contractility of the left ventricle. It is evident that the improvement of ventricular relaxation also plays a major role in those patients.

References

1. Ferlinz J, Easthope JL, Aronow WS (1979) Effects of verapamil on myocardial performance in coronary disease. Circulation 59:313–319
2. Brower RW, Hugenholtz PG, Ten Katen HJ, Meester GT, Serruys P (1979) Effect of nifedipine on regional ventricular shortening during pacing after coronary artery bypass grafting. Circulation [Suppl II] 59, 60:51
3. Bussmann W-D, Schöfer H, Kaltenbach M (1977) Hemodynamic effects of nifedipine in acute myocardial infarction. Herz/Kreislauf 9:140–147
4. Kaltenbach M, Hopf R, Keller M (1976) Calciumantagonistische Therapie bei hypertroph-obstructiver Kardiomyopathie. Dtsch Med Wochenschr 101:1284
5. Nayler WG, Szeto J (1972) Effect of verapamil on contractility, oxygen utilization and calcium exchangeability in mammalian heart muscle. Cardiovasc Res 6:120
6. Rosing DR, Kent KM, Borer JS, Seides SF, Maron BJ, Epstein SE (1979) Verapamil therapy: a new approach to the pharmacologic treatment of hypertrophic cardiomyopathy. I. Hemodynamic effects. Circulation 60:1201–1207
7. Serruys PW, Van den Brand M (1979) Effects of nifedipine on left ventricular isovolumic contraction following intravenous or intracoronary administration. Circulation [Suppl II] 59, 60:82
8. Serruys PW, Brower RW, Bom AH, Ten Katen HJ, Hugenholtz PG (1979) Contractility relaxation and regional wall motion following intracoronary injection of a Ca^{++} antagonist. Circulation [Suppl II] 59, 60:180
9. Mangiardi LM, Hariman RJ, McAllister RG jr, Bhargava V, Surawicz B, Shabetai R (1978) Electrophysiological and hemodynamic effects of verapamil. Circulation 57:366–372
10. Smith HJ, Goldstein RA, Griffith JM, Kent KM, Epstein SE (1976) Regional contractility – Selective depression of ischemic myocardium by verapamil. Circulation 54:629–635

Effect of Verapamil on Left Ventricular Isovolumic Relaxation Time and Regional Left Ventricular Filling in Hypertrophic Cardiomyopathy*

PETER HANRATH, DETLEF G. MATHEY, PETER KREMER, FRANK SONNTAG, and WALTER BLEIFELD

Hypertrophic obstructive and nonobstructive cardiomyopathy are often associated with an abnormal prolonged left ventricular isovolumic relaxation time and a disturbed left ventricular filling pattern [1–5]. Recent experimental studies revealed that calcium antagonists may improve impaired left ventricular relaxation caused by ischemia or hypoxia [6, 7]. Based on these experimental results, it was the purpose of the present study to examine whether the impaired left ventricular relaxation in patients with obstructive and nonobstructive hypertrophic cardiomyopathy can be improved by intravenous application of verapamil.

Methods

Patients

Eleven patients ($5\female, 6\male$) with hypertrophic cardiomyopathy were studied. In all patients the diagnosis was based on the typical angiographic, hemodynamic, and echocardiographic criteria. Six patients had left ventricular outflow obstruction at rest or after provocation and five patients had no intraventricular pressure gradient. The mean age was 39 ± 12 years (range from 19 to 54 years). All patients were in sinus rhythm and without any medication for at least 4 days prior to the study. Selective coronary angiography according to Judkin's technique revealed no significant narrowing of the extramural coronary arteries in any patients.

Echo- and Phonocardiographic Studies

Echocardiograms were recorded in a standard manner with a Picker "Echoview 80 C" ultrasoundscope using a 1.25-cm diameter, 2.25-MHz transducer, with a pulse repetition rate of 1000 cycles/s. The recordings were made with a multichannel Honeywell 1856 strip chart recorder at a paper speed of 50 mm/s along with an electro- and phonocardiogram. The phonocardiogram was recorded in order to define aortic valve closure (A_2). During the study the transducer was kept constant in that intercostal space near the left lateral border of the sternum, where clear and continous echograms of the ventricular septum, the posterior left ventricular wall, and the free margins of both leaflets of the mitral valve were recorded.

---

* Supported in part by the „Gesellschaft für Strahlen- und Umweltforschung mbH" München, Research grant: MMT 02

Simultaneous echo- and phonocardiographic baseline recordings and blood pressure measurements by cuff were performed immediately before intravenously injected verapamil (0.15 mg/kg body weight). After the intravenous injection of verapamil echo- and phonocardiograms were recorded and blood pressure measured every minute over a period of 10 min.

There was a short initial decrease in blood pressure and a compensatory increase in heart rate. These parameters usually returned to control values within 5 min after the injection of verapamil. The following echo- and phonocardiographic recordings were used for the evaluation of the effects of verapamil.

Computerized Analysis of the Combined Phono- and Echo-Cardiograms

Phono-echocardiograms of the control recording (C) and after verapamil (V) injection were digitized and processed by a computerized method as previously described [5, 8]. In each patient, three successive cardiac cycles were analyzed from the pre- and post-drug recordings. From these digitized data the following time and dimension calculations were performed by computer and printed out in an alphanumerical protocol.

Measurements and Calculations of Left Ventricular Time Intervals

Time intervals were referred to the beginning R wave of the first QRS complex as zero reference point. With respect to this reference point, the occurrence of the different time points within the cardiac cycle could be exactly determined. Time parameters of particular interest for this study were:
a) Cycle length (R-R): Time interval between two successive peak R-waves on the electrocardiogram.
b) Electromechanical systole (R-A_2): Time interval from the beginning of the R wave to aortic valve closure (A_2) (Fig. 1).
c) Time point of aortic cusp closure (A_2): The beginning of the first high frequency component of the second heart sound (Fig. 1).
d) Time point of mitral valve opening (MO): The onset of separation of both mitral leaflets (Fig. 1).
e) The left ventricular isovolumic relaxation time (IVR) was calculated as the time interval between the time points of aortic valve closure and mitral valve opening (Fig. 2).
f) The time interval of left ventricular filling (T_{LVF}) was measured as the difference between cycle length and the time point of mitral valve opening (Fig. 2).
g) The relative left ventricular filling period ($T_{LVF\%}$) was calculated according to the following formula:

$$T_{LVF\%} = \frac{T_{LVF}}{\text{cycle length}} \times 100$$

Measurements of Regional Left Ventricular Dimensions

End-diastolic left ventricular dimension (DD) was measured at the peak of the R wave and end-systolic dimension at the time point of aortic valve closure (D_{A2}).

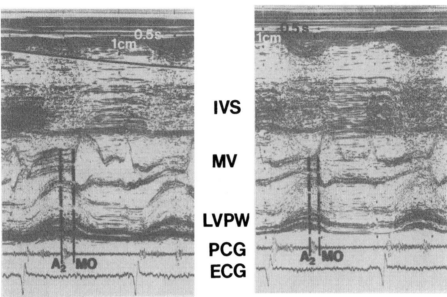

Fig. 1. Simultaneous recording of the echophonocardiogram of a patient with hypertrophic nonobstructive cardiomyopathy, before (*left*) and after intravenous injection of 10 mg verapamil (*right*) A_2, aortic valve closure; *IVS*, interventricular septum; *MO*, mitral valve opening; *MV*, mitral valve leaflets; *LVPW*, posterior wall of the left ventricle. (American Journal of Cardiology)

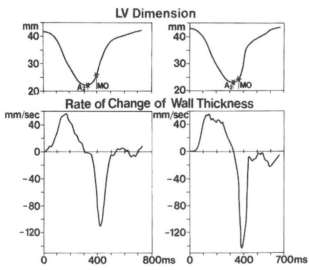

Fig. 2. Computer output of the echograms of the left ventricular cavity shown in Fig. 1 before (*left*) and after intravenous injection of verapamil (*right*). Prolonged isovolumic relaxation time is decreased and peak rate of diastolic wall thinning is increased after i.v. application of verapamil. A_2, aortic valve closure; *MO*, mitral valve opening (American Journal of Cardiology)

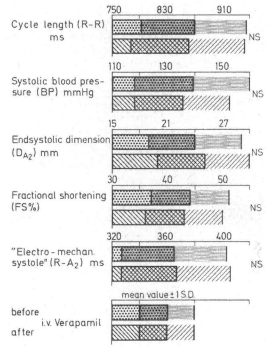

Fig. 3. Effect of verapamil on left ventricular systolic performance in hypertrophic cardiomyopathy

From these values the percentage shortening of the minor axis of the left ventricle (FS) was calculated.

The regional dimension change during isovolumic relaxation (ΔD_{IVR}) was measured as the difference between the left ventricular dimension at the time point of aortic valve closure and that of mitral valve opening (Figs. 2, 3). The dimension increase during left ventricular filling (ΔD_{LVF}) was measured as the dimension increase between the time point of mitral valve opening and that of the peak of the following R wave (Fig. 2). The peak rate of diastolic posterior wall thinning was calculated according to the following formula (Fig. 2):

$$\frac{d\,PW\,min}{dt} \quad (mm/s)$$

The statistical significance of the mean values ±1 S.D. was assessed by paired Student's t test. Studies concerning the interobserver variability and reproducibility have been already published elsewhere [9].

Results

Mean cardiac cycle length (R-R, 869±76 → 861±81 ms, NS) as well as systolic blood pressure (BP, 139±21 → 135±17 mmHg, NS) showed no statistical difference before and after treatment with verapamil. Furthermore, neither end-systolic dimension (ΔD_{A2}, 24±5 → 25±5 mm, NS), nor fractional shortening of the left

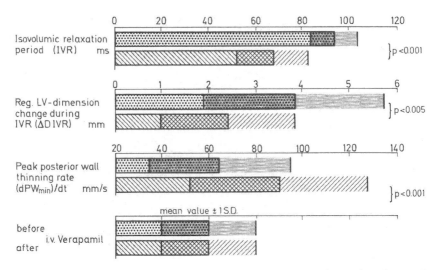

Fig. 4. Effect of verapamil on left ventricular isovolumic relaxation and peak posterior wall thinning rate in hypertrophic cardiomyopathy

ventricular minor axis (FS, $44\pm 7 \rightarrow 43\pm 7\%$, NS), nor the electromechanical systole (R-A_2, $365\pm 38 \rightarrow 366\pm 39$ ms, NS) showed any significant change (Fig. 3).

The duration of the isovolumic relaxation period (IVR) decreased significantly by an average of $29\pm 12\%$ from 93 ± 10 to 67 ± 15 ms ($P<0.001$), which was accompanied by a significant decrease in left ventricular dimension change during this time interval (ΔD_{IVR}, 3.8 ± 1.9 mm $\rightarrow 2.4\pm 1.4$ mm, $P<0.005$) (Fig. 4).

Verapamil significantly increased the peak rate of diastolic posterior wall thinning (dPW min/dt = $64\pm 30 \rightarrow 89\pm 38$ mm/s, $P<0.001$) compared to the baseline measurement (Fig. 4).

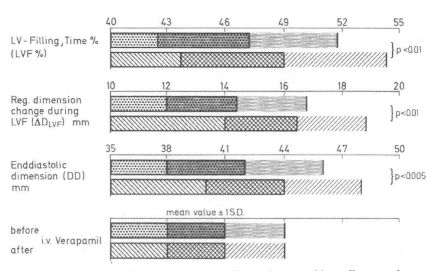

Fig. 5. Effect of verapamil on left ventricular filling in hypertrophic cardiomyopathy

The relative left ventricular filling period (LVF%, $47.2 \pm 4.6 \rightarrow 49 \pm 5.3$; $P<0.01$) was prolonged after the injection of verapamil and associated with an increase of the left ventricular dimension change during left ventricular filling (ΔD_{LVF}, $14.4 \pm 2.4 \rightarrow 16.4 \pm 2.4$; $P<0.01$) resulting in a greater end-diastolic left ventricular dimension after verapamil (DD, 44 ± 4 mm) compared with the control measurement (42 ± 4 mm; $P<0.005$) (Fig. 5).

Discussion

In the present study isovolumic relaxation time is defined as the time interval between the first high frequency component of the second heart sound measured by phonocardiography and the onset of mitral valve separation measured by echocardiography. The initial high frequency component of the second heart sound is synchronous with aortic valve closure as has been proven by echocardiography and by high fidelity pressure recordings [10–12]. Therefore A_2 can be taken as the start point of the isovolumic relaxation period. The beginning of the separation of the mitral cusps was taken as the endpoint of left ventricular isovolumic relaxation. In animal studies it has been proven that the onset of blood flow across the mitral valve is synchronous with the initial separation of the cusps [13]. In our laboratory isovolumic relaxation time, thus measured, is 55 ± 10 ms and agrees with recently reported values of Chen and Gibson [14].

After intravenous application of verapamil a $29 \pm 12\%$ shortening of the prolonged isovolumic relaxation time was observed in patients with hypertrophic cardiomyopathy. This shortening of the isovolumic relaxation time was associated with less increase in regional left ventricular dimension change during this period. We interpret these changes as an improvement in global and regional left ventricular relaxation.

Left ventricular relaxation can be influenced by several extramyocardial as well as myocardial factors [15–18]. Heart rate, systolic pressure, endsystolic volume, and left atrial pressure are regarded as important extramyocardial determinants of relaxation. Benchimol and Ellis reported a slight decrease in isovolumic relaxation period with increasing heart rate [17]. In the present study, however, cycle length before and after verapamil application showed no significant difference. Furthermore, no difference was found in end-systolic dimension and systolic aortic pressure. Although left atrial pressure was not measured in the present noninvasive study, recent hemodynamic studies in patients with coronary artery disease using a slightly smaller or equal dose (0.1 mg/kg or 10 mg, resp.) revealed only a small increase in left ventricular filling pressure or no change in the mean pulmonary artery pressure after intravenous application of verapamil [20, 21].

Viscous and elastic properties of the myocardium as well as certain biochemical processes are regarded as myocardial factors influencing ventricular relaxation. The biochemical factor of left ventricular relaxation is a complex energy-dependent process, which transports calcium away from the myofilaments to the sarcoplasmic reticulum [22–28]. Adenosintriphosphate is the principal energy source for this process of calcium sequestration by the sarcoplasmic reticulum. It is hydrolized by an ATPase distinct from that activating the sodium pump [23]. The fact that the biochemical process of relaxation is different from that of contraction explains why these processes may be influenced separately by different interventions or patho-physiological conditions.

Myocardial ischemia – induced experimentally by reduced regional myocardial blood flow [7, 26–29] or in the recovery phase after rapid atrial pacing in patients with coronary artery disease [28–31] – has been shown to impair left ventricular relaxation: isovolumic relaxation period is prolonged, and wall thinning as well as negative dp/dt are decreased.

Prolonged isovolumic relaxation time and abnormal diastolic filling pattern despite normal systolic function were reported in patients with hypertrophic cardiomyopathy [1–5] and were also observed in the present study. Left ventricular isovolumic relaxation time was prolonged to 93 ± 10 ms despite normal systolic function. The underlying cause of impaired left ventricular relaxation in patients with hypertrophic cardiomyopathy is thought to be ischemia in the subendocardial myocardium, caused by an imbalance between the oxygen demand of the exces-sively hypertrophied myocardium and the oxygen delivery.

The beneficial effect of verapamil on left ventricular isovolumic relaxation time seems, however, not related to the specific cause leading to myocardial hypertrophy. Observations in our laboratory indicate that a reduction of the prolonged isovolumic relaxation time and an improvement of left ventricular filling by verapamil can also be achieved in patients with secondary left ventricular hyper-trophy due to severe arterial hypertension [9].

Recent in vitro studies by Nayler [33] strongly support the idea that impaired relaxation of the heart muscle is primarily caused by a sudden depletion of the high energy phosphate reserves in the heart muscle due to hypoxia, followed consequently by disturbed intracellular calcium metabolism.

Experimental studies with different calcium antagonists, which have been performed in the last few years, have shown that these drugs are able to reduce the mechanical biochemical and histological defects caused by acute myocardial ischemia. A selective depression on regional contractility in ischemic myocardium by verapamil was reported by Smith and coworkers [34]. Other authors observed a protective effect of this drug in acute myocardial infarction measured by ST segment depression [35, 36] or by a combined biochemical and histological study [37, 38]. Recently Weishaar and coworkers reported upon beneficial metabolic effects of diltiazem, a new calcium antagonist, in ischemic myocardium [39]. In 1977, Henry observed in in vitro studies an inhibition of myocardial contracture and a decrease of left ventricular stiffness associated with a decreased intracellular calcium accumulation in those ischemic hearts that were pretreated with nifedipine [6]. Similar observations in animal experiments were recently made by Verdow and coworkers [7] based on ultrasonic measurements. After intracoronary adminis-tration of nifedipine a normalization of wall thickening and a loss of contrac-tion during isovolumic relaxation in ischemic pig hearts compared to untreated animals were observed. However, beneficial effects of verapamil on myocardial relaxation have so far not been reported in the literature.

In the present study, peak posterior wall thinning, left ventricular dimension change during the time interval of left ventricular filling, the relative filling period, and the end-diastolic dimension increased significantly after injection of verapamil. Due to the fact that the end-systolic dimension and the left ventricular fractional shortening were not altered compared with the control values, the increase in end-diastolic dimension cannot be the result of the negative inotrope effect of this drug. This increase must be considered as an improvement of left ventricular filling. The improvement of left ventricular filling is also expressed in the present study by the increase of the peak rate of posterior wall thinning during the early phase of diastolic filling as well as the increase in relative left ventricular filling period. Disturbed diastolic filling patterns in patients with hypertrophic cardiomyopathy, in terms of a shortened rapid filling period combined with a reduced dimension increase during this time interval, as well as a reduced rate of left ventricular posterior wall thinning, are thought to be expressions of increased resistance to left ventricular filling [1–3, 5]. Based on similar clinical observations in patients with coronary artery disease, these findings are considered to be caused primarly by impaired left ventricular relaxation due to myocardial ischemia, resulting in an increase in left ventricular stiffness [29–32].

The present observations of improvements in left ventricular isovolumic relaxation time and left ventricular filling by verapamil strongly support the theory that impaired left ventricular isovolumic relaxation may contribute to a decrease in left ventricular compliance [30, 32].

Recent observations of clinical improvement in patients with hypertrophic obstructive and nonobstructive cardiomyopathy who were chronically treated with high doses of verapamil may be in part due to the described mechanism of improved left ventricular relaxation and filling [40–42]. However, whether long-term oral treatment improves left ventricular relaxation and filling needs further investigation.

References

1. Sanderson JE, Traill TA, St John Sutton MG, Brown DJ, Gibson DG, Goodwin JF (1978) Left ventricular relaxation and filling in hypertrophic cardiomyopathy. An echocardiographic study. Br Heart J 40:596–601
2. Sanderson JE, Gibson DG, Brown DJ, Goodwin JF (1977) Left ventricular filling in hypertrophic cardiomyopathy. An angiographic study. Br Heart J 39:661–670
3. Martin G, St John Sutton MG, Tajik AJ, Gibson DG, Brown DJ, Seward IB, Giuliani E (1978) Echocardiographic assessment of left ventricular filling and septal and posterior wall dynamics in idiopathic hypertrophic subaortic stenosis. Circulation 57:512–520
4. Harmjanz D, Böttcher D, Scheitler CC (1971) Correlation of electrocardiogram pattern, shape of ventricular septum and isovolumic relaxation time in idiopathic hypertrophic subaortic stenosis. Br Heart J 13:928–937
5. Hanrath P, Mathey DG, Sigert R, Bleifeld W (1980) Left ventricular relaxation and filling pattern in different forms of left ventricular hypertrophy. An echocardiographic study. Am J Cardiol 45:15–23
6. Henry PD, Shuchleib R, Davis J, Weiss ES, Sobel BE (1977) Myocardial contracture and accumulation of mitochondrial calcium in ischemic rabbit heart. Am J Physiol 233/6:H 677–H 684

7. Verdow PD, Brown AH, Ten Cate FJ, Serruys PW (1979) Ventricular wall thickness changes during myocardial ischemia and after administration of Ca-antagonists (Abstr). In: Symposium quantification of myocardial ischemia, Goettingen, W Germany, May 13–15, 1979

8. Krebs W, Hanrath P, Bleifeld W, Effert S (1977) Rechnergestützte Auswertung von M-Mode-Echokardiogrammen. Herz/Kreislauf 9:519–525

9. Hanrath P, Mathey DG, Kremer P, Sonntag F, Bleifeld W (1980) Effect of verapamil on left ventricular isovolumic relaxation time and regional left ventricular filling in hypertrophic cardiomyopathy. Am J Cardiol 45:1258–1264

10. Rodbard S, Rathews N (1975) Valve closure and the second heart sound. Circulation 52:519–521

11. Leatham A, Leech 6 (1975) Observations on the relations between heart sounds and valve movement by simultaneous echo- and phonocardiography (Abstr). Br Heart J 37:557

12. Hirschhield S, Liebman J, Boskat G, Borsmith C (1977) Intracardiac pressure-sound correlates of echographic aortic valve closure. Circulation 55:602–604

13. Laniado S, Yellin E, Kottler M, Levy L, Stadler J, Terdiman R (1975) A study of the dynamic relations between the mitral echogram and phasic mitral flow. Circulation 51:104–113

14. Chen W, Gibson D (1979) Relation of isovolumic relaxation to left ventricular wall movement in man. Br Heart J 42:51–56

15. Cohn PE, Liedtke AJ, Senir J, Sonnenblick HE, Urschel CW (1972) Maximal rate of pressure fall (peak negative dp/dt) during ventricular relaxation. Cardiovasc Res 6:263–267

16. Weisfeldt ML, Seully HE, Frederiksen J, Rubenstein JJ, Pohost GM, Beierholm E, Bello AG, Daggelt WM (1974) Hemodynamic determinants of maximum negative dp/dt and periods of diastole. Am J Physiol 227:613–621

17. Benchimol A, Ellis JG (1967) A study of the period of isovolumic relaxation in normal subjects and in patients with heart disease. Am J Cardiol 19:196–206

18. Grossman W, McLaurin LP (1976) Diastolic properties of the left ventricle. Ann Intern Med 84:316–326

19. Papapietro HC, Coghlan W, Zissermann D, Russel RO, Rackley ChE, Rogers WJ (1979) Impaired maximal rate of left ventricular relaxation in patients with coronary artery disease and left ventricular dysfunction. Circulation 59:984–990

20. Ferlinz J, Easthope JL, Aronow WJ (1979) Effects of Verapamil on myocardial performance in coronary disease. Circulation 59:313–319

21. Singh BN, Roche AHG (1977) Effects of intraveneous verapamil on hemodynamics in patients with heart disease. Am Heart J 94:593–599

22. Fanburg BR, Finkel RM, Marjonosi A (1964) The role of calcium in the mechanism of relaxation of cardiac muscle. J Biol Chem 239:2298–2306

23. Weber A, Herz R, Reiss J (1967) The nature of cardiac relaxaing factor. Biochem Biophys Acta 131:188–194

24. Katz AM, Repke DJ (1973) Calcium membrane interactions in the myocardium: effects of ouaborin, epinephine and 3'.5' cyclic adenosine monophosphate. Am J Cardiol 31:193–201

25. Langer GA (1974) Ionic movements and the control of contraction in the mammalian myocardium. In: Langer GA, Brady AJ (eds) Wiley & Sons, New York, pp 193–218

26. McLaurin LP, Grossman W, Herdorn W (1975) Defective left ventricular relaxation during experimental myocardial ischemia (Abstr) Clin Res 23:1964

27. Mathey D, Bleifeld W, Franken G (1974) Left ventricular relaxation and diastolic stiffness in experimental myocardial infarction. Cardiovasc Res 8:583–592

28. Frist WH, Palacias J, Powell WMJ (1978) Effect of hypoxia on myocardial relaxation in isometric cat papillary muscle. J Clin Invest 61:1218–1224

Effect of Verapamil on Left Ventricular Isovolumic Relaxation Time

29. McLaurin LP, Rolette EL, Grossman W (1973) Impaired left ventricular relaxation during pacing induced ischemia. Am J Cardiol 32:751–757
30. Mann T, Brodie BR, Grossman W, McLaurin LP (1977) Effect of angina on left ventricular diastolic pressure-volume relationship. Circulation 55:761–766
31. Mann T, Goldberg S, Mudge GH, Grossman W (1979) Factors contribution to altered left ventricular diastolic properties during angina pectoris. Circulation 59:14–20
32. Grossman W, Mann JT (1978) Evidence impaired left ventricular relaxation during acute ischemia in man. Eur J Cardiol [Suppl] 7:239–249
33. Nayler WG, Williams A (1978) Relaxation in heart muscle: some morphological and biochemical considerations. Eur J Cardiol [Suppl] 7:35–50
34. Smith HJ, Goldstein RA, Griffith JM, Kent KM, Epstein SE (1976) Regional contractility. Selective depression of ischemic myocardium by verapamil. Circulation 54:629–635
35. Smith HJ, Singh BN, Nisketh HD, Norris RM (1973) Effects of verapamil on infarct size following experimental coronary artery occlusion. Cardiovasc Res 9:569–578
36. Wende W, Bleifeld W, Nayler J, Stuhlen HW (1975) Reduction of the size of acute, experimental myocardial infarction by verapamil. Basic Res Cardiol 70:198–208
37. Nayler WG, Grau A, Stade A (1976) A protective effect of verapamil on hypoxia heart muscle. Cardiovasc Res 10:650–662
38. Nayler WG, Szeto J (1972) Effect of verapamil on contractility, oxygen utilization, and calcium exchangeability in mammalian heart muscle. Cardiovasc Res 6:120–128
39. Weishaar R, Ashikawa K, Bingy RJ (1979) Effect of diltiazem, a calcium antagonist on myocardial ischemia. Am J Cardiol 43:1137–1143
40. Kaltenbach M, Hopf R, Kellner M (1976) Calciumantagonistische Therapie bei hypertropher-obstruktiver Kardiomyopathie. Dtsch Med Wochenschr 101:1284–1287
41. Rosing DR, Kent KM, Maron J, Epstein SE (1979) Verapamil treatment: a new approach to the pharmacologic treatment of hypertrophic cardiomyopathy. II. Effects on exercise capacity and symptomatic status. Circulation 60:1208
42. Kaltenbach M, Hopf R, Kober G, Bussmann D, Kellner M, Petersen Y (1979) Treatment of hypertrophic obstructive cardiomyopathy with verapamil. Br Heart J 42:35–42

Treatment of Hypertrophic Cardiomyopathy with Verapamil

Synopsis

H. Kuhn

Successful treatment of a disease implies improvement or complete relief of complaints and/or improvement of prognosis. What is the present therapeutic attitude in patients with hypertrophic cardiomyopathy?

Hypertrophic Obstructive Cardiomyopathy (HOCM)

Compared to untreated or medically treated patients the best clinical and hemodynamic results can apparently be achieved by surgical treatment. This has been shown by many studies in recent years [1]. Dr. Maron's paper (Efficacy of Operation for Obstructive Hypertrophic Cardiomyopathy: A 20-Year Experience with Ventricular Septal Myotomy and Myectomy, Chap. 5) and Dr. Lösse's paper (Functional results of exercise testing in medically and surgically treated patients with hypertrophic obstructive cardiomyopathy, Chap. 5) summarize the results and evaluate the efficacy of operation.

Unresolved clinical problems include the operative mortality which, although less than 10 years ago [1], is still too high for a general application of operation to patients with minimal or mild symptoms. Another question is whether the beneficial clinical effect observed during the first few months and years can be maintained. In this regard, the subsequent papers demonstrate that a small proportion of patients deteriorate after a relative long period of clinical improvement, and in some instances after operation progressive dilatation of left ventricle occurs, which is not seen in the natural course of the disease. Finally it is not known whether the prognosis of the disease can be definitely improved by operation, although some evidence suggesting an improved prognosis following operation has been published [1].

Considering the medical treatment of HOCM, the enthusiasm of treatment with beta blockers, which have been in use since 1965, has waned: the frequency of sustained benefit derived from the beta blockers in patients responding to such drugs is low and the prognosis does not seem to be improved [1]. Moreover, the incidence of severe cardiac arrhythmias and of sudden death does not appear to be reduced. Finally, beta blockers do not seem able to lower the abnormal elevated left ventricular end-diastolic pressure or to raise the depressed cardiac output (see Chap. 1).

In view of the limited efficacy of beta blockers in therapy in HOCM and of the limited indication for surgical therapy, it is of great clinical importance that new drugs for the treatment of HOCM are undergoing intensive study. Since the first introduction of verapamil by Kaltenbach and coworkers in 1976 [2] to treat patients

Synopsis

with HOCM, various groups have performed clinical, echocardiographic, and/or hemodynamic investigations. The papers given in sessions IV and V at this symposium by Dr. Hopf (Dr. Kaltenbach's group), Dr. Kaltenbach, Dr. Rosing (Dr. Epstein's group), Dr. Hirzel (the Zürich group), Dr. Kuhn (the Düsseldorf group), Dr. Kober (German multicentric study), and by Dr. Epstein characterize the present clinical status. Summarizing the results of these papers, it appears the following conclusions emerge:

There seems to be no doubt that verapamil improves clinical symptoms in many patients. The same holds true for the ECG, which in many patients changes (reduction of ST segment depression, decrease of the amplitude of QRS complex) in a way that in general indicates improvement of cardiac disease.

In addition, several intriguing problems raised and reported at this meeting will need further clarification: whether regression of cardiac hypertrophy occurs, what the incidence is and the severity of side effects, the mechanism of the beneficial clinical effect, the clinical use of the estimation of plasma levels of verapamil, and the selection of patients for this therapy. Despite these uncertainties, the clinical experience documented by the papers derived from this symposium indicate that verapamil treatment is a reasonable therapeutic option that can be considered before operation is contemplated in those many patients with pronounced complaints who show no clinical benefit from treatment with beta blockers. However, further controlled studies are necessary to determine criteria for selecting patients for the different therapeutic modalities currently available.

Hypertrophic Nonobstructive Cardiomyopathy (HNCM)

According to recent investigations, HNCM differs from HOCM in many aspects and is a more frequent disease than has been previously assumed [3]. To date, no medical therapy has been proven and surgical approaches are not applicable. The clinical results of our own study reported at this meeting in patients with HNCM suggest that verapamil also exerts a beneficial clinical effect in this form of hypertrophic cardiomyopathy. This seems to be of special interest because no outflow tract obstruction is present, thereby indicating that mechanisms other than reduction in intraventricular gradient must be operative. The small but significant reduction in thickness of the ventricular septum and posterior wall documented in our study by echocardiography can be interpreted as a regression of cardiac hypertrophy and/or a negative inotropic effect of verapamil. Further prospective studies in a large number of patients are needed to ascertain the clinical role of verapamil in patients with HNCM, and to clarify the exciting question of whether a drug can reduce the muscular hypertrophy of a disease in which the cause of hypertrophy is unknown.

References

1. Kuhn H, Krelhaus W, Bircks W, Schulte HD, Loogen F (1978) Indication for surgical treatment in patients with hypertrophic obstructive cardiomyopathy. In: Kaltenbach M, Loogen F, Olsen EGJ (eds) Cardiomyopathy and myocardial biopsy. Springer, Berlin Heidelberg New York p 308
2. Kaltenbach M, Hopf R, Keller M (1976) Calciumantagonistische Therapie bei hypertroph-obstruktiver Kardiomyopathie. Dtsch Med Wochenschr 101:1284
3. Kuhn H, Thelen U, Köhler E, Lösse B (1980) Die hypertrophische nicht obstruktive Kardiomyopathie (HNCM)-klinische, hämodynamische, elektro-, echo- und angiokardiographische Untersuchungen. Z Kardiol 69:457

Verapamil Treatment of Hypertrophic Cardiomyopathy

RÜDIGER HOPF and MARTIN KALTENBACH

Introduction

The natural course of hypertrophic cardiomyopathy is usually characterized by variable degrees of progression [10, 11, 18]. Long-term therapy with beta-blocking agents has proved to be disappointing [3, 11]. Surgical intervention led to initial improvement in many patients, but complaints may reappear with time [17]. These therapeutic strategies thus seem unable to influence either the progression or the long-term prognosis of the disease.

The calcium ion has been found to play an important role for myocardial hypertrophy and necrosis in certain types of hereditary cardiomyopathy [1, 12]. In experimentally induced hypertrophy, following internal cellular calcium accumulation after isoproterenol administration, calcium antagonists were potent in preventing this process of hypertrophy [7]; similarly, hypoxia-induced cardiac hypertrophy could be inhibited with verapamil [4]. In human hypertrophic cardiomyopathy, the calcium ion may have the same important influence. Plasma membrane processes were found to extend into the cytoplasm of adjacent cells and sometimes terminated in the vicinity of longitudinally oriented T tubules [2], where the "calcium-channels" are thought to be localized [14].

The use of calcium antagonists might therefore also be expected to influence the mechanism of hypertrophy in human hypertrophic cardiomyopathy.

Since 1973 this principle has been applied in the treatment of hypertrophic cardiomyopathy at our institution [6, 9]. The results obtained in 50 patients during long-term treatment with calcium antagonists, reflecting a total of 134 patient treatment years, are presented in this study.

Patients and Methods

Patients

Fifty patients with hypertrophic cardiomyopathy, 38 men and 12 women, ranging from 14 to 60 years of age (mean 41.86 years) participated in the study. In all patients diagnosis was established by noninvasive and invasive methods, including right and left heart catheterization with selective coronary arteriography and biplane left ventricular angiography. In 23 of the 50 patients left ventricular myocardial biopsies had been obtained.

Forty-one patients were found to have typical hypertrophic obstructive cardiomyopathy (HOCM) with a left ventricular outflow tract gradient at rest and/or after provocation; 13 of these had a coexisting right ventricular outflow tract gradient. The other nine patients had hypertrophic nonobstructive cardiomyopathy (HCM): six had no or minor gradients (up to 30 mmHg even following provocation) and three had isolated right ventricular obstruction (Table 1).

Table 1. Characterization of 50 patients with hypertrophic cardiomyopathy treated with calcium antagonists

50 patients with hypertrophic cardiomyopathy

$\delta : 38 \qquad \varphi : 12 \qquad \delta : \varphi = 3 : 1$

age 14–60 years (mean 42 years)

mean observation period prior to verapamil treatment: 20 months
duration of verapamil treatment: 3–56 months   mean: 32 months

gradient:	left ventricle only:	28 patients ⎫ HOCM
	both ventricles:	13 patients ⎭
	right ventricle only:	3 patients ⎫ HCM
	LV gradient < 30 mmHg:	6 patients ⎭
LV gradient:	rest:	0–136 (mean 46) mmHg
	provocation:	32–290 (mean 99) mmHg

RV gradient (when present): 5–25 (mean 11.5) mmHg

Methods

Electrocardiogram

Before the start of the study repeated 12-lead electrocardiograms were made in all patients. For each patient the same unit was used for all tracings. No filter was employed and scrupulous attention was paid to exact calibration. The sum of the largest R and S amplitudes in the precordial leads was calculated to assess changes before and during treatment. In addition, Holter monitor electrocardiograms over 4 h on 2 or 3 different days were recorded in 19 patients.

Echocardiogram

M-mode echocardiograms were obtained using the Picker echoview system 80 C with a 2.25 megahertz focused transducer (diameter 13 mm). In 26 patients the study was carried out before the initiation of calcium antagonist therapy. Twenty-four patients had already been treated with verapamil for 2 or more years at the time of the first echocardiogram.

X-ray Findings

Standard chest X-rays were taken in the standing position. Heart volume determinations were calculated from X-rays obtained in the horizontal position

Verapamil Treatment of Hypertrophic Cardiomyopathy 165

according to the method of Rohrer [16] and Kahlstorf [8] modified by Mushoff and Reindell [13]. Heart volume is expressed in ml/1.73 m² body surface area.

Cardiac Catheterization

Cardiac catheterization was performed in all patients. Initial pressure readings were followed by the administration of nitrates. Coronary arteriography (Sones technique) and ventricular angiography were then performed. To permit an accurate comparison of coronary artery diameter, identical doses of nitrates were given during the initial and follow-up studies in those patients who were re-catheterized.

After left ventricular angiography in 60° LAO and 30° RAO projection, the patient was moved over a distance of 6 cm with the catheter in the ventricle. This procedure, filmed like a conventional angiogram, allowed exact correction for X-ray magnification. Projected cineangiograms and catheter tip displacement were traced. Employing Simpson's rule, volume calculations were performed using a Siemens Volumat computer. In the same manner, coronary artery diameters were calculated at defined measuring points. Left ventricular muscle mass was derived from end-diastolic volume and wall thickness [15] and is expressed as in ml/1.73m² body surface area. Left ventricular biopsy was performed in 23 patients during the same catheterization procedure.

Medication

In 49 patients, verapamil treatment was started with the standard oral dose of 480 mg/day. In eight instances, doses of up to 720 mg were given. In one patient the dose was reduced to 320 mg because of a first degree AV-block. The average verapamil dose was 500 mg/day. One patient received 30 mg nifedipine/day.

Treatment with calcium antagonists was conducted over a mean period of 32 months (3–56 months). Twenty-five of the 50 patients had been observed prior to therapy with calcium antagonists for an average of 20 months (1–100 months). During this observation period, 14 of the 25 patients had been maintained with beta-blocking agents, whereas the remaining 11 patients received no therapy.

Follow-up Studies

After initiation of calcium antagonistic therapy, patients were followed up closely during the first 3 months. Thereafter, the patients were seen approximately every 6 months, when physical examination, ECG, echocardiogram, standard chest X-rays, and heart volume determinations were carried out. In 45 patients verapamil plasma levels were determined before and after a single oral dose of 160 mg.

Patients were followed up during calcium antagonistic therapy for a mean period of 32 months (3–56 months). Fourteen patients were treated for 4 or more years. Patients followed for the same interval were grouped together; their mean follow-up values were compared to mean baseline value of the same group. A second method of analysis was devised based on the mean of all follow-up values obtained for each single patient. Then the patients with the same duration of therapy were grouped together, and mean treatment values versus mean pre-treatment values were compared.

166 Rüdiger Hopf and Martin Kaltenbach

Cardiac catheterization, performed in all patients before therapy, was repeated in 18 cases after a mean treatment period of 26 months (8–51 months), including repeated myocardial biopsy in five patients.

Results

Symptoms

Prior to treatment, 44 of the 50 patients had complaints. Dyspnea was reported by 30 patients (60%), chest pain in 26 (52%), dizziness in five (10%), and collapse and/or syncope in 11 (22%) cases. Six patients never had complaints.

Thirty-seven of the 44 symptomatic patients improved during verapamil therapy. Twelve patients, including the six asymptomatic cases, reported no change during the treatment, and one felt worse. Dyspnea was less pronounced or eliminated in 22 (preexisting in 30 patients) and chest pain in 23 (preexisting in 26 patients) patients. In all 16 cases of preexisting dizziness as well as syncope and/or collapse, improvement or elimination was reported (Table 2).

Table 2

Prior to therapy		During therapy			
		increased	unchanged	decreased	eliminated
dyspnea:	30	1	7	18	4
chest pain:	26	1	2	19	4
syncope/collapse:	11			6	5
arrhythmias:	6		1	1	4
weakness:	6		2	3	1
dizziness:	5			4	1
palpitations:	4			1	3
diaphoresis:	3		1	1	1
edema:	3	1	2		
no complaints:	6		6		

Diminution of complaints was accompanied by improved physical capacity. Based on criteria of the New York Heart Association in all patients, an average improvement from functional class 2.6 to 1.9 was noted (Fig. 1).

Four patients interrupted therapy for various reasons. In all of them complaints reappeared or deteriorated.

Physical Findings

Physical findings did not change dramatically. In some cases the systolic murmur decreased in intensity or disappeared.

Verapamil Treatment of Hypertrophic Cardiomyopathy

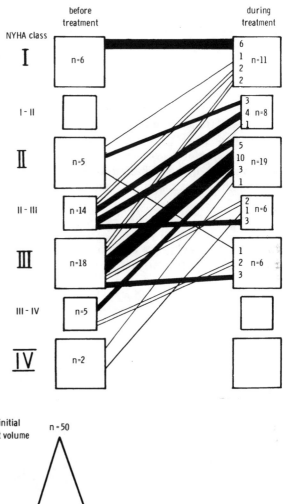

Fig. 1. Clinical course of 50 verapamil-treated patients with hypertrophic cardiomyopathy after a mean therapy period of 32 months

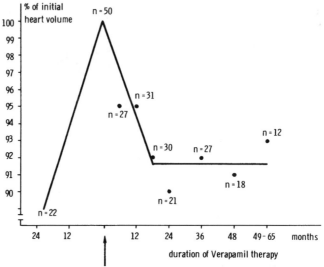

Fig. 2. Changes in heart volume before in 22 and during therapy with verapamil in 50 patients with hypertrophic cardiomyopathy. Under therapy with verapamil, heart volume decreased by more than 8%. Results are based on the mean values of all patients followed during the same 6-month period and compared to these patients' initial pretreatment values

No significant change in average blood pressure was observed. However, blood pressure normalized in one patient with moderate hypertension. The mean heart rate of all patients was 74 beats per min before verapamil. During the first 6 months of therapy, heart rate was reduced to 66 per minute, and remained 3% below the initial value.

Abnormal carotid pulse tracings with a typical bisfireous contour were found in 32 of the 50 patients before therapy. In eight, the tracings normalized during therapy; in 14 small improvement was noticed while the remaining showed no change. In no patient did pulse tracings deteriorate.

No patient developed heart failure during verapamil treatment. The occasional occurrence of mild pretibial or ankle edema was attributed to changes in vessel permeability following vasodilatation.

Chest X-Rays

Standard chest X-rays revealed no change in heart configuration and size. Signs of cardiac failure, particularly lung congestion, neither appeared nor worsened during therapy.

Heart Volume

Heart volume determinations, based on horizontal tele-chest X-rays, showed an increase during the period prior to therapy in 22 of 25 patients (average from 857 to 955 ml/1.73 m²). During treatment with calcium antagonists, heart volume decreased in 35 of 50 patients. The average decrease in all 50 patients was 8%. This

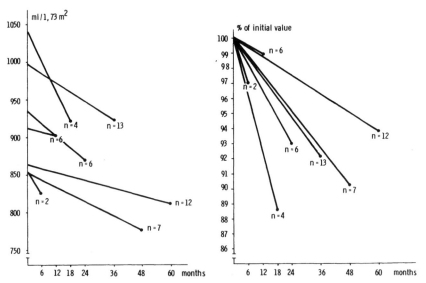

Fig. 3. Changes in heart volume in groups of patients treated for equal lengths of time. Heart volume during therapy was derived from the mean of all heart volume determinations during the treatment period. Changes in absolute values (*left*) and in percent (*right*)

Table 3. ECG and heart volume in four patients with hypertrophic cardiomyopathy during verapamil treatment and a drug-free interval (duration in months)

	Patient	Therapy Value Before	End	Duration	Interruption Value	Duration	Renewed therapy Value	Duration
ECG	1	3.4	3.4	30	3.7	14	2.8	21
$S_{max}+R_{max}$	2	4.5	3.9	15	4.5	15	4.0	15
(mV)	3	6.8	6.0	5	6.9	6	6.2	17
	4	4.0	2.6	22	4.0	28	–	–
	$\bar{x}$	4.7	4.2	18	4.8	15.8	4.3	17.7
	s	1.5	1.8	11	1.5	9	1.7	3.1
Heart volume	1	855	765	30	800	14	740	21
(ml/1.73 m²)	2	1030	830	15	925	15	860	15
	3	955	865	5	890	6	860	17
	4	900	775	22	880	28	–	–
	$\bar{x}$	945	808	18	874	15.8	820	17.7
	s	81	47	11	53	9	69	3.1

After interruption of verapamil therapy in all patients deterioration occurred. Following renewed therapy in three, subjective and objective improvement was reestablished. In the fourth patient renewed beginning of treatment lies ahead.

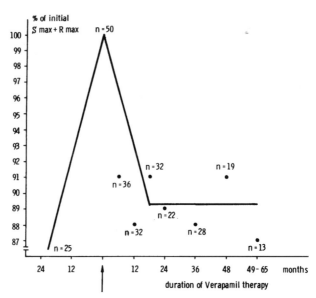

Fig. 4. ECG findings in 25 patients with hypertrophic cardiomyopathy before and in 50 during therapy with verapamil. During the pretreatment period, QRS amplitude in the 25 patients increased by 14% even though 14 had received beta blockers. During verapamil treatment QRS amplitude decreased by a mean of 11%. Results are based on the mean values of all patients followed over the same 6-month period and compared to these same patients' pretreatment values

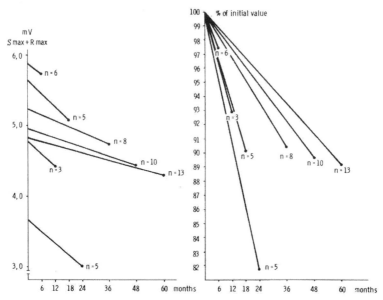

Fig. 5. Changes in QRS amplitude in groups of patients treated for equal lengths of time. QRS amplitude during therapy was derived from the mean of all heart volume determinations during the treatment period. Shown are absolute changes in mV (*left*) and changes from baseline values (100%) expressed in percent (*right*)

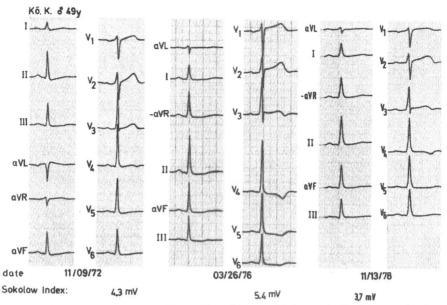

Fig. 6. Development of electrocardiographic evidence of left ventricular hypertrophy in a patient with hypertrophic cardiomyopathy. Despite beta blockade, the Sokolow Index increased from 4.3 mV to 5.4 mV between 1972 and 1976, when verapamil treatment was begun. By 1978, the Sokolow Index had receded to 3.7 mV

effect has persisted for more than 4 years (Figs. 2, 3). Heart volume showed a renewed increase in the four patients who discontinued taking verapamil (Table 3).

Electrocardiogram

Calculated as the sum of the largest R and S amplitude in the precordial leads, QRS amplitude increased during the 20 months observation period prior to therapy from 4.47 to 5.08 mV. These observations included 11 untreated patients and 14 receiving beta blockers (Figs. 4, 6). During calcium antagonistic therapy, QRS amplitude decreased in 31 patients. The average decrease of all 50 patients within the first 6-12 months was 11%. Improvement was maintained over 4 or more years (Figs. 4-6). A prolonged interruption of therapy in four patients led to a slight reincrease in QRS amplitude (Fig. 7, Table 3).

Based on the results of repeated ECG registrations and especially the HOLTER monitor electrocardiograms, rhythm disorders were found in 11 patients. In four cases, atrial fibrillation was documented. In one patient, a first degree AV block was seen, and, in another patient, AV dissocation could be observed. The five remaining patients displayed atrial and/or ventricular premature beats. Atrial fibrillation as well as premature beats were not influenced by verapamil therapy. Preexisting AV conduction disturbances, seen in two patients, could no longer be observed during treatment.

Echocardiogram

Mean left ventricular end-diastolic and end-systolic diameter did not change markedly. On average, end-diastolic diameter changed insignificantly from 4.19 to

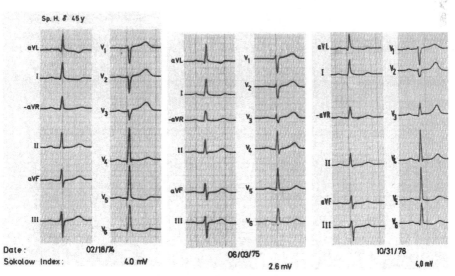

Fig. 7. ECG normalization under verapamil therapy in a 45-year-old patient with hypertrophic cardiomyopathy. Hypertrophy reappeared after the patient refused further medication because subjective symptoms had disappeared

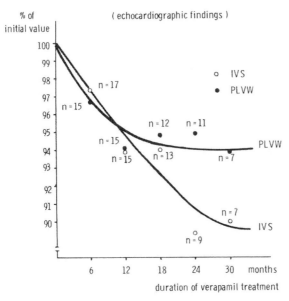

Fig. 8. Reduction of ventricular septum (*IVS*) and posterior wall (*PLVW*) thickness in patients with hypertrophic cardiomyopathy during verapamil therapy

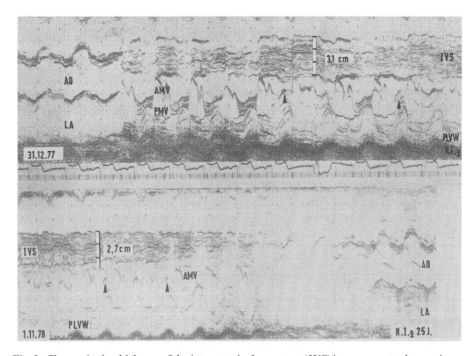

Fig. 9. Change in the thickness of the interventricular septum (*IVS*) in response to therapy in a 25-year-old woman with hypertrophic cardiomyopathy

Verapamil Treatment of Hypertrophic Cardiomyopathy

4.12 cm, and end-systolic diameter from 2.84 to 2.88 cm. By contrast, left atrial diameter declined markedly, paralleling the reduction in heart volume. Repeated and surveyable echocardiographic findings of interventricular septum and left ventricular posterior wall were available in 40 patients. The interventricular septum was reduced in 33 and the posterior wall in 19 patients during 18–24 months of calcium antagonistic therapy. In the average of the 40 patients septum and posterior wall thickness receded significantly by 10% and 5% respectively (Figs. 8, 9).

Heart Catheterization

Before initiation of calcium antagonistic therapy, heart catheterization was performed in all patients, including selective coronary angiography and cineangiography of the left – in some cases also the right – ventricle. In order to verify therapeutic results and establish a correlation between invasive and clinical findings, cardiac catheterization was repeated in 18 patients after a mean treatment period of 26 months.

Twelve of the recatheterized patients had previously been judged clinically improved in terms of heart volume and Sokolow Index. Four were considered unchanged, and two to have worsened.

Eight of the 12 patients classified as clinically improved had typical hypertrophic obstructive cardiomyopathy. They showed a decrease in left ventricular filling pressure from 20 to 17 mmHg. Left ventricular outflow tract gradient at rest fell from 15 to 6 and, after provocation, from 74 to 40 mmHg. Left ventricular muscle mass declined significantly from 201 to 169 ml/1.73 m² and coronary artery diameter was reduced significantly from 4.05 to 3.64 mm, that is, by

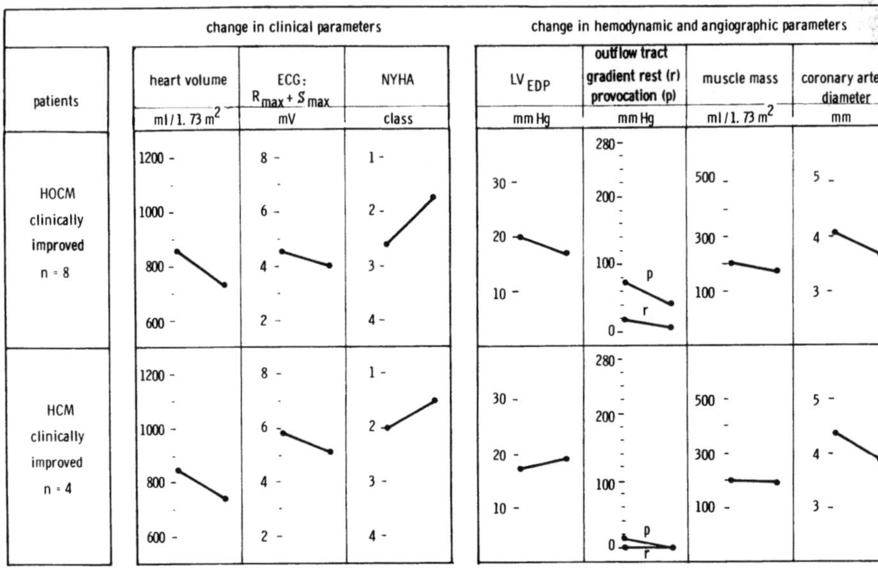

Fig. 10. Comparison between clinical and hemodynamic-angiographic findings in 12 clinically improved patients (*HOCM* [n = 8] and *HCM*, [n = 4])

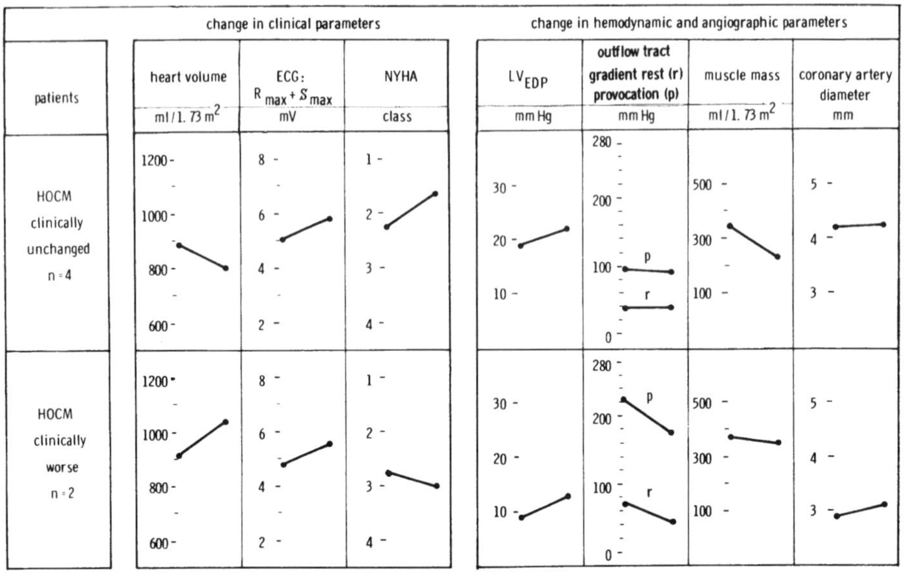

174 Rüdiger Hopf and Martin Kaltenbach

Fig. 11. Comparison between clinical and hemodynamic-angiographic findings in 6 clinically unchanged (n = 4) or worsened (n = 2) patients with HOCM

10%. The remaining four of the 12 improved patients had hypertrophic (non-obstructive) cardiomyopathy. They showed less pronounced, insignificant changes. Left ventricular filling pressure increased from 17 to 19 mmHg. Left ventricular muscle mass decreased from 196 to 189 ml/1.73 m² and coronary artery diameter from 4.37 to 3.75 mm (Fig. 10).

In four patients in whom clinical parameters remained essentially unchanged, invasive studies also failed to detect any significant alterations. A slight increase in filling pressure and coronary artery diameter was found, whereas outflow tract gradient and left ventricular muscle mass declined.

Two patients had worsened clinically. Left ventricular filling pressure increased from 9 to 13 mmHg, coronary artery diameter from 2.87 to 3.09 mm. Left

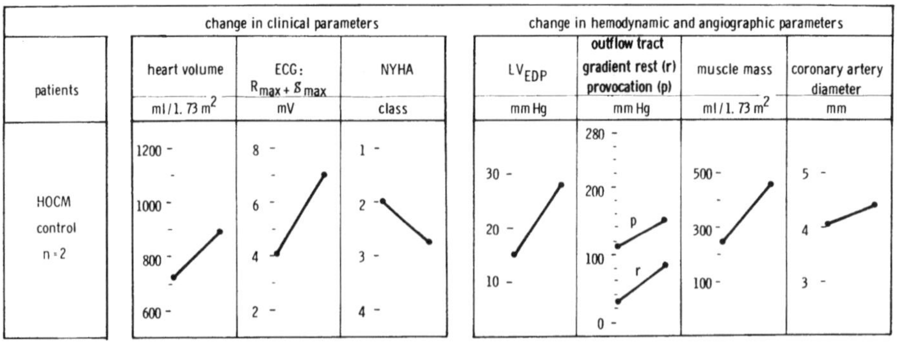

Fig. 12. The natural course of two untreated patients with HOCM. Shown are clinical and hemodynamic-angiographic findings

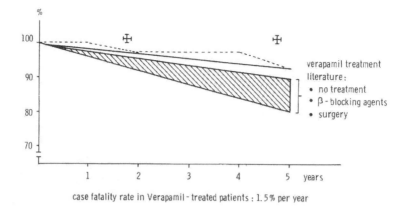

Fig. 13. Five-year survival rate in 50 verapamil-treated patients with hypertrophic cardiomyopathy compared to the natural course of the disease and other forms of treatment as described in the literature

ventricular muscle mass declined from 375 to 350 ml/1.73 m². Left ventricular outflow tract gradient was reduced at rest and after provocation from 73 to 45 and 223 to 177 mmHg, respectively (Fig. 11).

Two untreated patients were catheterized twice at a mean interval of 64 months. They showed an increase in heart volume and QRS amplitude and clinical deterioration according to New York Heart Association criteria from 2.0 to 2.75. Left ventricular filling pressure increased from 15 to 28 mmHg, left ventricular muscle mass from 245 to 465 ml/1.73 m². A marked increase was also seen in left ventricular outflow tract gradient at rest and after provocation from 30 to 84 and from 112 to 151 mmHg, respectively. Coronary artery diameter increased from 4.04 to 4.41 mm (Fig. 12).

Survival Rate

Sudden death occurred in two patients. One instance involved the only patient who was treated with nifedipine, a 44-year-old woman with atrial fibrillation and ventricular premature beats; the other was a 20-year-old man with atrial and ventricular premature beats unresponsive to treatment. Overall 5-year survival rate therefore was 96%. Expressed in terms of 134 patient treatment years, a case fatality rate of 1.5%/year may be assumed. This is lower than survival data from the literature for other forms of treatment as well as the natural course of the disease [10, 11] (Fig. 13).

Side Effects

During the first months of therapy, some patients reported the presence of slight tremor, increased diaphoresis, and constipation. These problems generally subsided spontaneously despite continued therapy. In one patient edema occurred and required diuretics. Side effects necessitating discontinuation of the drug were not observed. A dose reduction to 320 mg of verapamil per day became necessary in only one patient because of a first degree AV block with a P-R interval of 300 ms. Conduction time subsequently normalized. In two patients preexisting AV conduction disturbances normalized during treatment.

Discussion

The natural course of the disease could be followed in 25 of 50 patients for 1 to 100 months prior to the start of verapamil therapy (mean 20 months). A slow progression of the condition could be observed on the basis of symptoms, QRS amplitude in the ECG, and radiographically determined heart volume. The course of the 14 patients who had been pretreated with the beta-blocking agents propranolol or pindolol did not differ from that of the 11 untreated patients. In two patients the progression of the disease was reflected in the hemodynamic and angiographic findings, as shown by repeated heart catheterization after an interval of 64 months. One of these patients had been treated with pindolol.

Therapeutic results during verapamil therapy did not appear suddenly. Subjective improvement of 37 patients occurred within the first weeks or months, but objective improvement, such as the reduction in heart volume and regression in QRS amplitude, was noted only after 6–18 months. Acute changes in the state of health and objective findings might have suggested an acute electrophysiological and hemodynamic response. But the present study implies that improvement progresses gradually over several months with a maximum between 18 and 24 months. This course can best be explained by an influence of verapamil on the hypertrophic process of the myocardium.

In addition, the effectiveness of treatment is demonstrated in those four patients who stopped taking verapamil. In all of them a slow, but progressive deterioration could be seen. In three of them renewed improvement upon resumption of therapy occurring within nearly 18 months was seen (the fourth one was not treated again).

The favorable effects of the calcium antagonistic therapy persisted in all 14 patients treated for 4 or more years. This observation is important in comparison with the pretreatment findings of these patients, showing a progressive deterioration even in patients treated with beta-blocking agents. With time, therefore, it appears that the course of patients treated with calcium antagonists may diverge progressively from that of patients without medication or those maintained on beta blockers.

The therapeutic response cannot be explained by peripheral effects, that is, a reduction in afterload. In this instance an increase in intraventricular outflow tract gradient could be expected. Owing to the fact that obstruction declines despite reduced filling pressure and despite reduced afterload, calcium antagonists must have direct influences on the myocardium.

One of the predominant characteristics of hypertrophic cardiomyopathy is the impairment of ventricular filling [5]. The observations during long-term verapamil treatment and additional hemodynamic investigations appear to be attributable to the following mechanisms of action: improvement of ventricular filling and decline of contractility lead to reduced obstruction (and perhaps less mitral insufficiency). By means of reduced calcium ion availability these hemodynamic changes are accompanied by a slow regression of myocardial hypertrophy.

Summary

Fifty patients with hypertrophic cardiomyopathy were treated with calcium antagonists; 49 of them with a mean oral dose of 500 mg verapamil per day and one with 30 mg nifedipine. This therapy was conducted over 3–56 months (mean 32 months).

1. Forty-three of 50 patients, that is 86%, showed symptomatic improvement or remained free of complaints.
2. Heart volume decreased in 35 patients. In all 50 patients the average decrease was 8%.
3. QRS amplitude decreased in 33 patients. In all 50 patients the average decrease was 11%.
4. Echocardiographic studies demonstrated a diminution of left atrial diameter in 25 of 45 patients. In 40 patients thickness of interventricular septum was reduced by an average of 10%. Posterior left ventricular wall decreased on average by 5%.
5. Improvement in subjective and objective findings persisted over more than 4 years.
6. Changes in noninvasive findings were confirmed by hemodynamic and angiographic findings.
7. In contrast to other forms of treatment, calcium antagonists may improve the prognosis of hypertrophic cardiomyopathy.

References

1. Bajusz E, Lossnitzer K (1968) Ein neues Krankheitsmodell: Erbliche nicht vaskuläre Myokarddegeneration mit Herzinsuffizienz. Muench Med Wochenschr 31:1756
2. Ferrans VJ, Roberts WC, Shugoll GI (1972) Plasma membrance extensions in intercalated discs of human myocardium and their relationship to partial dissociations of the discs. J Mol Cell Cardiol 5:161
3. Frank MJ, Abdulla AM, Canedo MI, Saylors RE (1978) Long-term Medical Management of Hypertrophic Obstructive Cardiomyopathy. Am J Cardiol 42:993
4. Genovese A, Chiariello M, Cacciapuoti AA, De Alfieri W, Latte S, Condorelli M (1980) Inhibition of hypoxia-induced cardiac hypertrophy by verapamil in rats. Basic Res Cardiol 75:757
5. Goodwin JF (1973) Treatment of the Cardiomyopathies. Am J Cardiol 32:341
6. Hopf R, Keller M, Kaltenbach M (1976) Die Behandlung der hypertrophen obstruktiven Kardiomyopathie mit Verapamil. Verh Dtsch Ges Innern Med 82:1053
7. Jahnke J, Fleckenstein A, Frey M (1975) Schutzeffekt von Ca^{++}-Antagonisten bei der Isoproterenol-induzierten hypertrophischen Kardiomyopathie der Ratte (Abstr). Z Kardiol 67:230
8. Kahlstorf A (1932) Über eine orthodiagraphische Herzvolumenbestimmung. Fortschr Röntgenstr 45:123
9. Kaltenbach M, Hopf R, Keller M (1976) Calciumantagonistische Therapie bei hypertroph-obstruktiver Kardiomyopathie. Dtsch Med Wochenschr 101:1284
10. Loogen F, Krelhaus W, Kuhn H (1976) Verlaufsbeobachtungen der hypertrophischen obstruktiven Kardiomyopathie (HOCM). Z Kardiol 65:5121

11. Loogen F, Kuhn H, Krelhaus W (1978) Natural history of hypertrophic obstructive cardiomyopathy and the effect of therapy. In: Kaltenbach M, Loogen F, Olsen EGJ (eds) Cardiomyopathy and myocardial biopsy. Springer, Berlin Heidelberg New York, p 286
12. Lossnitzer K (1975) Genetic induction of cardiomyopathy. In: Schmier J, Eichler O (eds) Heart and circulation. Springer, Berlin Heidelberg New York (Handbuch der experimentellen Pharmakologie, vol XVI/3, p 309)
13. Mushoff K, Reindell H (1956, 1957) Zur Röntgenuntersuchung des Herzens in vertikaler und horizontaler Körperstellung. Dtsch Med Wochenschr 81:1001, 82:1075
14. Nayler WG, Krikler DM (1975) Depolarisation, repolarisation and conduction. In: Krikler DM, Goodwin F (eds) Cardiac arrhythmias. The modern electrophysiological approach. Saunders, London Philadelphia Toronto, p 1
15. Rackley CE, Dodge HT, Coble YD, Hay RE (1964) A method for determining left ventricular mass in man. Circulation 29:666
16. Rohrer F (1916) Volumenbestimmung von Körperhöhlen und Organen auf orthodiagraphischem Wege. Fortschr. Roentgenstr 24:285
17. Rothlin M, Arbenz N, Krayenbuehl HP, Turina J, Senning A (1976) Spätresultate nach Operationen bei muskulärer subvalvulärer Aortenstenose. Z Kardiol 65:501
18. Shah PM, Adelmann AG, Wigle ED, Gobel FL, Burchell HB, Hardarson T, Curiel R, De la Calzada C, Oakley CM, Goodwin JF (1975) The natural (and unnatural) history of hypertrophic obstructive cardiomyopathy. Circ Res [Suppl II] 34, 35:179

Volume Parameters of the Heart During Long-Term Verapamil Treatment in Patients with Hypertrophic Cardiomyopathy

M. KALTENBACH and R. HOPF

Volume changes during verapamil treatment are of particular interest because verapamil (v) has negative inotropic properties and therefore may lead to an enlargement in ventricular volumes. A diminished intraventricular gradient and even a clinical improvement could be the consequence of a cardiac dilation finally converting hypertrophic into congestive cardiomyopathy. Therefore three types of volume measurements were performed before and during long-term verapamil treatment in patients with hypertrophic cardiomyopathy:

1. Heart volume from tele chest X-rays in supine position

2. Left ventricular volumes from cineangiograms

3. Left atrial diameter from M-mode echograms

Methods and Patients

Heart Volume

Heart volume was determined according to the method of Rohrer and Kahlstorf, modified by Klepzig and Reindell [4, 5, 6, 8]. 2 m tele chest X-rays were taken in supine position in lateral and posteroanterior projection. The patient was lying on his front side. Before lying down he had swollowed contrast material so that the contrast filled esophagus delineated the posterior wall of the heart (Fig. 1).

Volume was calculated from three diameters (l, b, t) according to the formula:

$$V = 1 \times b \times t \times 0.4$$

(Fig. 2).

Twenty-two patients had repeated volume measurements at an interval of 22 (1–40) months with either no specific medication (n = 11) or beta-blocker treatment (n = 11). If on beta blockers, this medication was stopped 48 h before heart volume determination.

Fifty patients (38 males, 12 females) had heart volume determination before and after different periods of verapamil treatment. The average dose of verapamil was 480 mg orally per day. The drug was stopped 48 h before volume determination.

In all patients the diagnosis of hypertrophic cardiomyopathy was confirmed clinically, by right and left heart catheterization including left ventricular angiograms and selective coronary angiograms as well as by echogram.

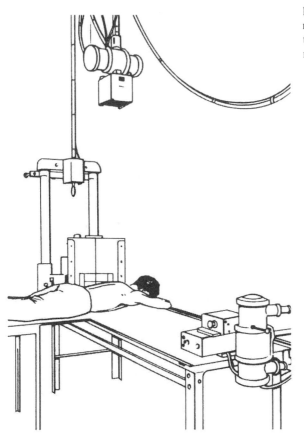

Fig. 1. Heart volume determination from tele chest X-rays taken in posteroantero and right to left lateral projection

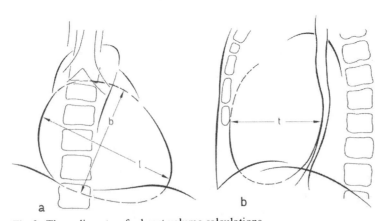

Fig. 2. Three diameters for heart volume calculations

Left Ventricular Volume

Eighteen patients had repeated left ventricular volume measurements from cineangiograms. Cineangiograms were performed in 50° LAO and 30° RAO projection at an exposure rate of 33 frames per second. 30–40 ml Urografin 76% were injected into the left ventricle. The X-ray magnification was determined by moving the patient over a distance of 6 cm and comparing the movement of the catheter tip seen on the screen with the real movement. During displacement of the patient over 6 cm the X-ray amplifier remained in the same position as during the angiogram. During projection of the film on a screen the left ventricular contours were outlined together with the displacement of the catheter tip while the patient was moved over a distance of 6 cm. X-ray magnification was calculated from the ratio:

$$\frac{\text{displacement of the catheter tip seen on the screen}}{\text{real displacement over 6 cm}}$$

The same procedure was done in RAO and LAO projection. Left ventricular contours in RAO and LAO projection as well as the respective X-ray magnification derived from the catheter tip displacement were fed into a computer (Volumat Siemens). Volume calculations were performed according to Simson's rule.

In all patients the diagnosis was confirmed by noninvasive and invasive methods. Verapamil treatment with a dose of 480 mg/day was conducted over a period of 26 (8–52) months. Before catheterization the drug was stopped for 48 h.

Left Atrial Diameter

Left atrial diameters were determined from repeated M-mode echograms in 14 patients with the diagnosis confirmed by noninvasive and invasive methods before and after verapamil treatment with 480 mg/day over a period of 6–36 months. Only echograms of excellent quality were evaluated.

Results

Heart Volume

22 patients had repeated heart volume determination before verapamil treatment. Among the 22 patients with hypertrophic cardiomyopathy 12 had no specific treatment while ten received beta blockers. In both groups a comparable increase in heart volume was observed which averaged 11% (from 857 to 956 ml/1.73 m²) over a mean period of 22 months.

In 50 patients the heart volume determination prior to treatment averaged 935 ml/1.73 m². The normal value of 620 ± 170 ml/1.73 m² for males and 570 ± 120 ml/1.73 m² for females ($\pm \mp 2$ s) was exceeded in 39 of the 50 patients. This finding reflects the fact that in many patients the heart volume is significantly increased in contrast to an apparently normal cardiac silhouette on conventional standing tele chest X-ray.

During various intervals of verapamil treatment heart volume determination was repeated in the 50 patients. The decrease in heart volume averaged 9–10%. This decrease was in sharp contrast to the increase of 11% seen in the 22 patients receiving no specific therapy or beta blockade.

Decrease in heart volume appeared maximal after a treatment period of 18 months (Fig. 3).

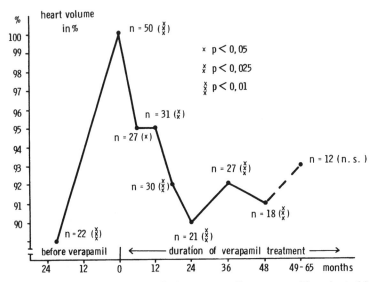

Fig. 3. Heart volume before and after verapamil treatment. 22 patients (*p*) showed during a pretreatment period of 18 months an increase of 11% (from 837 to 956 ml/1.73 m²). In 50 *p* during a treatment period of 6–65 months, a decrease in heart volume of 10% was seen

Left Ventricular End-Diastolic Volume

Left ventricular end-diastolic volume averaged 127 ± 39 ml/1.73 m² and was found unchanged after verapamil treatment with an average of 126 ± 24 ml/1.73 m². Also left ventricular end-systolic volume remained unchanged ($82 \pm 7.7\%$ before and $85 \pm 7.6\%$ after treatment over a mean period of 26 months). Left ventricular ejection fraction (82 ± 7.7 before $85 \pm 7.6\%$ after) remained somewhat supernormal (Fig. 4).

LVEDV 127 ± 39 → 126 ± 24 ml/1.73 m²
LVEF 82 ± 7.7 → $85 \pm 7.6\%$

Duration of verapamil treatment 26 (8–52) months

n = 18

Fig. 4. Unchanged left ventricular end-diastolic volume, systolic volume, and ejection fraction during verapamil treatment

Left Atrial Diameter

Left atrial diameter decreased at an average of about 10%. The maximal decrease was achieved about 12–18 months after the beginning of verapamil treatment (Fig. 5).

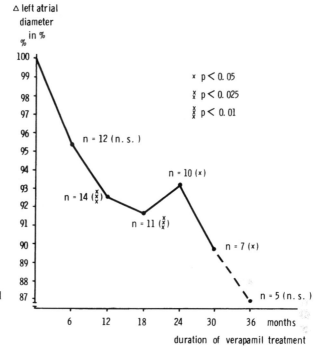

Fig. 5. Decrease in left atrial diameter and duration of verapamil treatment

Discussion

Heart volume as well as left atrial diameter decreased during verapamil treatment while left ventricular volume remained unchanged. The decrease in heart volume was in contrast to an increase seen in patients receiving no treatment or beta blocker therapy.

The findings confirm that despite its apparent negative inotropic efficacy verapamil does not convert hypertrophic into dilative cardiomyopathy. This conclusion can be drawn from the fact that left ventricular volume remained unchanged. Also there were no signs of pulmonary congestion or left ventricular failure on chest X-rays in standing position taken every 6 months during verapamil treatment.

Between heart volume and left atrial diameter a positive correlation was found (Fig. 6). The decrease in heart volume paralleled the decrease in left atrial diameter (Fig. 7). Both measurements reflect a decreased atrial volume. If verapamil has a predominant effect on left atrial volume, a change in left ventricular diastolic properties must be postulated. The echographic findings of Hanrath et al. [1] and the

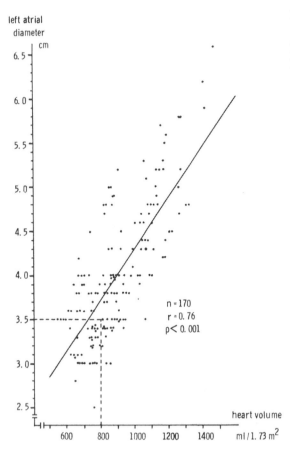

Fig. 6. Positive correlation between left atrial diameter derived from M-mode echograms and heart volume derived from chest X-rays

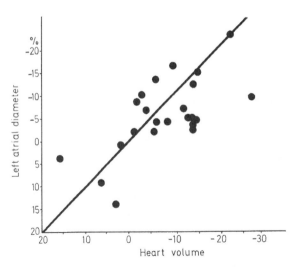

Fig. 7. Changes in left atrial diameter and in heart volume during verapamil treatment

Volume Parameters of the Heart During Long-Term Verapamil Treatment

preliminary findings of the National Institute of Health with gated blood pool technique point toward an increased diastolic ventricular compliance and thus may explain the described decrease in atrial volume occurring with no simultaneous change of ventricular volumes and ejection fraction.

On the other hand a reduction in ventricular muscle mass during verapamil treatment seems to occur as documented by a decrease in septal thickness in the echogram and in posterior free wall thickness in the angiogram (2, 3, 9). The decrease in coronary artery diameter [2, 3] can also best be explained by a reduced heart muscle mass. It is therefore likely that the reduction in heart volume is the consequence of both a reduction in ventricular muscle mass as well as a reduction in left atrial size.

Summary

Three types of volume measurement were performed to evaluate verapamil therapy in hypertrophic cardiomyopathy:
1. Heart volume determination from tele chest X-rays showed an increase of 11% (from 837 to 956 ml/1.73 m²) in a pretreatment period of 18 months. During verapamil treatment a decrease was seen of 9–10% persisting over a treatment period of up to 65 months.
2. Left ventricular enddiastolic volume, systolic volume, and ejection fraction determined from left ventricular angiograms in two planes remained unchanged during verapamil treatment.
3. Left atrial diameter determined from M-mode echograms decreased at an average of 10%.

It is concluded that the diminished heart volume during long-term verapamil treatment of hypertrophic cardiomyopathy is due to a decrease in atrial volume – most likely as a consequence of increased diastolic left ventricular compliance *and* to a reduced ventricular muscle mass. The results exclude conversion of hypertrophic into dilative cardiomyopathy by this form of treatment.

References

1. Hanrath P, Mathey DG, Kremer P, Sonntag F, Bleifeld W (1980) Effect of verapamil on left ventricular isovolumic relaxation time and regionel left ventricular filling in hypertrophic cardiomyopathy. Am J Cardial 45:1258
2. Kaltenbach M, Hopf R, Kober G, Rietbrock N, Woodcock B (1979) Treatment of Hypertrophic Obstructive Cardiomyopathy with Verapamil (Abstr). Circulation 60/II:76
3. Kaltenbach M, Hopf R, Kober G, Bussmann W-D, Keller M, Petersen Y (1978) Treatment of Hypertrophic Obstructive Cardiomyopathy with Verapamil. Br Heart J 42:35–42
4. Kaltenbach M, Klepzig H (1966) Röntgenologische Herzvolumenbestimmung. In: Opitz H, Schmid F (eds) Springer, Berlin Heidelberg New York (Handbuch der Kinderheilkunde, pp 258–261)
5. Kahlstorf A (1932) Über eine orthodiagraphische Herzvolumenbestimmung. Fortschr Roentgenstr 45:123

6. Klepzig H, Fritsch P (1965) Röntgenologische Herzvolumenbestimmung in Klinik und Praxis. Thieme, Stuttgart
7. Lemke R, Hopf R, Kober G, Kaltenbach M (to be published) Echokardiographische Befunde unter calciumantagonistischer Therapie der hypertroph-obstruktiven Myokardiopathie. Z Kardiol
8. Rohrer F (1916) Volumenbestimmung von Körperhöhlen und Organen auf orthodiagraphischem Wege. Fortschr Roentgenstr 24:285
9. Troesch M, Hirzel HO, Jenni R, Krayenbühl HP (1979) Reduction of septal thickness following verapamil in patients with asymmetric septal hypertrophy (ASH) (Abstr) Circulation 60/II:155

Long-Term Clinical Effects of Verapamil in Patients with Hypertrophic Cardiomyopathy*

DOUGLAS R. ROSING, JOHN R. CONDIT, BARRY J. MARON, KENNETH M. KENT, MARTIN B. LEON, ROBERT O. BONOW, LEWIS C. LIPSON, and STEPHEN E. EPSTEIN

For many years beta adrenergic receptor blocking drugs have been the primary pharmacologic agents for treating symptomatic patients with hypertrophic cardiomyopathy [1–3]. Although effective, not all patients respond adequately to this type of therapy and many experience unpleasant side effects. Recent studies from our laboratory have demonstrated that verapamil administration to patients with hypertrophic cardiomyopathy reduces left ventricular outflow obstruction [4], increases exercise capacity [5], and reduces subjective symptomatology (see below [5]). Kaltenbach and associates have also reported chronic verapamil administration improves symptoms in patients with hypertrophic cardiomyopathy [6]. In addition, angiographic, electrocardiographic, and echocardiographic data have been interpreted as suggesting that verapamil reduces left ventricular muscle mass or ventricular septal thickness in these patients [6, 7]. In the present study, we report the results of continued examination of the clinical effects of verapamil in patients with hypertrophic cardiomyopathy discharged from the hospital on chronic therapy.

Methods

Between September 1977 and September 1979, we initiated verapamil therapy in 78 patients with hypertrophic cardiomyopathy. The diagnosis of hypertrophic cardiomyopathy was based on echocardiographic demonstration of a nondilated, hypertrophied left ventricle in the absence of other acquired or congenital heart disease that produces left ventricular hypertrophy [8]. The 78 patients consisted of 38 men and 40 women, ages 13–77 years (mean = 46 years). Sixty-seven fulfilled our criterion for obstructive hypertrophy cardiomyopathy (basal or provocable subaortic peak systolic pressure gradient ≥ 30 mmHg, or, in the six patients where catheterization was not performed, the presence of systolic anterior motion of the anterior mitral valve leaflet with the leaflet contacting the septum in the basal state, or with provocation); seven did not and were classified as nonobstructive hypertrophic cardiomyopathy. Four patients had undergone previous septal

---

* This paper has previously been published (see 1 below)

1 Rosing DR, Condit J, Maron BJ, Kent KM, Epstein SE (1981) Verapamil therapy: A new approach to the pharmacologic treatment of hypertrophic cardiomyopathy. III. Effects of chronic administration. Am J Cardiol 48:545–553

myotomy-myectomy; one had no postoperative left ventricular outflow tract gradient and three had basal gradients greater than 30 mmHg.

Despite what was considered to be optimal medical treatment, six patients were classified as functional class IV (New York Heart Association criteria) and 56 functional class III. Of the remaining patients, 15 were in functional class II, and one, who had freqent premature ventricular beats including multiple episodes of ventricular tachycardia, was in functional class I. Sixty-seven patients were taking propranolol and three metoprolol when admitted to the National Heart, Lung, and Blood Institute. Seven patients who had taken beta receptor blocking agents at one time had discontinued them; four because of adverse effects and three because the drug was ineffective. The maximal daily dose of propranolol treatment was 40–1600 mg/day (median dose 320 mg/day). Seventy-one patients were in normal sinus rhythm and six had atrial fibrillation. One patient had a fixed rate ventricular pacemaker and another had a demand sequential atrioventricular pacemaker in place.

Seventy-two patients underwent cardiac catheterization either at the NIH or the referring institution and 50 patients had radionuclide cineangiographic studies at the NIH, employing techniques as previously described [9].

Thirty-one of the patients underwent coronary angiography. Of these, 27 had no obstruction greater than 75% of the cross sectional area (50% luminal diameter) in any coronary vessel. Of the 47 remaining patients who did not have coronary angiography, 13 were men under 40 years of age and 18 were women under 50.

Drug Administration

At the onset of the study, each patient received verapamil, 80 mg every 6 h for eight doses. If this dose was well-tolerated, the dose was increased to 120 mg every 6 hours for 3 days. If a patient had tolerated this dose, they were discharged on it. As a result of occasional adverse electrocardiographic effects and marked postural blood pressure changes with this regimen, the dosing interval (therefore total daily dose) was reduced midway through the study to every 8 hours. The administration of 120 mg verapamil three or four times per day has previously been found to be an effective dose for patients with hypertrophic cardiomyopathy [5]. Patients were discharged on this dosage if it was well tolerated and reasonably controlled the patient's symptoms in the hospital environment. If this dose was not well tolerated, the highest tolerated dose was selected. If symptoms were not controlled in hospital, verapamil was discontinued. Discharge dose was 80 mg three times per day in four patients, 80 mg four times per day in 11, 120 mg three times per day in 24, and 120 mg four times per day in 29. In six patients whose symptoms were not controlled, and who experienced no adverse drug effects, the dose was increased after discharge to 160 mg four times per day.

Upright Exercise Testing

Patients underwent exercise testing according to one of two protocols: (1) starting at 2.2 mph and 0% grade, the speed is held constant and the grade increased 2.5% every 2.5 minutes (Standard Protocol); and (2) starting at 1.9 mph and 10% grade,

Long-Term Clinical Effects of Verapamil

speed and incline are increased every 2.5 minutes to 2.3 mph, 12%; 2.7 mph, 14%; 3.1 mph, 16%; 3.5 mph, 18%; 3.9 mph, 20%, and 4.7 mph, 20% (Augmented Protocol).

Protocol selection was determined by the patient's symptoms and with the goal that a symptomatic end point be reached after 2.5–12.5 min of exercise. Symptomatic end points were defined as the onset of chest pain, lightheadedness, or sufficient dyspnea or fatigue that the patient requested exercise be discontinued. The Augmented Protocol was used in 60 of the 78 patients. The first exercise study was usually conducted with patients taking the medications they were on at the time of admission. A second study was performed with all cardiac medications stopped for at least five drug half-lifes. A final study took place after the patients had received the verapamil dose that was felt to be optimal for at least eight doses. Repeat testing was performed at 6-month intervals. Patients in normal sinus rhythm were also studied approximately 1 year after discharge after verapamil had been discontinued for at least 48 h.

In order to examine the reproducibility of exercise testing in patients with hypertrophic cardiomyopathy, exercise capacity in 19 patients on placebo was examined twice, 48 h apart. These patients included two who were not part of the present group, and in all cases the exercise testing took place as part of a previously reported study [5].

Echocardiographic Studies

M-mode echocardiograms were obtained with a 2.25-MHz, 1.2-cm diameter transducer connected to a Hoffrel 201 ultrasound unit employing methods previously described [10]. The ultrasound signal was connected via a custombuilt video amplifier to a Honeywell 1856 Visicorder and recorded continuously on light sensitive paper. Thickness of the ventricular septum was measured below the tips of the mitral valve leaflets just prior to atrial systole. Thickness of the posterobasal left ventricular wall was measured at the level of the tips of the mitral valve leaflets during the same phase of the cardiac cycle. Left atrial dimension was measured in early diastole from the damped portion of the record by recording the distance from the posterior aortic wall to the posterior left atrial wall. The magnitude and duration of systolic anterior motion of the anterior mitral leaflet (SAM) was qualitatively graded from 1+ (slight anterior motion) to 4+ (prolonged contact between anterior leaflet and ventricular septal endocardium consistent with marked obstruction to left ventricular outflow) in each echocardiogram. Echocardiographic measurements were obtained without knowledge of which of the echocardiographic studies was obtained before, and which after, institution of verapamil.

Plasma Verapamil Levels

Blood samples to determine plasma verapamil levels were drawn at the time of exercise testing just prior to hospital discharge and at all follow-up visits. A high pressure liquid chromatographic assay utilizing a commercially available column and fluorometric detection was employed for the analysis of verapamil plasma levels [11].

Statistical Analysis

Data were analyzed using either the two-tailed t test for paired data or unpaired data.

Results

Subjective Symptomatic Response

During the initial hospitalization, verapamil administration was discontinued in 10 of the 78 patients treated (Table 1). Two patients suffered sinus arrest after one

Table 1. Reasons for discontinuing verapamil therapy[a]

	In hospital	Post discharge
Therapeutic failure	8	23
Recurrent or persistent symptoms	3	20
Sinus node arrest	2	–
Death	1	2
Congestive heart failure	1	–
Gastrointestinal side effects	1	1
Noncompliance by patient	2	3
Total	10	26

[a] From Rosing et al. (see front page)

verapamil tablet and the drug was discontinued. One patient, also on quinidine, developed hypotension and pulmonary edema, necessitating discontinuation of verapamil. Hypotension and atrioventricular block limited dosage in two patients who remained significantly symptomatic on the highest tolerated dose, even in a hospital environment. One patient experienced no relief of symptoms, while in another the drug was discontinued because nausea and vomiting developed. Two patients chose not to continue with the study protocol before reaching discharge dosage.

Among the 68 patients discharged on verapamil, 24 decided to discontinue the drug from 1 week to 14 months (median = 5 months) after leaving the hospital, and two patients died. The remaining 42 patients have continued taking the medication for 6–30 months (median = 14 months) (Fig. 1). The reasons for discontinuing verapamil in the 26 patients are listed in Table 1.

All 42 patients who have continued taking verapamil have done so because they feel their life style is acceptable on the drug. Although 17 patients have not improved their symptomatic status by an entire functional class (Fig. 2), all but three describe an improvement in symptoms. The three whose symptomatology

Long-Term Clinical Effects of Verapamil

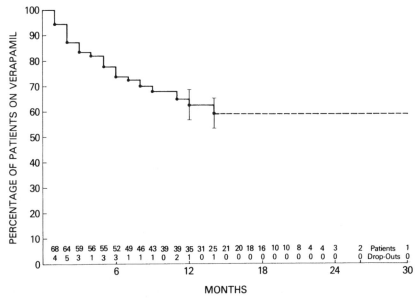

Fig. 1. Plot of percentage of patients still on verapamil after being discharged from the hospital on the medication. The curve, obtained using the method of Kaplan and Meier [12], is shown by a *broken line* after 14 months because no patient of the 21 on the drug has discontinued taking the medication after that time. "Drop-outs" depict patients in whom the medication was discontinued as described in Table 1. (Rosing DR, Condit J, Maron BJ, Kent KM, Epstein SE, Verapamil therapy: A new approach to the pharmacologic treatment of hypertrophic cardiomyopathy. III. Effects of administration, see front page)

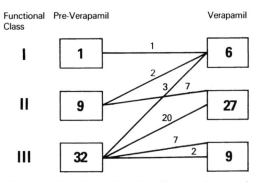

Fig. 2. Change in functional class in 42 patients who described their style of living as improved on verapamil and thus have continued taking the medication (6–30 months). Upsloping lines connecting the same functional class indicate persons who described a decrease in symptoms, but whose functional class remained unchanged. The two patients who were still functional class III and had no change in the severity of symptoms stated that they felt "better" on verapamil and chose to continue on the medication. The patient who was functional class I when started on verapamil was begun on the medication because it decreased the incidence of ventricular tachycardia in her. (Rosing et al., see Fig. 1)

remains the same find their style of life more acceptable because bothersome side effects from beta-blocking agents have been eliminated. The effectiveness of verapamil in relieving chest pain, dyspnea, or syncope was similar.

Of the original 78 patients, 53 who had obstructive hypertrophic cardiomyopathy were referred for operative intervention because of severe symptoms refractory to conventional therapy. Twenty-five (47%) of these patients experienced sustained improvement in symptoms and achieved a sufficiently satisfactory life style on verapamil that they decided to forego operation for the time being. Of the remaining 28 patients who were initially operative candidates, 25 (47%) have subsequently undergone ventricular septal myectomy because of unsatisfactory symptomatic control with verapamil. Three patients died while on verapamil treatment.

Exercise Testing

The results of exercise testing are depicted in Table 2. During the initial hospitalization, there was no difference in exercise capacity between studies performed on no medication and on beta-blocking agents. Verapamil treatment in hospital significantly improved exercise capacity by 3.1 ± 0.6 (SEM)[2] min ($53 \pm 10\%$) compared with no medication and 2.0 ± 0.7 min ($32 \pm 12\%$) compared with beta-blocking agents. Exercise capacity at the time of last study, while on verapamil, 6–25 (median = 12) months after discharge from the hospital, was also significantly greater than that of in-hospital control (Fig. 3), and was further increased compared to the initial study on verapamil (Fig. 3).

Repeat exercise testing in 19 patients on placebo medication was undertaken to determine test reproducibility. The standard deviation of the mean difference, –11 s,

Table 2. Exercise capacity on no medication, beta adrenergic blocking agents, and verapamil[a]

	N	Exercise duration	% difference	P value
No medication[b]	31	5.7 ± 0.7	$+ 6 \pm 9$	NS
Beta blockers[b]	31	5.9 ± 0.6		
Beta blockers[b]	32	6.2 ± 0.7	$+32 \pm 12$	<0.01
Verapamil[b]	32	8.2 ± 0.8		
No medicine[b]	35	5.9 ± 0.6	$+53 \pm 10$	<0.001
Verapamil[b]	35	9.0 ± 0.8		
Verapamil initial[b]	37	8.7 ± 0.8	$+25 \pm 7$	<0.0025
Verapamil last study	37	10.9 ± 0.8		

[a] From Rosing et al.
[b] During initial hospitalization.

2 All statistics are expressed as mean $\pm$ SEM except where indicated

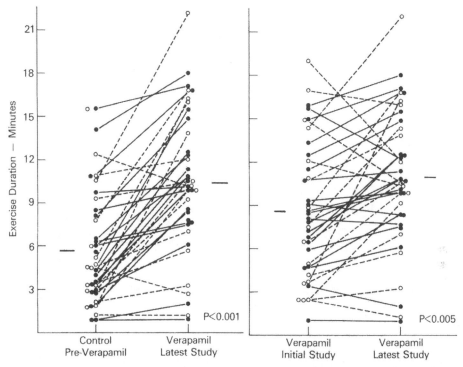

Fig. 3. Exercise capacity in patients remaining on chronic verapamil therapy. Comparison between control period with patients on no medication and latest study on verapamil (*left*). Comparison between initial exercise test, patients had been on verapamil treatment for approximately 5 days, and latest study, patients had been on medication for 6–25 months (right). *Horizontal bars* indicate mean values. *Open circles* and *broken line* depict Standard Protocol exercise test and *closed circles* and *solid line* Augmented Protocol exercise test. (Rosing et al., see Fig. 1)

in exercise capacity between the results of the two tests was ± 15% or ± 50 s. Hence, a change in exercise capacity was considered to have taken place in an individual patient if exercise duration changed by at least 30% or 100 s (± 2 SD). Employing this type of analysis, 28 of the 42 patients (67%) who remained on verapamil showed a significant increase in their exercise capacity at the time of their latest evaluation on verapamil, compared to their in-hospital control study. Twenty of the 38 patients (53%) who underwent exercise testing on verapamil during their initial hospitalization, and have remained on verapamil, showed a significant increase in their exercise capacity at the time of their latest study on verapamil compared to the initial verapamil study.

In 24 patients who had been on verapamil for 1 year, exercise duration was determined after the medication had been stopped for 48–72 h. Although exercise duration while off medication 1 year after starting verapamil was greater than before starting the drug (8.3 ± 1.1 vs 6.7 ± 0.8 min), the difference did not achieve statistical significance. We found 12 patients improved their baseline exercise

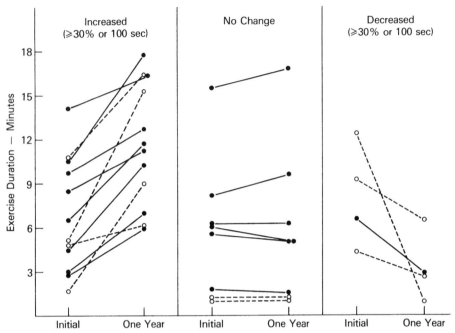

Fig. 4. Exercise capacity on no cardiac medication 1 day prior to starting verapamil ("initial") and 1 year later on no cardiac medication after verapamil had been discontinued for 48 h ("one year"). Twelve patients showed an increase in exercise capacity that could not be ascribed to variability inherent in the testing technique and was thus considered significant (*left*). Eight patients showed no change (*center*). Four patients showed a significant decrease in exercise capacity greater than would be expected by random variation (*right*). *Open circles* and *broken line* depict Standard Protocol exercise test and closed circles and solid line Augmented Protocol exercise test. (Rosing et al., see Fig. 1)

Table 3. Echocardiographic findings in 31 patients with hypertrophic cardiomyopathy[a]

	Control Mean ± SEM	Verapamil (1 year) Mean ± SEM	
Ventricular septal thickness (mm)	22 ± 0.8	21 ± 0.7	NS
Posterior LV free wall thickness (mm)	11 ± 0.3	12 ± 0.4	NS
Septum: free wall thickness ratio	1.9 ± 0.1	1.8 ± 0.1	NS
Left atrial transverse dimension (mm)	48 ± 1.6	48 ± 1.6	NS

[a] From Rosing et al. (see first page or previous table)

performance after taking the drug for 1 year (Fig. 4). Exercise performance was unchanged in eight and decreased in four.

Echocardiographic Studies

In the 31 patients followed for at least 1 year, there were no differences between measurements of ventricular septal or posterior left ventricular free wall thicknesses, septal: free wall thickness ratios, or left atrial transverse dimension obtained before starting on verapamil and at the time of the 1-year study (Table 3). There was a qualitative decrease in the magnitude or duration of systolic anterior motion of the anterior mitral valve leaflet between these studies in nine patients, no change in 15, and an increase in two. In the subgroup of 12 patients who both increased their exercise capacity by at least 30% or 100 s and improved their functional classification by at least one category, there was no significant change in echocardiographic measurements.

Plasma Verapamil Levels

Plasma verapamil levels obtained at the time of exercise testing before discharge revealed no difference between 11 of the patients in whom the drug was discontinued because of lack of clinical improvement (153 ± 23.9 ng/ml) and 28 of the patients on continued therapy (127 ± 12.3 ng/ml). After further analysis of these two groups with regard to exercise and/or subjective symptomatic responses, measurement of plasma verapamil levels, at hospital discharge or during follow-up, did not differentiate between responders and nonresponders[3].

All patients had verapamil levels greater than 25 ng/ml at all follow-up visits.

Clinical Successes Versus Failures

Comparison of exercise capacity on and off medication, ventricular septal thickness, septal: free wall ratio, left atrial size, left ventricular ejection fraction at rest and with exercise (obtained by radionuclide cineangiography [9]), sex, basal and provocable left ventricular outflow tract gradients, and mean pulmonary artery and pulmonary artery wedge pressures between those patients continuing on verapamil and those in whom the drug had been discontinued because of lack of clinical benefit failed to demonstrate any significant differences between the two groups. In hospital, 55% of the patients who are still taking the medication were stopped by angina pectoris during exercise tests while on no medication, a figure similar to that of patients judged to be clinical failures (65%; NS). The patients who were clinical failures were significantly younger (39 ± 3 vs 49 ± 2 years, $P<0.01$).

Side Effects of Verapamil

Table 4 lists the cardiovascular and noncardiovascular side effects encountered during verapamil administration in the 78 patients in this study.

---

3 Leon MB, Rosing DR, Jaouni TM, Fales HM, Epstein SE, Correlation of plasma verapamil levels with clinical responses, unpublished work

Deaths

Description of the first patient who died after the acute development of electrical mechanical dissociation has appeared previously [5]. The other two deaths occurred in patients who initially had experienced symptomatic improvement with verapamil for periods of 5 weeks and 8 months, respectively. One developed increasing dyspnea over several hours and was found to be in pulmonary edema upon arriving at an emergency room. The other had increasing symptoms of dyspnea on exertion over several weeks. She was scheduled for septal myotomy-myectomy, but

Table 4. Adverse effects encountered during verapamil treatment in 78 patients [a]

Cardiovascular	19 [b]
Hemodynamic	9 [b]
Death	3
Pulmonary congestion	5
Hypotension	3
Electrophysiologic	10
Sinus arrest or pauses	2
Junctional rhythm	5
Wenkeback 2° heart block	3
Noncardiovascular	
Gastrointestinal	
Upper abdominal discomfort	2
Constipation	frequent
Hair loss	infrequent

[a] From Rosing et al.
[b] Two patients developed both pulmonary congestion and hypotension.

experienced a sudden episode of dyspnea at rest and was found to be in pulmonary edema when she arrived at an emergency room. Both died shortly after admission to the hospital. Of note, both patients had demonstrated previous evidence of marked left ventricular outflow tract obstruction, as well as either an elevated pulmonary artery wedge pressure at catheterization or a history compatible with pulmonary venous hypertension.

Electrophysiological Abnormalities

The development of a junctional rhythm was always transient and occurred at the time of peak verapamil blood levels, 1–3 h after the previous dose; it never lasted more than 1 or 2 h, and the junctional rate was always 50–70 beats/min. No patient experienced detectable compromise in cardiac function, and all patients remained on verapamil, usually at reduced dosages. The basic abnormality usually appeared to be due to sinus slowing to rates just below that of the AV junction, leading to isorhythmic dissociation.

All but two of the electrophysiologic abnormalities were encountered during the initial hospitalization. Two instances of transient junctional rhythm were detected at the time of 1-year evaluation. The two episodes of sinus node dysfunction occurred after the administration of one 80 mg tablet of verapamil; in one patient the rhythm disturbance necessitated administration of phenylephrine to maintain blood pressure until the drug effect dissipated.

Pulmonary Congestion

One episode of marked pulmonary congestion occurred during initial hospitalization in a patient with the obstructive form of the disease and was corrected by placing the patient at bed rest, discontinuing verapamil and administering a diuretic and nasal oxygen. A patient with nonobstructive hypertrophic cardiomyopathy and atrial fibrillation also developed marked pulmonary congestion 5 months after discharge while on digoxin, furosemide, and verapamil. Verapamil was discontinued after this episode. Three other instances of gradually increasing dyspnea on exertion developed in patients during the first month after discharge and were improved with the administration of diuretics without discontinuing verapamil.

Postural Hypotension

Three patients developed postural hypotension on verapamil; two of the patients were also taking quinidine at the time. One of these patients exhibited acute pulmonary congestion simultaneous with the postural blood pressure changes and both drugs were stopped. The third patient, taking only verapamil, responded well to a decrease in the verapamil dose. She later developed increasing dyspnea on exertion. Verapamil was increased and diuretic added without further episodes of hypotension or pulmonary congestion. However, she did not receive adequate benefit from the drug, and eventually underwent successful ventricular septal myectomy.

Noncardiovascular Side Effects

These included two instances of upper abdominal discomfort necessitating discontinuation of the drug. Constipation was a common complaint; patients occasionally needed to take laxatives and stool softeners. An occasional patient complained of hair loss, but this was difficult to attribute to the drug. No patient had to discontinue their medication because of either of these complaints.

Discussion

Beta-blocking agents effectively control symptoms in the large majority of patients with hypertrophic cardiomyopathy [13] and operation has resulted in symptomatic improvement in most of those patients with left ventricular outflow obstruction who have responded inadequately to medical management [14]. The major problem that still confronts the physician in caring for patients with this disease, therefore, is whether alternative nonsurgical therapeutic approaches can effectively control symptoms in those patients who are refractory to, or cannot tolerate, beta-blocking agents. Hence, it was not the purpose of the present investigation to conduct a randomized double-blinded study on the relative efficacy of verapamil versus propranolol or operative therapy. Rather, the primary question this study was designed to answer is whether verapamil improves exercise capacity and symptoms during long-term chronic therapy in a group of patients with hypertrophic cardiomyopathy who previously had demonstrated inadequate symptomatic response to conventional medical therapy.

The results of this investigation are encouraging, and demonstrate that verapamil was frequently effective in reducing symptoms and improving exercise capacity in patients with hypertrophic cardiomyopathy. Most importantly, the salutary effects of verapamil occurred despite the fact that most of our patients were selected for verapamil therapy *because* they proved refractory to conventional medical measures. Thus, 62 of 78 patients (79%) were either functional class III or IV and found their style of living unacceptable even after having been treated with beta-adrenergic blocking agents. When verapamil was administered chronically for 6–30 months, either a sustained significant increase in exercise capacity, or an improvement in functional classification by one group, was exhibited by 32 of 42 (76%) patients. Thus, 47% of all patients discharged from the hospital on verapamil showed either a significant improvement in exercise capacity or subjective symptomatology, while 29% demonstrated a significant improvement in both areas. In addition, 54% of all patients evaluated and 63% of those discharged from hospital on verapamil regarded their style of living as acceptable and improved over what it had been on their former medical program (as also observed by Kaltenbach [6]). Moreover, approximately half of the patients, who had obstruction to left ventricular outflow and were judged to be candidates for operation because of severe symptoms unresponsive to medical therapy, improved sufficiently in response to verapamil so that operation was no longer considered necessary. The improvement we found, however, was manifest by patients who had no more than moderately severe symptoms; no patient who was functional class IV when verapamil was initiated benefitted enough from the medication for it to be continued.

Because verapamil undergoes extensive first-pass metabolism in the liver [15], we considered the possibility that the first-pass effect might cause a variation in plasma drug levels and be responsible for some of the patients' failure to respond to the drug. Although marked variation in the random plasma concentrations did occur in the present study, there was no consistent relation between plasma verapamil levels and the clinical response to the drug.

Sixty-seven (86%) of the patients in this study had obstruction to left ventricular outflow, seven (9%) did not have obstruction and four (5%) had previously undergone ventricular septal myotomy and myectomy. Although the latter two subgroups consist of too few subjects to draw definite conclusions about them, the same tendencies regarding benefits from the drug were demonstrated; four of the

Long-Term Clinical Effects of Verapamil

seven nonobstructive patients and two of the four operated patients received good symptomatic benefits for at least 6 months.

As part of this study, an attempt was made to determine whether chronic verapamil administration alters the patient's underlying functional capacity. To accomplish this, exercise capacity prior to starting verapamil was compared to exercise capacity achieved 1 year later, 48 h after discontinuation of verapamil. Although no consistent trends were observed, 12 of the 24 patients who underwent repeat testing off verapamil 1 year after starting the drug manifested an increase in exercise performance that could not be ascribed to variability inherent in the testing technique (Fig. 4). This improvement could have been caused by a training effect due to a general increase in physical activity secondary to a decrease in symptomatology. Alternatively, it is intriguing to postulate that these 12 patients experienced an improvement in the underlying intrinsic cardiomyopathic process; however, their ventricular septal, left ventricular free wall, and left atrial echocardiographic dimensions were unchanged when compared with those studies obtained prior to beginning verapamil.

The results of the 1-year studies performed after discontinuation of verapamil may also have been affected by the fact that these tests were performed only 48 h after the last dose had been administered. Although blood levels were negligible by this time, rebound hemodynamic events may have occurred that adversely affected exercise capacity, thereby accounting for the decrease in exercise capacity experienced by four patients. However, it is also possible that functional deterioration in these patients was due to intrinsic progression of the disease.

Our findings that ventricular wall thickness did not change significantly in either the entire group of patients who had been on verapamil for 1 year, or in the subgroups who improved symptomatically and with exercise testing, appear to differ from the results of other studies [6, 7]. However, although Kaltenbach and associates described a reduction in left ventricular muscle mass by angiography, these changes did not attain statistical significance [6]. Furthermore, the measurements made by these investigators were calculated from cineangiograms, and the reproducibility of this methodology is uncertain. Troesch and associates have presented preliminary M-mode echocardiographic data indicating that verapamil significantly reduces ventricular septal thickness [7], but the magnitude of the decrease they reported for the entire group of 28 patients was only 1 mm. Whether this small change represents a biologically important difference, remains to be determined. Most importantly, recent two-dimenional echocardiographic studies [16] have demonstrated the heterogenous distribution of hypertrophy in patients with hypertrophic cardiomyopathy, a finding that raises questions as to whether M-mode echocardiography is an entirely reliable technique for measuring changes in wall thickness or muscle mass in this disorder.

Adverse drug effects to verapamil could be grouped into two categories: (1) those which were bothersome, but not life threatening, and (2) those which definitely posed a risk to the well-being of the patient. Verapamil caused very few clinically important problems of the first type. Although approximately one-third of patients on chronic treatment reported the presence of occasional constipation, no one discontinued the drug because of this development, and an increased dietary fiber content and/or the use of stool softeners and laxatives usually corrected the problem. Other gastrointestinal side effects included one patient experiencing intolerable upper abdominal discomfort and another nausea and vomiting soon after starting the drug. In both cases these side effects necessitated the discontinuation of the medication. Other tolerable side effects included a small group of patients describing changes in hair texture or loss of hair, but this type of complaint in predominantly middle-aged patients is difficult to attribute to a drug effect and was usually not a persistent finding in a given patient. The lack of other significant adverse effects of this category makes verapamil a well-tolerated medication.

The more serious adverse effects secondary to verapamil administration result from either accentuated hemodynamic or electrophysiologic responses to the drug. The three deaths in patients on verapamil occurred as a result of pulmonary edema and inadequate cardiac output. All three had the obstructive form of the disease. It is not absolutely clear, however, whether these fatal complications occurred as a result of verapamil-induced drop in systemic blood pressure with resultant increase in obstruction to left ventricular outflow [4], to the negative inotropic action of the drug [7], or were, in fact, entirely unrelated to the drug. This latter possibility cannot be entirely dismissed, since verapamil was being administered to a group of patients with a life-threatening disease which has a spontaneous annual mortality of about 3% [18].

As a result of this experience, we presently do not initiate verapamil therapy in patients with obstructive hypertrophic cardiomyopathy who had a previous history of significant congestive heart failure. In all patients who are candidates for verapamil treatment we perform a right heart catheterization if one has not been performed in the last 6 months. We do not administer the drug to anyone with a mean pulmonary artery wedge pressure greater than 22 mmHg (one and one-half times the upper limits of normal for our laboratory). Exceptions to this rule only occur if a patient is not a candidate for operative intervention, and then only after it has been demonstrated that the intravenous administration of the drug does not adversely effect the mean pulmonary artery wedge pressure or the left ventricular outflow tract gradient in these patients.

The electrophysiologic side effects produced by verapamil led to loss of sequential atrial-ventricular depolarization, which in a patient with hypertrophic cardiomyopathy, could seriously compromise cardiac function ([4] and [19]). Adverse electrophysiologic effects of verapamil were usually transient, and only infrequently necessitated discontinuation of the drug. However, they occasionally prevented the use of higher doses, which might have provided more optimal symptomatic relief.

The mechanism by which verapamil produces its beneficial effects in patients with hypertrophic cardiomyopathy is unknown. We have demonstrated that its administration can acutely decrease left ventricular outflow tract obstruction [4], and it is assumed that this action is probably related to the ability of the drug to inhibit slow channel ion flux [20, 21]. Preliminary work also indicates that verapamil improves diastolic function in this disease ([5] and [22]). Both of these actions probably contribute to the symptomatic improvement described by many of our patients.

Long-Term Clinical Effects of Verapamil

201

In summary, on the basis of this and other [7] studies, it appears that administration of verapamil improves exercise capacity and symptomatic status in many patients with hypertrophic cardiomyopathy. These benefits occur both acutely and chronically in patients, including those who have persistent severe symptoms despite the administration of beta-adrenergic blocking agents. We therefore conclude verapamil can be an excellent alternative to the use of beta-blocking agents in the treatment of this disease. As with other potent drugs, however, its administration does carry with it the potential for serious complications. Thus, patients should be carefully selected and therapy should be initiated under properly controlled conditions [4].

Acknowledgment. We thank Knoll Pharmaceutical Company, Whippany, New Jersey, for supplying us with verapamil (Isoptin).

References

1. Cohen LS, Braunwald E (1967) Amelioration of angina pectoris in idiopathic hypertrophic subaortic stenosis with beta-adrenergic blockade. Circulation 35:847–851
2. Swan DA, Bell B, Oakley CM, Goodwin J (1971) Analysis of symptomatic course and prognosis and treatment of hypertrophic obstructive cardiomyopathy. Br Heart J 33:671–685
3. Adelman AG, Wigle ED, Ranganathan N, Webb GD, Kidd BSL, Bigelow WG, Silver MD (1972) The clinical course in muscular subaortic stenosis: a retrospective and prospective study of 60 hemodynamically proved cases. Ann Intern Med 77:515–525
4. Rosing DR, Kent KM, Borer JS, Seides SF, Maron BJ, Epstein SE (1979) Verapamil therapy: A new approach to the pharmacologic treatment of hypertrophic cardiomyopathy. I. Hemodynamic effects. Circulation 60:1201–1207
5. Rosing DR, Kent KM, Maron BJ, Epstein SE (1979) Verapamil therapy: A new approach to the pharmacologic treatment of hypertrophic cardiomyopathy. II. Effects on exercise capacity and symptomatic status. Circulation 60:1208–1213
6. Kaltenbach M, Hopf R, Kober G, Bussman W-D, Keller M, Petersen Y (1979) Treatment of hypertrophic obstructive cardiomyopathy with verapamil. Br Heart J 42:35–42
7. Troesch M, Hirzel HO, Jenni R, Kayenbühl HP (1979) Reduction of septal thickness following verapamil in patients with asymmetric septal hypertrophy (Abstr). Circulation [Suppl 2] 60:II–155
8. Maron BJ, Epstein SE (1979) Hypertrophic cardiomyopathy: A discussion of nomenclature. Am J Cardiol 43:1242–1244
9. Borer JS, Bacharach SL, Green MV, Kent KM, Epstein SE, Johnston GS (1977) Real-time radionuclide cineangiography in the noninvasive evaluation of global and regional left ventricular function at rest and during exercise in patients with coronary artery disease. N Engl J Med 296:839–844
10. Henry WL, Clark CE, Epstein SE (1973) Asymmetric septal hypertrophy: Echocardiographic identification of the pathognomonic anatomic abnormality of IHSS. Circulation 47:225–233

---

4 Epstein SE, Rosing DR (1981) Verapamil: Its potential for causing serious complications in patients with hypertrophic cardiomyopathy. Circulation 64:432–441
5 Bonow RO, Rosing DR, Bacharach SL, Green MB, Kent KM, Lipson LC, Maron BJ, Leon MB, Epstein SE (1981) Left ventricular systolic function and diastolic filling in patients with hypertrophic cardiomyopathy; Effect of verapamil. Circulation 64:787–796

11. Jaouni TM, Leon MB, Rosing DR, Fales HM (1980) Analysis of verapamil in plasma by liquid chromatography. J Chromatogr 182:473–477
12. Kaplan EL, Meier P (1958) Non-parametric estimation for incomplete observations. J Am Stat Assoc 53:457–481
13. Epstein SE, Henry WL, Clark CE, Roberts WC, Maron BJ, Ferrans VJ, Redwood DR, Morrow AG (1974) Asymmetric septal hypertrophy. Ann Intern Med 81:650–680
14. Maron BJ, Merrill WH, Freier PA, Kent KM, Epstein SE, Morrow AG (1978) Long-term clinical course and symptomatic status of patients after operation for hypertrophic subaortic stenosis. Circulation 57:1205–1213
15. Schomerus M, Spiegelhalder B, Stelren B, Eichelbaum M (1976) Physiological disposition of verapamil in man. Cardiovasc Res 10:605–612
16. Maron BJ, Gottdiener JS, Epstein SE (1981) Patterns and significance of distribution of left ventricular hypertrophy in hypertrophic cardiomyopathy: A wideangle, twodimensional echocardiographic study of 125 patients. Am J Cardiol 48:418–428
17. Singh BN, Ellrodt G, Peter CT (1978) Verapamil: A review of its pharmacological properties and therapeutic use. Drugs 15:169–197
18. Shah PM, Adelman AG, Wigle ED, Gobel FL, Burchell HB, Hardarson T, Curiel R, De La Calzada C, Oakley CM, Goodwin JF (1973) The natural (and unnatural) course of hypertrophic obstructive cardiomyopathy. A multicenter study. Circ Res [Suppl II] 24, 25:179–195
19. Glancy DL, Shepherd RL, Beiser GD, Epstein SE (1971) The dynamic nature of left ventricular outflow obstruction in idiopathic hypertrophic subaortic stenosis. Ann Intern Med 75:589–592
20. Kohlhardt M, Bauer B, Krause H, Fleckenstein A (1972) New selective inhibitors of the transmembrane Ca conductivity in mammalian myocardial fibers. Studies with the voltage clamp technique. Experientia 28:288–289
21. Shigenobu K, Schneider JA, Sperelakis N (1974) Verapamil blockade of slow Na^+ and Ca^{++} responses in myocardial cells. J Pharmacol Exp Ther 190:280–288
22. Hanrath P, Mathey DG, Kremer P, Sonntag F, Bleifeld W (1980) Effect of verapamil on left ventricular isovolumic relaxation time and regional left ventricular filling in hypertrophic cardiomyopathy. Am J Cardiol 45:1258–1268

Effects of Verapamil on Ventricular Wall Thickness of Patients with Hypertrophic Cardiomyopathy*

HEINZ O. HIRZEL, MICHEL P. TROESCH, ROLF JENNI, and HANS P. KRAYENBUEHL

Introduction

It still remains a matter of debate whether the clinical terms of hypertrophic obstructive cardiomyopathy and asymmetric nonobstructive septal hypertrophy are referring to one single disease entity [1, 2]. Despite the fact that vast amounts of knowledge have been gained in the past regarding the special diagnostic features, the natural history, and prognosis of the disease, little is known so far about the etiology of the localized hypertrophy of the interventricular septum. This is certainly due to the fact that comparable disease states in animals are uncommon. Further knowledge about the development of abnormal hypertrophy may be gained, however, from the findings of Witzke and Kaye [3], who were able to induce a hypertrophic cardiomyopathy in newborn puppies by administration of nerve growth factor. Another clue to this disease may be derived from observations in nonhypertrophic hereditary or experimentally induced cardiomyopathies of various animal species which have focused on the important role of calcium ions in the pathogenesis of myocardial damage [4–6].

In treating patients with hypertrophic obstructive cardiomyopathy with the calcium antagonist verapamil, Kaltenbach et al. [7, 8] observed a reduction of heart size in the chest roentgenogram and a diminution of the electrocardiographic signs of left ventricular hypertrophy. It remains unclear, however, whether these changes reflected a true reduction in septal muscle mass or whether they were simply due to hemodynamic or ionic changes induced by the drug.

In the present study we thus determined left ventricular septal and posterior wall thickness and cavity size by use of M-mode echocardiography in 32 patients with either obstructive or nonobstructive septal hypertrophy in the course of a long-term treatment with verapamil.

Patient Population

The study group comprised 32 patients, 24 men and eight women, with a mean age of 44 years (range 19 to 63 years). An obstructive form of the disease was present in 25 patients, a nonobstructive form in seven. The diagnosis was confirmed by heart catheterization and angiocardiography in 19/25 patients with outflow tract obstruction and in 5/7 patients without obstruction. In fifteen out of the 19

---

* This paper has already been presented in part in abstract form in Circulation 60 (Suppl. II): II–155, 1979

catheterized patients with obstruction a pressure gradient was present at rest, averaging 36 ± 8 mmHg (mean $\pm$ SEM), whereas it was demonstrable only during provocation in four patients, amounting to 101 ± 13 mmHg in either the postextrasystolic beat or during isoproterenol infusion. The five patients without obstruction showed a markedly thickened interventricular septum at angiography. In the remaining eight patients (six with the obstructive form, two with the nonobstructive form of the disease) the diagnosis was based on the typical clinical findings and the pathognomonic features of the single beam and the two-dimensional echocardiogram.

In the M-mode echocardiogram a thickened septal muscle mass with a septum to posterior wall ratio exceeding 1.3 [9] was present in all cases. Systolic anterior motion of the anterior mitral leaflet and early closure of the aortic valve [9, 10] were the typical features of the patients with obstruction. No noticeable associated heart lesions were present in any of the patients nor did arterial blood pressure exceed 140/95 mmHg as measured repeatedly before entering the study [11].

Five out of the 25 patients with outflow tract obstruction had been operated upon prior to entering the study but remained symptomatic. This necessitated recatheterization in two patients which revealed a significant pressure gradient at rest in one patient and residual asymmetric septal hypertrophy without obstruction in the other. The remaining three patients showed echocardiographically a markedly thickened interventricular septum despite the surgical intervention, two of whom had the additional signs of outflow tract obstruction.

Two patients had to be operated on during the study after 6 months of therapy because of insufficient response to medical management.

Methods

At least 7 days before entering the study all previous medication, including beta-blocking agents, were stopped. Following the control examination treatment with verapamil[1] at an average dose of 320 mg (240 mg–360 mg) per day was instituted. First examination took place at 6.2 ± 0.5 (SEM) months after initiation of therapy. Thereafter the dose of verapamil was increased to an average of 360 mg (320 mg–480 mg) per day and a second examination was performed at 12.4 ± 0.9 months.

The study protocol comprised the following parameters: The clinical symptomatology of the patients was assessed according to the NYHA classification. In the standard 12-lead electrocardiogram the Sokolow Index ($S_{V1} + R_{V5,6}$) was determined. Moreover, the repolarization disturbances which were present in the absence of left bundle branch block in 27/32 patients were assessed as the sum of the maximal ST-T negativity in the precordial leads measured in millimeters.

M-mode echocardiographic tracings were recorded with an Organon Teknika Echokardiovisor equipped with a 2.2 mHz transducer with a repetition frequency of 1000 pulses per second. The output was displayed on a Honeywell strip chart

---

1 We would like to thank Dr. E. Vogt, Knoll AG, CH-4410 Liesthal, for providing large samples of verapamil

recorder together with the simultaneously recorded electro- and phonocardiogram. All recordings were performed with the patient in the supine AP or RAO position and the transducer located at the left sternal edge in the third or fourth intercostal space. Utmost care was given to repeat all the recordings in a standardized fashion and the measurements were always carried out in the aorto-apical sweep.

The thickness of the interventricular septum in the outflow tract was measured in end-diastole (as defined by the R-wave in the electrocardiogram) from the echocardiograms obtained at the plane of the mitral valve, where both mitral leaflets were visible. Just below the plane of the mitral valve (i.e., when only the echos arising from the chordae tendineae were recorded) the thickness of the septum in the corpus, the thickness of the posterior wall of the left ventricle, and the end-diastolic and end-systolic dimensions of the left ventricle were measured. In addition, the size of the left atrium was assessed from the tracings in the plane of the aortic root [10]. The reason for measuring the thickness of the interventricular septum at two different sites emerges from the fact that the hypertrophied muscle mass can be located at various levels of the septum [2, 12], as shown schematically in Fig. 1. Thus, the septal thickness was always measured at both levels, i.e., in the outflow tract (upper portion of the septum) and in the corpus (lower or mid-septal portion).

In deciding which signals represent the true surfaces of the septum and the posterior wall, the criteria developed by Henry and coworkers [13] were adopted.

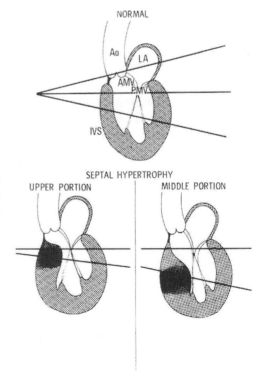

Fig. 1. Schematic drawing of a longitudinal section through the left ventricle of a normal heart (*above*) and hearts with septal hypertrophy either located in the upper portion of the septum (outflow tract) (*below on the left side*) or in the midseptal portion (corpus) (*below on the right side*). *Ao,* aorta; *LA,* left atrium; *AMV,* anterior mitral leaflet; *PMV,* posterior mitral leaflet; *IVS,* interventricular septum. The different lines indicate the planes of the echo beam at which the different echocardiographic measurements were performed (for further explanation see text)

Thus, only parallel lines on the anterior and posterior surfaces which were present continuously throughout an entire cardiac cycle moving relative to the stationary transducer were considered to be representative of the true borders (Fig. 2). All measurements were performed by two independent observers who did not know at which stage of the study the echo recordings were taken. The respective correlation coefficients ranged between 0.85 and 0.90.

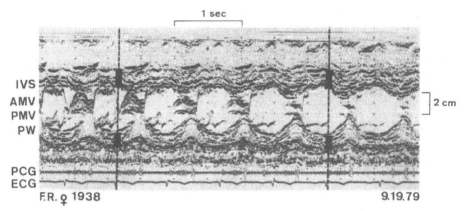

Fig. 2. M-mode echo sweep through the left ventricular cavity of a patient with hypertrophic obstructive cardiomyopathy. Starting in the plane of the mitral valve (*left side*) where both mitral leaflets and the systolic anterior motion of the anterior leaflet are clearly visible, the echo beam is continuously tilted toward the apex of the heart (*right side*). The thickened interventricular septum is measured in end diastole defined by the R wave in the electrocardiogram in the plane of the mitral valve (*outflow tract*) and just below the mitral valve (corpus) as indicated by the *black bars*. In the latter position the thickness of the posterior wall was also measured

Occasionally, the examination was completed by two-dimensional echocardiograms performed with a Varian V-3000 model phased array 84° ultrasonic sector scanner equipped with either a 2.2 or a 3.5 mHz transducer. Since serial studies, however, were done in only a few patients, these examinations were not used to measure wall thicknesses.

Statistics

The results are presented as means ± 1 SEM. Paired comparisons with Student's t test were used to evaluate the statistical significance of differences of the data.

Results

During treatment with verapamil the NYHA class of the patients improved significantly. The respective values amounted to 1.9 ± 0.1 before treatment, to 1.3 ± 0.1 at the first ($P < 0.001$) and to 1.3 ± 0.1 at the second examination.

With regard to *electrocardiography* the following observations were made: In the 27 patients without left bundle branch block the Sokolow Index decreased from 3.7±0.2 mV before treatment to 3.4±0.2 mV (*P*<0.05) at the first and to 3.2±0.2 mV (*P*<0.01 as compared to the control value) at the second examination. Moreover, the repolarization disturbances also improved. The sum of the maximal ST-T negativity in the precordial leads decreased from 5.1±0.2 mm before treatment to 4.0±0.2 mm (*P*<0.05) at the first examination and showed no further change at the second examination, in which it averaged 4.1±0.2 mm. AV nodal conduction abnormalities or significant increases in the P-R interval were never observed during the time of treatment.

Echocardiographic Measurements. At *control,* maximal septal thickness measured either in the outflow tract or in the corpus exceeded 13 mm in all 32 patients. The respective mean values were 18.8±0.1 mm in the outflow tract and 17.1±0.1 mm in the corpus in the 25 patients with obstruction, and 15.7±0.1 mm in the outflow tract and 14.1±0.1 mm in the corpus in the seven patients without obstruction. The ratio of septal to posterior wall thickness averaged 1.64±0.01 (the septum measured in the outflow tract) and 1.50±0.01 (the septum measured in the corpus) in the 25 patients with obstructive disease, and 1.54±0.04 (the septum measured in the

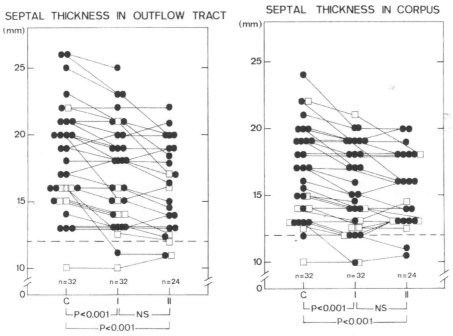

Fig. 3. Echocardiographic measurements of the septal thickness in the outflow tract and in the corpus before initiation of the treatment with verapamil (*C*), at the first examination (*I*) 6 months after therapy and at the second examination (*II*) performed after 12 months of therapy in the 32 patients with hypertrophic cardiomyopathy. The *black dots* represent the 25 patients with an obstructive form of the disease, the *open squares* the seven patients with a nonobstructive form. The interrupted lines indicate the upper limits of normal. In both regions a uniform trend of a decrease in septal thickness is noted during the treatment

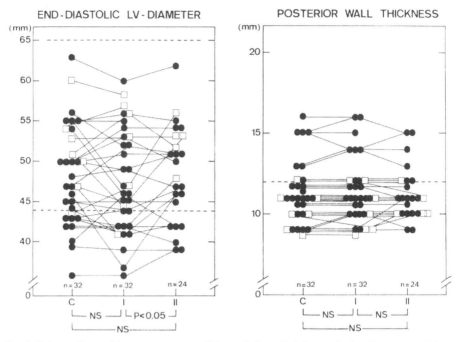

Fig. 4. Echocardiographic measurements of the end-diastolic left ventricular diameter and the posterior wall thickness before therapy (*C*), at the first (*I*) and at the second (*II*) examination during the treatment with verapamil in the same patient group. The *black dots* represent the 25 patients with an obstructive form of the disease, the *open squares* the seven patients with a nonobstructive form. The interrupted lines indicate the limits of normal. The end-diastolic left ventricular diameter did not change noticeably during the time of treatment nor did the posterior wall thickness

outflow tract) and 1.37 ± 0.04 (the septum measured in the corpus) in the seven patients with asymmetric nonobstructive cardiomyopathy.

During *treatment with verapamil* the thickness of the septum decreased significantly in both regions. For the entire group of 32 patients the respective mean values of septal thickness in the outflow tract decreased from 18.2 ± 0.1 mm before treatment to 17.1 ± 0.1 mm ($P<0.001$) at the first, and to 16.2 ± 0.1 mm (NS as compared to the first examination) at the second examination. In the corpus the respective mean values were 16.6 ± 0.1 mm before treatment, 15.3 ± 0.1 mm ($P<0.001$) at the first, and 15.3 ± 0.1 mm at the second examination (Fig. 3). The thickness of the posterior wall did not change during the time of therapy, averaging 11.3 ± 0.1 mm prior to initiation of the treatment, 11.4 ± 0.1 mm at the first, and 11.3 ± 0.1 mm at the second examination. In addition, left ventricular end-diastolic diameter also did not change noticeably; it averaged 48.3 ± 1.1 mm before treatment, 47.6 ± 1.1 mm (NS) at the first, and 48.8 ± 1.3 mm (NS as compared to the value before therapy, $P<0.05$ as compared to the value at the first examination) at the second examination (Fig. 4). In contrast, left atrial diameter decreased slightly from 41.4 ± 1.2 mm before treatment to 40.2 ± 1.3 mm ($P<0.05$) at the first examination. At the second examination it amounted again to 41.0 ± 1.6 mm. The heart rates were similar at all three examinations, averaging 69 ± 2 beats per minute at the control, 71 ± 2 beats per minute (NS) at the first, and 69 ± 3 beats per minute at the second examination.

In general treatment with verapamil at the moderate dose levels of 240–480 mg daily was well tolerated and side effects were noted in only a few patients at the beginning of therapy. Thus, three patients complained of intercurrent constipation and four patients of ache and fatigue. Dizziness attributable to systemic hypotension was never reported. Repeated blood pressure measurements revealed no changes either in systolic or in diastolic blood pressure. The respective mean values amounted to $126 \pm 2 / 78 \pm 1$ mmHg before treatment, to $128 \pm 2 / 78 \pm 1$ mmHg at the first and to $127 \pm 3 / 77 \pm 2$ mmHg at the second examination. Severe complications or adverse effects of the drug including excessive bradycardia, conduction abnormalities, or congestive heart failure were never observed. In no instance were side effects evident that forced us to interrupt the treatment or to reduce the dose of verapamil administered.

Two patients, however, did not respond satisfactorily to verapamil therapy. Since they both presented with severe outflow tract obstruction – the pressure gradient exceeding 150 mmHg in the postextrasystolic beat in both patients – they were operated on 6 months after initiation of therapy.

No deaths occurred in the 32 patients during the time of treatment.

Since the dosages of verapamil used in this study were smaller than the dosages used by others [7, 8], plasma concentrations of the drug were examined in a subgroup of 13 patients to evaluate whether the dosages would have been sufficiently high to be considered as therapeutically effective. Plasma concentrations determined 12 h after the last drug intake ranged between 20 and 180 ng/ml in 12 patients, whereas no measurable concentrations of verpamil were found in one patient. Moreover, these studies conducted in a randomly selected subgroup of patients at the time of the second examination (i.e., 12 months after initiation of therapy) permitted some insight into patient compliance, which still amounted to 83% at that time.

Discussion

This study demonstrates a beneficial effect of long-term treatment with the calcium antagonist verapamil (at dose levels of 240 to 480 mg/day) on the clinical symptomatology of patients with obstructive and nonobstructive hypertrophic cardiomyopathy. Furthermore it confirms the observations made earlier by Kaltenbach and associates [7, 8] that this specific treatment leads to a reduction of the electrocardiographic signs of left ventricular hypertrophy. The most important findings of this study, however, concern the echocardiographic measurements of the thickened interventricular septum. We found septal thickness decreased in the portion located in the left ventricular outflow tract as well as that located in the corpus. Posterior wall thickness, which was not hypertrophied in any patient, remained unaffected by treatment. In contrast to the findings reported by Schmid et al. [14], who noted an increase in left ventricular end-diastolic and end-systolic

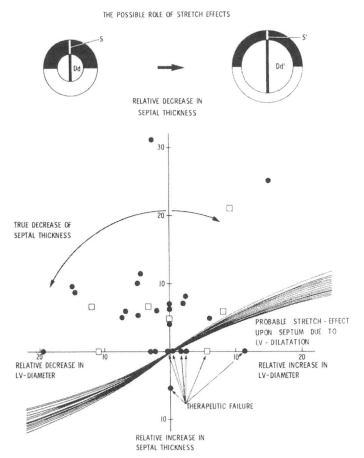

Fig. 5. Calculation of the relative changes in septal thickness which would have to be expected if a stretch effect upon the septum due to left ventricular dilatation occurred for each individual case as based on the two-dimensional model of the left ventricle cross-sectioned at its short axis and assuming that the septal muscle mass comprises half of the circumference as shown schematically (*top*). In comparing the actual values measured during the first period of treatment with the corresponding calculated changes (*curvilinear lines*) it is evident that the decrease in septal thickness cannot be explained by an increase in left ventricular diameter in 25 cases. Seven cases, however, show no response to the treatment and have thus to be regarded as therapeutic failures. The *black dots* represent the cases with an obstructive form of the disease, the open squares a nonobstructive form. *Dd*, end-diastolic left ventricular diameter; *S*, septal diameter

diameter following acute administration of verapamil, no enlargement of the left ventricular cavity was detected.

We recognize that the observed changes in septal thickness are small; but it would be unrealistic to expect an abundant shrinking of the thickened septum within a 6- or 12-month period of treatment. Although the trend of the decrease of septal thickness was uniform, and hence appeared to be valid, a critical evaluation of these striking results is mandatory. Since posterior wall thickness remained unaltered, as did left ventricular end-diastolic diameter during therapy, a thinning of the septum caused simply by a stretch effect upon the thickened muscle mass due to an increase in left ventricular volume seems unlikely. Nevertheless, we calculated the relative changes in septal thickness that would be expected if a stretch effect upon the septum due to left ventricular dilatation occurred for each individual patient. Calculations were based on a two-dimensional model of the left ventricle cross-sectioned at its short axis, assuming that the septal muscle mass comprises half of the circumference (Fig. 5, curvilinear lines). In comparing the actual values measured during the first period of treatment with the corresponding calculated changes it becomes evident that in 25 patients the decrease in septal thickness cannot be explained by an increase in left ventricular diameter. In seven cases, however, no response to the treatment is apparent, and these patients therefore have to be regarded as therapeutic failures.

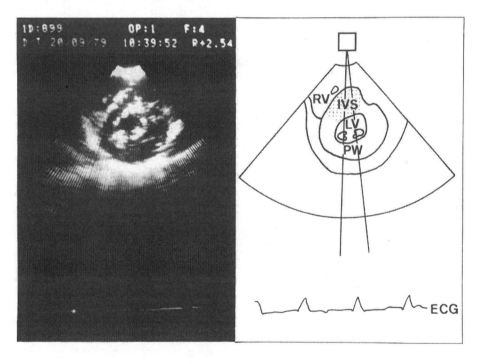

Fig. 6. Two-dimensional echocardiographic cross section through the left ventricle just below the plane of the mitral valve in a patient with a hypertrophic obstructive cardiomyopathy. *LV*, left ventricular cavity; *IVS*, interventricular septum; *PW*, posterior wall; and *RV*, right ventricular cavity. The two echo signals located within the left ventricular cavity arise from the papillary muscle tips. As is clearly visible the interventricular septum (*dotted area*) is not uniformly thickened throughout its cross section in this case. This, of course, could be of influence in measuring the diameter of the septum by single beam technique. A slight angulation of the transducer perpendicular to the plane of its rotation to record an aorto-apical sweep tracing as illustrated schematically by the two vertical lines originating from the same transducer results in a slightly different septal diameter

212   Heinz O. Hirzel et al.

More objections may concern the echocardiographic method itself. First, one has to be aware of the general difficulties related to the measurement of isolated septal hypertrophy by M-mode echocardiography. From pathology as well as from two-dimensional echo scans (Fig. 6), it is known that the pathologically hypertrophied septal mass may not be evenly distributed throughout the septum from base to apex and from anterior to posterior [11, 12]. Whereas sweeping of the echo beam from the aortic root to the apex of the heart definitely permits the localization of the thickened portion within the septum in its longitudinal axis, i.e., in the outflow tract region or in the corpus of the septum, a slightly altered angulation of the transducer perpendicular to the plane of the aorto-apical sweep could direct the echo beam more toward the lateral borders of a ball-shaped hypertrophy and thus result in an apparent smaller septal diameter. This could seriously affect serial measurements. Secondly, the resolution capability of the method may not be neglectable in measuring changes of the magnitude of 1–2 mm. And thirdly, detection of the true endocardial surfaces may sometimes become an additional problem [13].

Thus, further studies will certainly be needed to confirm these findings.

The fact that no severe complications or adverse effects of the drug were observed during the time of treatment might have been due in part to the policy of including in the study only those patients whose clinical symptomatology was mild to moderate and who did not need any additional medications. Patients with severe symptoms due to excessive outflow tract obstruction were referred to surgery. According to the experiences gained during the study it seems advisable to confine treatment with verapamil only to patients with hypertrophic obstructive and nonobstructive cardiomyopathy who are moderately symptomatic.

Summary

The results of this study show that long-term treatment with the calcium antagonist verapamil at moderate dose levels in patients with obstructive and nonobstructive hypertrophic cardiomyopathy favorably influences clinical symptoms and leads to a decrease of the electrocardiographic signs of left ventricular hypertrophy. Moreover, they demonstrate a reduction in septal thickness following therapy but no effect of the drug on posterior wall thickness or left ventricular end-diastolic diameter.

Acknowledgment. We wish to thank Miss Ruth Wegmueller for her careful assistance in the preparation of the manuscript.

References

1. Bulkley BH (1977) Idiopathic hypertrophic subaortic stenosis afflicted: Idols of the cave and the marketplace. Am J Cardiol 40:476–479
2. Goodwin JF (1980) Hypertrophic cardiomyopathy: A disease in search of its own identity. Am J Cardiol 45:177–180

Effects of Verapamil on Ventricular Wall Thickness 213

3. Witzke DJ, Kaye MP (1976) Hypertrophic cardiomyopathy induced by administration of nerve growth factor. Circulation [Suppl II] 54:II–88
4. Lossnitzer K (1975) Genetic induction of cardiomyopathy. In: Schmier J, Eichler O (eds) Heart and circulation. Springer, Berlin Heidelberg New York (Handbook of experimental Pharmacology, vol 16, p 309)
5. Fleckenstein A (1969) Myokardstoffwechsel und Nekrose. In: Heilmeyer L, Holtmeier HJ (eds) Herzinfarkt und Schock. Thieme, Stuttgart, p 94
6. Wrogemann K, Pena SDJ (1976) Mitochondrial calcium overload. A general mechanism for cell necrosis in muscle diseases. Lancet I:672–674
7. Kaltenbach M, Hopf R, Keller M (1976) Calciumantagonistische Therapie bei hypertroph-obstruktiver Kardiomyopathie. Dtsch Med Wochenschr 101:1284–1287
8. Kaltenbach M, Hopf R, Kober G, Bussmann WD, Keller M, Petersen Y (1979) Treatment of hypertrophic obstructive cardiomyopathy with verapamil. Br Heart J 42:35–42
9. Epstein SE, Henry WL, Clark CE, Roberts WC, Maron BJ, Ferrans VJ, Redwood DR, Morrow AG (1974) ASH. Ann Intern Med 81:650–680
10. King JF, De Maria AN, Reis RL, Bolton MR, Dunn MI, Mason DT (1973) Echocardiographic assessment of IHSS. Chest 64:723–731
11. Maron BJ, Gottdiener JS, Goldstein RE, Epstein SE (1978) Hypertrophic CMP: The great masquerader. Chest 6:659–670
12. Henry WL, Chester EC, Roberts WC, Morrow AG, Epstein SE (1974) Differences in distribution of myocardial abnormalities in patients with obstructive and nonobstructive asymmetric septal hypertrophy (ASH). Circulation 50:447–455
13. Henry WL, Clark CE, Epstein SE (1973) Asymmetric septal hypertrophy (ASH): Echocardiographic identification of the pathognomonic anatomic abnormality of IHSS. Circulation 47:225–233
14. Schmid P, Pavek P, Klein W (1979) Echokardiographische und haemodynamische Untersuchungen zur Beeinflussung der hypertrophischen obstruktiven Kardiomyopathie durch Verapamil. Z Kardiol 68:89–92

Long-Term Verapamil Treatment in Patients with Hypertrophic Nonobstructive Cardiomyopathy *

H. KUHN, U. THELEN, C. LEUNER, E. KÖHLER, V. BLUSCHKE, and F. LOOGEN

Summary

It was shown by different investigators that verapamil improves symptoms and possibly reduces myocardial hypertrophy in patients with hypertrophic obstructive cardiomyopathy. In order to study the effect in patients with hypertrophic nonobstructive cardiomyopathy (HNCM) the clinical course, the ECG, and the M-mode echocardiographic data were analyzed in patients with (group I, 14 patients) and without (group II, 18 patients) verapamil treatment ((group I: mean age 41 years, follow-up 16 ± 9 months, dosage of verapamil 240–480 mg (average $= 389$ mg); group II: mean age 39 years, follow-up 23 ± 7 months)). Clinical improvement occurred in three patients of group I and in no patient of group II. Six patients of group II and one patient of group I deteriorated by one clinical class (criteria of NYHA). One patient of group I (age 15 years) died after a traffic accident (heart weight at autopsy 1020 g). There were no significant changes in the ECG in both groups. The thickness of septum, however, decreased from 23.3 ± 6.6 mm to 21.6 ± 6.6 mm ($P<0.01$) in group I and was nearly unchanged (18.7 ± 4.6 mm/19.2 ± 3.4 mm) in group II. The posterior wall in group I was 14.3 ± 3.9 mm before treatment and decreased to 13.5 ± 5.3 mm after treatment ($P<0.05$). The corresponding values in group II were 13.2 ± 3.9 mm at the first examination and 12.9 ± 3.1 mm at the latest examination (not significant). The left ventricular end-diastolic diameter increased in both groups, i.e., from 40.2 ± 5.5 to 42.4 ± 4 mm ($P<0.05$) in group I and from 43.0 ± 5.4 to 45.4 ± 6.2 mm ($P<0.05$) in group II. The fractional shortening of the left ventricular end-diastolic diameter and the diameter of the left atrium did not change significantly.

Although the changes are very small and must be confirmed by additional studies before definitive conclusions can be drawn, the results suggest verapamil reduces left ventricular septal and free wall thickness. This could have occurred as a result of either a verapamil-induced regression of myocardial hypertrophy or dilatation of the left ventricle, caused perhaps by the negative inotropic effect of verapamil. Further prospective studies will have to show to what degree the present clinical and echocardiographic results reflect a definite therapeutic effect of verapamil in patients with HNCM.

It was shown by different investigators [1–4] that verapamil improves symptoms and possibly reduces myocardial hypertrophy in patients with hypertrophic obstructive cardiomyopathy (HOCM). The underlying mechanism of the

---

* With the technical assistance of M. Bosilj, MTA

apparently beneficial effect of verapamil in patients with HOCM is unknown (predominant effect on the myocardium of the left ventricle or clinical improvement by reduction of outflow tract obstruction?). Based on the favorable clinical effect of verapamil in HOCM and the unknown mechanism of this effect, a study was designed to evaluate the effect of verapamil in patients with the nonobstructive form of the disease (hypertrophic nonobstructive cardiomyopathy HNCM). Such a study was believed to be of interest for two reasons: First, in our experience patients with HNCM do not respond to beta blockers and, because of the absence of obstruction to left ventricular outflow, operation would be of no help; and second, because of the absence of an intraventricular pressure gradient, clinical improvement would suggest verapamil was exerting a direct effect on the hypertrophied myocardium.

Patients and Methods

The study comprised two groups of patients. Detailed technical, clinical, and diagnostic data of patients with HNCM have been published elsewhere [5, 6]. A schematic view of HNCM is shown in Fig. 1.

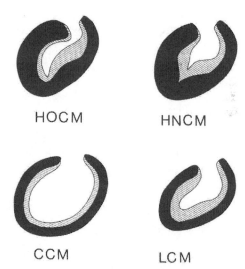

Fig. 1. Classification of idiopathic cardiomyopathies with a schematic view of the lateral projection of the left ventricle. The diastolic (*dark*) and the systolic (*hatched*) face of the ventriculogram is shown. In the LCM (latent cardiomyopathy) the ventriculogram and the shape of the left ventricle is normal; however, there is an impairment of ventricular function during exercise. The CCM (congestive cardiomyopathy or dilated cardiomyopathy) is characterized by a dilated left ventricle and reduced ejection fraction. In hypertrophic cardiomyopathy the septum and mostly also the ventricular wall are thickened because of muscular hypertrophy. In addition, there is intraventricular obstruction in HOCM (hypertrophic obstructive cardiomyopathy) and usually a funnel-like muscular obliteration of the apex in HNCM (hypertrophic nonobstructive cardiomyopathy)

216 H. Kuhn et al.

Group I consisted of 14 patients (mean age was 41 years, follow-up period was 16 ± 9 months and dosage of verapamil was 240–480 mg (average 389 mg). Group II consisted of 18 patients (control group, no verapamil treatment). Mean age was 39 years and follow-up time was 23 ± 7 months (mean $\pm$ SD).

The following criteria for the selection of patients were applied. Group I consisted of consecutive patients studied in whom good quality M-mode echocardiograms were obtained that allowed for quantitative analysis; in addition, patients were only accepted if they received no additional medical therapy and their place of residence was near Düsseldorf.

Group II included all consecutive patients studied who had a good quality echocardiogram and who (1) did not wish to undergo verapamil treatment using a high dosage (n = 5), (2) originally belonged to the verapamil group but in whom verapamil therapy had to be stopped (6–14 days after the onset of verapamil therapy) because of drug side effects (this subgroup consisted of three patients, who were included in group II 12–17 weeks after removal from group I), and (3) had been treated with other drugs (propranolol in six and digitalis in four).

The patients were examined every 3 months by physical examinations, ECG, phonocardiogram and carotid pulse tracing, and every 6 months in addition by M-mode echocardiography and X-ray of the chest.

The echocardiograms were analyzed by at least three independent physicians who did not know whether patients were in the verapamil or control group, or the date on which the echocardiograms were performed.

For statistical analysis the Wilcoxon test for paired data was used.

Results

Clinical Course

The results of the long-term follow-up studies are shown in Fig. 2. Seven patients deteriorated, six of whom were in the control group (group II); one patient treated with verapamil (group I) deteriorated. One additional patient of group I died. She was a 15-year-old girl (heart weight at autopsy 1020 g) who died immediately after a severe traffic accident [6]. Three patients improved by one functional class (NYHA criteria): Each of these was in the verapamil treatment group. The cardiothoracic ratio during follow up was unchanged: 0.5 ± 0.06 (mean $\pm$ SD) and 0.51 ± 0.07 in group I, and 0.51 ± 0.06 and 0.52 ± 0.07 in group II.

Severe clinical complications during treatment with verapamil were not observed. Because of side effects (headache, dizziness, nausea, heartburn) the dosage of verapamil had to be reduced in three patients and the treatment had to be stopped in three additional patients. The patients with reduced dosage remained in group I. However, the patients in whom treatment had to be stopped were excluded from group I and put in group II (see patients and methods).

Heart rate and blood pressure (cuff method) did not change significantly. The heart rate was 72 ± 3 before the verapamil treatment was started and 70 ± 3 beats/min at the end of the trial (group I). The corresponding values in group II were 70 ± 2 and 68 ± 4 beats/min. The blood pressure was $133 \pm 4/83 \pm 2$ mmHg

Fig. 2. Long-term follow up studies in patients with HNCM ———, verapamil group (n = 14, follow-up 16 ± 9 months); – – – –, control group (n = 18, follow-up 23 ± 7 months)

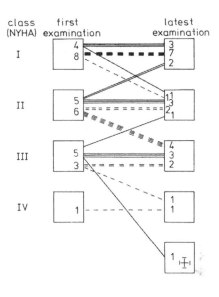

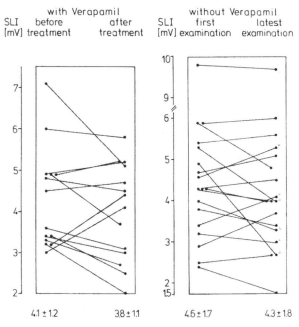

Fig. 3. Changes of Sokolow Lion index during follow-up in patients with HNCM with and without verapamil treatment. The asterisks represent the patients who were treated with propranolol

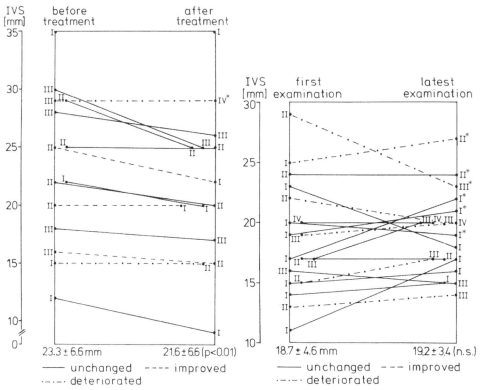

Fig. 4. Echocardiographic data and functional class (related to each patient) (NYHA criteria) in the course of patients with HNCM with treatment with verapamil. ─────, patients whose functional class was unchanged; ─ ─ ─ ─, patients who improved; ─·─·─·─, patients who deteriorated (n = 14, x̄ = 16 months). *Asterisks* represent the patients who were treated with propranolol. On the bottom of the figure the mean values ± SD of the different echocardiographic data are shown. Thickness of intraventricular septum (*IVS*)

Fig. 5. Echocardiographic data and functional class (related to each patient) (NYHA criteria) in the course of patients with HNCM without treatment with verapamil. ─────, patients whose functional class was unchanged; ─ ─ ─ ─, patients who improved; ─·─·─·─, patients who deteriorated (n = 18, x̄ = 23 months). *Asterisks* represent the patients who were treated with propranolol. On the bottom of the figure the mean values ± SD of the different echocardiographic data are shown. Thickness of intraventricular septum (*IVS*)

before therapy and 134±3/85±2 mmHg at the latest examination in group I. In group II these values were 138±3/84±3 mmHg and 140±5/85±3 mmHg respectively (mean ±SD).

Electrocardiogram

The Sokolow Lion index declined, but not significantly, in both groups: in group I from 4.1±1.2 to 3.8±1.1 mV and in group II from 4.6±1.7 to 4.3±1.8 mV (Fig. 3).

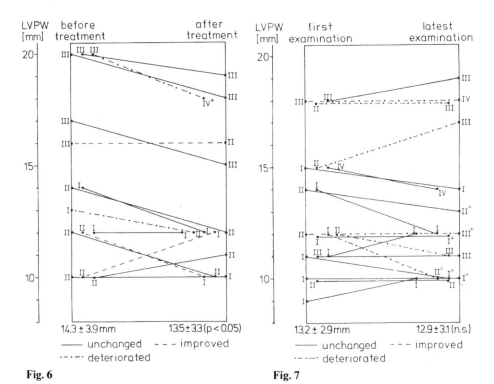

Fig. 6. Echocardiographic data and functional class (related to each patient) (NYHA criteria) in the course of patients with HNCM with treatment with verapamil. ———, patients whose functional class was unchanged; — — — —, patients who improved; — · — · — · —, patients who deteriorated (n = 14, x̄ = 16 months). *Asterisks* represent the patients who were treated with propranolol. On the bottom of the figure the mean values ± SD of the different echocardiographic data are shown. Thickness of left intraventricular posterior wall (*LVPW*)

Fig. 7. Echocardiographic data and functional class (related to each patient) (NYHA criteria) in the course of patients with HNCM without treatment with verapamil. ———, patients whose functional class was unchanged; — — — —, patients who improved; — · — · — · —, patients who deteriorated (n = 18, x̄ = 23 months). *Asterisks* represent the patients who were treated with propranolol. On the bottom of the figure the mean values ± SD of the different echocardiographic data are shown. Thickness of left intraventricular posterior wall (*LVPW*)

The amplitude of T-waves increased, decreased, or remained unchanged to the same degree in both groups. The depression of ST-segment remained unchanged.

Echocardiogram

In Figs. 4–9 and in Tab. 1 the echocardiographic data of both groups are shown. There was a very small but significant decrease of the thickness of the intraventricular septum and of the posterior wall of left ventricle in group I, and a

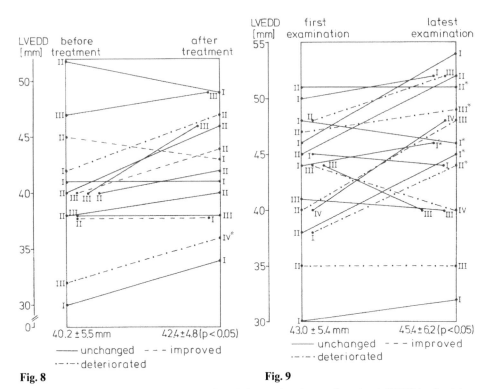

Fig. 8. Echocardiographic data and functional class (related to each patient) (NYHA criteria) in the course of patients with HNCM with treatment with verapamil. ———, patients whose functional class was unchanged; — — — —, patients who improved; —·—·—·—, patients who deteriorated (n=14). *Asterisks* represent the patients who were treated with propranolol. On the bottom of the figure the mean values ±SD of the different cardiographic data are shown. Left ventricular end-diastolic diameter (*LVEDD*)

Fig. 9. Echocardiographic data and functional class (related to each patient) (NYHA criteria) in the course of patients with HNCM without treatment with verapamil. ———, patients whose functional class was unchanged; — — — —, patients who improved; —·—·—·—, patients who deteriorated (n=18, $\bar{x}$=23 months). *Asterisks* represent the patients who were treated with propranolol. On the bottom of the figure the mean values ±SD of the different echocardiographic data are shown. Left ventricular end-diastolic diameter (*LVEDD*)

significant increase of left ventricular end-diastolic diameter in group I and in group II. No relations between clinical and echocardiographic changes were observed.

Discussion

In the present paper we evaluated the effects of verapamil on the clinical and echocardiographic changes found during long-term follow-up of patients with hypertrophic nonobstructive cardiomyopathy (HNCM). The following alterations in the clinical course were observed. Seven patients deteriorated, – only one of these belonging to the verapamil group, and six to the control group. Three patients improved by one functional class and all of those were in the verapamil treatment group. In addition, these three patients are the only ones who improved out of a total of 37 patients with HNCM in whom long-term follow-up studies have been performed (mean follow-up: 5.7 years), including eight patients treated with propranolol (six of these eight patients being in the control group of this trial) (Fig. 10) [5].

These results indicate that verapamil treatment could turn out superior to no treatment and to propranolol treatment in patients with HNCM (in our experience patients with HNCM do not improve with beta blocker therapy). However, one has to consider that to date no randomized studies using beta blockers in patients with HNCM have been performed and that in this study some conditions of the verapamil group and the control group were different: the mean follow-up period was 16 months in group I and 23 months in group II; the thickness of intraventricular septum was 23.3 mm and 18.7 mm respectively, which indicates a different state of the disease; no patients in group II were treated with verapamil; however, some were treated with beta blockers or digitalis, whereas in group I the only drug administered was verapamil.

The Sokolow Lion index in the ECG tended to decrease in patients with HNCM treated with verapamil – a finding similar to that in patients with HOCM being treated with verapamil [1]. However, this decline was also observed in the control group, and in each the change was not statistically significant. Although one cannot exclude the possibility that significant differences will become evident after the

Table 1. Echocardiographic data in patients with (group I) and without (group II) verapamil treatment before and after treatment and at the first and at the latest examination respectively

	Group I (Verapamil) (n = 14, follow-up 16 ± 9 months)				Group II (Control) (n = 18, follow-up 23 ± 7 months)			
	Before treatment		After treatment		First examination		Latest examination	
	$\bar{x}$	$\pm$ SD	$\bar{x}$	$\pm$ SD	$\bar{x}$	$\pm$ SD	$\bar{x}$	$\pm$ SD
IVS (mm)	23.3	6.6	21.6	6.6[a]	18.7	4.6	19.2	3.4 ns
LVPW (mm)	14.3	3.9	13.5	3.3[b]	13.2	2.9	12.9	3.1 ns
IVS/LVPW	1.7	0.8	1.7	0.7 ns	1.5	0.4	1.6	0.3 ns
LVEDD (mm)	40.2	5.5	42.4	4.8[b]	43.0	5.4	45.4	6.2[b]
FS (%)	41.9	8.7	37.5	5.8 ns	38.1	8.1	37.5	8.3 ns
LA (mm)	42.1	8.2	42.7	4.8 ns	41.6	7.3	43.1	6.4 ns

IVS, intraventricular septum; LVPW, left ventricular posterior wall; LVEDD, left ventricular end-diastolic diameters; FS, fractional shortening of LVEDD; LA, diameter of left atrium; ns, not significant.
[a] $P<0.01$ [b] $P<0.05$

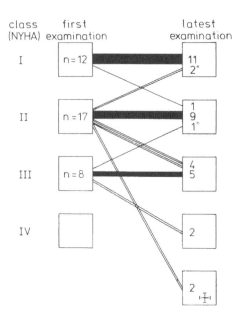

Fig. 10. Changes of functional class (criteria of NYHA) during long-term follow-up studies in patients with HNCM (n=37, mean follow-up time=5.1 years (range 1–20 years) [5])

verapamil group is followed for as long as the control group, our study does not permit such a conclusion to be drawn.

Pronounced "improvement" of the ECG, as was found in patients with HOCM being treated with verapamil [1] or in very rare patients with propranolol [7], were not observed in our patients with HNCM. In addition, there were no different changes in the ST segment or the T waves in either group. These data demonstrate that verapamil does not seem to influence the ECG in the same way in patients with HNCM as it does in patients with HOCM.

The echocardiographic data, however, did reveal differences between the treated and control group. The only significant change in the control group was an increase of left ventricular end-diastolic diameter, whereas in the verapamil group, besides the significant increase of left ventricular end-diastolic diameter, a significant reduction of the thickness of the intraventricular septum and of the posterior wall of the left ventricle was seen. No significant changes in fractional shortening were observed in either group.

Unfortunately, a definitive interpretation of these findings is not possible. The echocardiographic alterations between the beginning and the end of the study cannot be ascribed to heart rate and blood pressure changes, as these remained unaltered in both groups. However, it is possible that the increase of left ventricular end-diastolic diameter may have been caused by an ellipsoid deformation or a compensatory dilatation of the left ventricle during the natural course of the disease. If so, these changes could result from an increase of heart muscle hypertrophy in the apex of the left ventricle (i.e., the site where the muscular thickening of the ventricular wall is often most pronounced in patients with HNCM (Fig. 1) [5, 8]). However, this explanation does not account for the significantly smaller left ventricular end-diastolic diameter found in patients showing a more advanced clinical stage of the disease (functional class II and III) (Table 2). Hence, it is unlikely that the decrease in intraventricular septal and of posterior wall thickness is due to the dilatation of the left ventricle during the natural course of patients with HNCM. Alternatively, it appears more likely that these changes in the verapamil group are the consequence of either a verapamil-induced regression of cardiac

Table 2. Correlation of echocardiographic and hemodynamic data to the functional class (NYHA) in patients with HNCM (n = 41) [5]

		Class		Class	P
IVS/PW	1.9 ± 0.7	I + II	1.2 ± 0.4	III + IV	< 0.01
PW (mm)	12 ± 3	I + II	17 ± 3	III + IV	< 0.01
LVEDD (mm)	46 ± 6	I	40 ± 6	II + III	< 0.05
LVEDP (mmHg)	14 ± 4	I + II	18 ± 9	III + IV	< 0.025
EDVI (ml.m^{-2})	82 ± 15	I	70 ± 16	II + III	< 0.05
C-T ratio	0.50 ± 0.05	I + II	0.54 ± 0.04	III + IV	< 0.025

IVS, intraventricular septum; LVEDP, left ventricular end-diastolic pressure; EDVI, end-diastolic volume index; C-T ratio, cardiothoratic ratio

hypertrophy or of a negative inotropic effect of verapamil. The possibility of a negative inotropic effect is supported by the tendency for left ventricular fractional shortening to diminish, a change, however, that was not statistically significant.

In summary, the clinical and echocardiographic data demonstrate that verapamil treatment in patients with HNCM leads to changes that are not observed in patients untreated with verapamil. However, additional prospective studies will be needed to show whether the present clinical results reflect an actual therapeutic effect of verapamil and whether the small echocardiographic changes observed are consistent and indicative of an actual decrease in muscle mass.

References

1. Kaltenbach M, Hopf R, Kober G, Bussmann W-D, Keller M, Petersen Y (1979) Treatment of hypertrophic obstructive cardiomyopathy with Verapamil. Br Heart J 42:35
2. Milazzotto F, Ceci V, Romei E, Malinconico U, Massini V (1980) Treatment of hypertrophic obstructive cardiomyopathy: Comparison between Verapamil and Pindolol therapy. Eur Congr Cardiol, Abstract Nr 350, Paris
3. Rosing DR, Kent KM, Maron BJ, Epstein SE (1979) Verapamil therapy: A new approach of the pharmacologic treatment of hypertrophic cardiomyopathy. II. Effects on exercise capacity and symptomatic status. Circulation 50:1208
4. Troesch M, Hirzel HO, Jeussi R, Krayenbühl P (1979) Reduction of septal thickness following Verapamil in patients with asymmetric septal hypertrophy (ASH). Circulation [Suppl II] 59, 60:604
5. Kuhn H, Thelen U, Köhler E, Lösse B (1980) Die hypertrophische nicht obstruktive Kardiomyopathie (HNCM) – Klinische, hämodynamische, elektro-, echo- und angiokardiographische Untersuchungen. Z Kardiol 69:457

6. Kuhn H, Thelen U, Leuner C, Köhler E, Bluschke V (1980) Langzeitbehandlung der hypertrophischen nicht obstruktiven Kardiomyopathie (HNCM) mit Verapamil. Z Kardiol 69:669
7. Loogen F, Gleichmann U, Krelhaus W (1971) Die obstruktive Myokardiopathie. Z Kreislf 60:1044
8. Yamaguchi H, Ischimura T, Nishiyama S, Nagasaki F, Nakanishi S, Takatsu F, Nishija T, Umeda T, Machii K (1979) Hypertrophic nonobstructive cardiomyopathy with giant negative T-waves (apical hypertrophy) Ventriculographic and echocardiographic features in 30 patients. Am J Cardiol 44:401

Verapamil: Its Potential for Causing Serious Complications in Patients with Hypertrophic Cardiomyopathy *

STEPHEN E. EPSTEIN and DOUGLAS R. ROSING

Verapamil is an important drug in the symptomatic treatment of patients with hypertrophic cardiomyopathy [1–3]. As with many potent drugs, however, the potential exists for the occurrence of adverse actions. These adverse actions might be further potentiated in patients with hypertrophic cardiomyopathy by the dynamic nature of the left ventricular outflow obstruction peculiar to such patients.

In the past 3 years we have administered verapamil to 120 patients with hypertrophic cardiomyopathy. Although the incidence of serious or potentially serious complications we have observed is relatively low, the fact that they have occurred has caused us concern. The impetus for this particular review, therefore, derives both from our concern about these occasional clinically important hemodynamic complications, and from the fact that verapamil is being used with rapidly increasing frequency for the treatment of patients with this disorder.

Because the absolute number of verapamil-induced complications we have observed is small, the basic format of this paper consists of (1) a theoretical analysis of how the known electrophysiologic and hemodynamic actions of verapamil *might* result in deleterious effects in patients with hypertrophic cardiomyopathy, and (2) brief, largely anecdotal presentations of the *actual* complications we have observed, which serve to illustrate the point that the theoretical potential for verapamil to cause deleterious effects may indeed lead to serious complications in the susceptible patient.

Patient Selection and Verapamil Dosage

Our criteria for deciding which patients with hypertrophic cardiomyopathy should receive the drug have been detailed previously [2], and are based mainly on unsatisfactory control of symptoms with propranolol. Verapamil dosages employed have also been detailed previously [2, 3]. Patients usually are started in hospital on 80 mg every 8 h; if no adverse side effects occur after 48 h, the dose is increased to 120 mg every 8 h. Higher doses (up to 640 mg/day) are employed during follow-up if complications have not occurred and if symptoms have not been adequately controlled on the standard dose.

---

* This paper has already been published in *Circulation*, September 1981

Suppression of Sinus Node Automaticity and Inhibition of AV Nodal Conduction

The incidence and type of these complications in our series is depicted in Table 1. Verapamil directly suppresses sinus node pacemaker activity and is one of the most potent inhibitors of AV nodal conduction [4–6]. Under usual circumstances, depression of the sinus node is not evident since the hypotensive actions of the drug lead to baroreceptor mediated reflex changes of autonomic tone to the sinus node

Table 1. Hypertrophic cardiomyopathy. Nonfatal electrophysiologic and hemodynamic complications associated with oral verapamil treatment (120 patients)

Electrophysiologic complications	Incidence of complications
Sinus arrest	2%
Sinus bradycardia with JER and ID	11%
Type I 2nd Degree AV block	3%
Type II 2nd Degree AV Block	1%
Hemodynamic complications	
Postural Hypotension[a]	3%

JER, junctional escape rhythm; ID, isorhythmic dissociation; AV, atrioventricular.
[a] Exclusive of patients who died (WG, Table 2) or developed pulmonary edema (PS, Table 2) in association with hypotension, and those who experienced hypotension when also taking quinidine (patients J.JE, J.J.U, and I.L; Table 3).

(sympathetic stimulation and parasympathetic withdrawal), thereby minimizing any tendency toward sinus slowing. Not uncommonly, however, sinus node depression becomes evident. Most often it manifests itself as mild bradycardia, usually associated with a junctional escape rhythm that superficially resembles complete heart block, but which on further analysis can be identified as isorhythmic dissociation (Fig. 1). Rarely, sinus arrest appears [2], although this complication probably occurs largely in patients with underlying abnormalities of sinus node pacemaker activity.

The first clinical sign of electrophysiologic effect usually is prolongation of AV nodal conduction, manifest by PR prolongation on the ECG [7, 8]. If given in high enough doses, however, verapamil can lead to complete heart block [6, 9, 10]. Since verapamil does not appear to inhibit all forms of junctional automaticity [6], it can be expected that a junctional rhythm will emerge at a reasonable rate. Nonetheless, patients with hypertrophic cardiomyopathy are singularly susceptible to abnormalities producing AV dissociation. Because of the diminished compliance of the left ventricle in this disease, loss of a synchronized contribution of atrial contraction to ventricular filling can lead to hypotension which, in turn, could cause

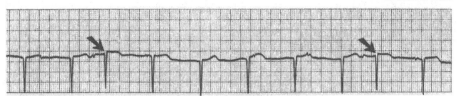

Fig. 1. Electrocardiogram demonstrating atrioventricular dissociation with occasional captured ventricular beats (*arrows*) appearing following the initiation of verapamil treatment

an increase in obstruction to left ventricular outflow. A vicious cycle is thereby established, leading to further hypotension, further obstruction, etc. The potent vasodilatory actions of verapamil would only exacerbate this sequence of events.

Vasodilatation

We have shown that verapamil, administered intravenously to patients in the cardiac catheterization laboratory, usually diminishes the gradient present in patients with hypertrophic cardiomyopathy who have obstruction to left ventricular outflow [8]. However, excessive vasodilatation can lead to serious hemodynamic consequences. Thus, if verapamil causes a marked drop in blood pressure, a paradoxical *increase* in left ventricular outflow obstruction can occur. The mechanisms responsible for this presumably derive from both the decrease in afterload and the resulting reflex increase in sympathetic stimulation to the heart. Each of these actions, by increasing the velocity of left ventricular ejection, can exacerbate the gradient [11].

Fig. 2 is an example of this occurring in the catheterization laboratory following i.v. administration of verapamil. As systemic systolic blood pressure decreased from 160 to 105 mmHg, left ventricular outflow tract gradient increased from 35 to approximately 80 mmHg. While the gradient quickly returned to control values in this particular patient after cessation of verapamil infusion, it is easily appreciated how the combination of a large decrease in blood pressure (with associated decrease in coronary perfusion pressure) and high intraventricular pressures could either lead directly to cardiac arrest, or cause progressive elevation of left ventricular filling pressures, which ultimately might deteriorate into frank pulmonary edema.

This same sequence of events probably was operative in at least two patients in whom verapamil was given orally. Patient J. J. U. (Table 3) developed lightheadedness and near syncope when arising from bed. Systolic blood pressure was 70 mmHg and shortly thereafter frank pulmonary edema developed. This occurred in the hospital after his thirteenth dose of oral verapamil (80 mg three times per day for six doses, and 120 mg three times per day for seven doses). This patient also was taking quinidine at the time verapamil was begun. Patient PS had a similar episode. When this patient's blood pressure decreased on verapamil (from control values of 150/100 to 110/70 mmHg) the intensity of his murmur increased (suggesting increased left ventricular outflow obstruction). These changes were accompanied by more severe shortness of breath and elevation of his pulmonary artery wedge pressure from 20 to 32 mmHg. In addition to these more serious complications, administration of verapamil orally was associated with postural hypotension, which did not lead to any congestive symptoms, in another three (3%) of our patients.

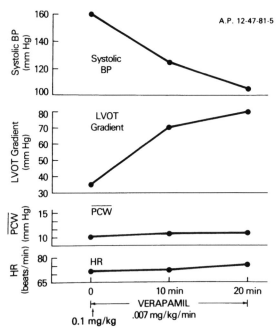

Fig. 2. Increase in left ventricular outflow tract gradient occurring following a verapamil-induced marked fall in systemic arterial pressure

Negative Inotropic Effects

Verapamil has been shown to be capable of decreasing myocardial contractility in vitro at high concentration [12, 13]. Although some studies have demonstrated verapamil-induced depression in contractility in vivo [9, 14], other studies have failed to elicit such an effect [15–17]. These conflicting results may be a consequence of different drug doses used, different experimental models, and differences in the relative contributions of the direct and indirect actions of verapamil in the various studies.

Whether hemodynamically important negative inotropic effects occur in patients with hypertrophic cardiomyopathy is uncertain. We have employed radionuclide cineangiography to measure change in contractile function and found that neither left ventricular ejection fraction nor rate of ejection was altered by verapamil in patients with hypertrophic cardiomyopathy studied [18]. Hence, although the negative inotropic activity of verapamil may theoretically result in major hemodynamic complications in patients with hypertrophic cardiomyopathy, no evidence currently exists suggesting that such complications have followed administration of the drug.

Sudden Death

Fig. 3 summarizes the potential mechanisms by which verapamil could lead to sudden death in patients with hypertrophic cardiomyopathy. The major factor predisposing to verapamil-induced fatal consequences is based on the sensitivity of patients with the obstructive form of the disease to hypotension; a fall in systemic pressure can increase obstruction to left ventricular outflow by both decreasing afterload and reflexly increasing sympathetic stimulation to the heart. The result is systemic hypotension with persistently high left ventricular pressures. These high intraventricular pressures would make the left ventricle particularly vulnerable to the decrease in coronary perfusion pressure occurring as a result of the systemic hypotension. As a consequence, primary arrhythmic death, or increased left ventricular filling pressures and pulmonary edema might be precipitated.

That these mechanisms by which verapamil might potentially lead to serious complications are not entirely theoretical is suggested by the eleven patients who experienced fatal (three patients) or serious (eight patients) hemodynamic complications while taking oral verapamil (Tables 2, 3). It should be emphasized that patients with hypertrophic cardiomyopathy die as a natural consequence of their disease, often making it difficult to attribute unequivocally a causal role of any drug in the death of a patient. In this regard, one (W. G.) of the three deaths seemed to be a direct consequence of the initiation of verapamil. This one patient was stable

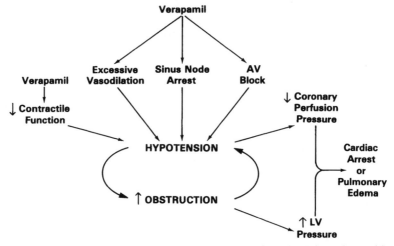

Fig. 3. Potential mechanisms by which verapamil could lead to sudden death in patients with hypertrophic cardiomyopathy

Table 2. Hypertrophic cardiomyopathy. Deaths and serious hemodynamic complications associated with oral verapamil treatment

Pt	Hx	PCW (mmHg)	LVOT Gradient (mmHg)	Verapamil dose (Blood level)	Outcome
WG	SOB at rest	14	110	120 qid (75 ng/ml)	Hypotension → Pulm edema → Death
FK	Pulm edema	22–26	62	120 tid	Pulm edema → Death
ME	Orthopnea	–	100	120 qid (50 ng/ml)	Pulm edema → Death
JH	Pulm edema	–	0	80 qid (165–230 ng/ml)	Pulm edema → Survival
PS	–	20	Marked SAM	80 qid (540 ng/ml)	Relative hypotension → Pulm edema → Survival
LO	PND	11	30 (→90)	120 tid (210 ng/ml)	Pulm edema → Survival
HF	Orthopnea	20	100	80 tid	Pulm edema → Survival
FN	–	14	50	120 tid	Pulm edema → Survival

SOB, shortness of breath; Pulm edema, pulmonary edema; PND, paroxysmal nocturnal dyspnea; Pt, patient; HX, history; PCW, mean pulmonary capillary wedge pressure; LVOT, left ventricular outflow tract; SAM, systolic anterior motion of the mitral valve; CHF, congestive heart failure; (→90), effect of provocation on gradient.

clinically and died in hospital after receiving only four 120 mg doses of verapamil. The other two patients died out of hospital, 5 weeks and 9 months after initiation of drug therapy. Whether they died *because* of verapamil or *despite* it cannot of course be determined. However, the clinical setting strongly suggested that most of the 11 patients with serious complications (Tables 2, 3) experienced a complication of drug therapy. In seven of the 11 patients the complication occurred in hospital. Each of these seven patients had been clinically stable at the time of admission; symptoms appeared in hospital shortly following initiation of verapamil treatment alone in four patients, after the addition of verapamil to quinidine in one patient, and after the addition of quinidine to verapamil in two patients.

Although it is difficult to generalize from such a small series of patients, the following features bear emphasis. Most importantly, all but three of the 11 patients had either a history indicative of severely elevated pulmonary venous pressures, or had pulmonary venous pressures of 20 mmHg more as measured at catheterization. This proportion of patients with evidence of elevated pulmonary venous pressures represents a disproportionately high percentage of patients who were treated

Verapamil: Its Potential for Causing Serious Complications 231

chronically with verapamil. In addition, of the six patients in whom verapamil blood level measurements were made, only one patient experiencing a serious complication believed to be due to verapamil exhibited an excessively high level of the drug. Although all but one patient with serious complications had marked obstruction to left ventricular outflow either at rest or with provocation, firm conclusions cannot be drawn from this observation, since most of the patients we have treated thus far have had the obstructive form of the disease.

In our current series of 120 patients given oral verapamil, other potentially less catastrophic complications have occurred, which we believe were due to verapamil (Table 1): these include sinus arrest, sinus bradycardia with junctional escape rhythm and isorhythmic dissociation, and types I and II second degree heart block. In all, approximately 17% of patients manifested electrophysiologic side effects during initiation of verapamil treatment. Moreover, three patients (3%) developed postural hypotension (without associated pulmonary edema) during oral administration of verapamil (in the absence of quinidine). Because of the close relation between onset of hypotension and initiation of verapamil treatment, as well as disappearance of hypotension upon reduction of verapamil dosage, the hypotension appears likely to be drug regulated. Although patients may experience significant symptoms in association with these electrophysiologic and hemodynamic effects, only rarely does the drug have to be discontinued because of persisting abnormalities despite decrease in dosage. However, each of these side effects, by predisposing to hypotension, has the potential of causing more serious hemodynamic complications (Fig. 3).

Of note, three patients developed significant hypotension when verapamil was administered in conjunction with quinidine, and two of the three developed acute pulmonary edema concident with the hypotension (Table 3). Further studies must

Table 3. Serious complications associated with concomitant administration of verapamil and quinidine

Pt	Hx	PCW	LVOT Gradient	Quinidine	Verapamil	Pulm edema	hypotension
J.JE	–	18	80	320 mg for 3 doses	120 mg tid	No	Blood pressure unobtainable when standing, lightheaded, diaphoretic, short burst of VT
J.JU	–	15	80	300 mg qid	120 mg qid for 13 doses	Yes	Yes
IL	PND	10	130	600 mg for 3 doses; 200 mg for 1 dose	120 mg qid	Yes	Yes

▢ ,drug added to first drug (verapamil to quinidine or quinidine to verapamil), following which the adverse effect occurred. Abbreviations as for Table 2; VT, ventricular tachycardia.

be performed to determine whether quinidine and other antiarrhythmic drugs do exacerbate the deleterious hemodynamic effects of verapamil. Until definitive studies are available, however, their concomitant use should be undertaken only with extreme caution.

Conclusions

The considerations presented in this paper suggest that verapamil may lead to serious hemodynamic complications in patients with hypertrophic cardiomyopathy. Such serious complications probably occur rarely, but their incidence may be further reduced by careful selection of patients. Based on our series of observations, we have tentatively adopted the following policy regarding the administration of verapamil to patients with hypertrophic cardiomyopathy.

The drug probably is contraindicated in patients who have:

1. High pulmonary capillary wedge pressures in the presence of obstruction to left ventricular outflow
2. A previous history of paroxysmal nocturnal dyspnea or orthopnea in the presence of obstruction to left ventricular outflow
3. Sick sinus syndrome without an implanted pacemaker
4. Significant atrioventricular junctional disease without an implanted pacemaker

The drug should be given only when other alternatives are unavailable and only with extreme caution to patients with:

1. High pulmonary capillary wedge pressures in the absence of obstruction to left ventricular outflow
2. A previous history of paroxysmal nocturnal dyspnea or orthopnea in the absence of obstruction to left ventricular outflow
3. Low systolic blood pressure, particularly in the presence of left ventricular outflow obstruction

The drug can probably be given, but with caution, to patients with:

1. Systolic hypertension and marked obstruction to left ventricular outflow (see Fig. 2)
2. Moderate prolongation of the PR interval on the ECG

In summary, we believe verapamil is extremely important to the treatment of patients with hypertrophic cardiomyopathy. However, the basic physiologic actions of the drug can lead to serious adverse effects. An appreciation of this fact, in addition to an understanding of the situations in which these mechanisms would most likely be operative, will minimize any potential of verapamil to cause serious complications in patients with hypertrophic cardiomyopathy.

References

1. Kaltenbach M, Hopf R, Kober G, Bussman W-D, Keller M, Peterson Y (1979) Treatment of hypertrophic obstructive cardiomyopathy with verapamil. Br Heart J 42:35–42
2. Rosing DR, Kent KM, Maron BJ, Epstein SE (1979) Verapamil therapy: A new approach to the pharmacologic treatment of hypertrophic cardiomyopathy. II. Effects on exercise capacity and symptomatic status. Circulation 60:1208–1213
3. Rosing DR, Condit J, Maron BJ, Kent KM, Leon MB, Bonow RO, Lipson LC, Epstein SE (1981) Verapamil therapy: A new approach to the pharmacologic treatment of hypertrophic cardiomyopathy. III. Effects of long-term administration. Am J Cardiol 48:545–553
4. Zipes DP, Fischer JC (1974) Effects of agents which inhibit the slow channel on sinus node automaticy and atrioventricular conduction in the dog. Circ Res 34:184
5. Wit AL, Cranefield PG (1974) The effect of verapamil on the sinoatrial and atrioventricular nodes of the rabbit and the mechanism by which it arrests in reentrant AV nodal tachycardia. Circ Res 35:413
6. Urthaler F, James TN (1979) Experimental studies on the pathogenesis of asystole after verapamil in the dog. Am J Cardiol 44:651–656
7. Heng MK, Singh BN, Roche AHG, Norris RM, Mercer CJ (1975) Effects of intravenous verapamil on cardiac arrhythmias and on the electrocardiogram. Am Heart J 90:487–498
8. Rosing DR, Kent KM, Borer JS, Seides SF, Maron BJ, Epstein SE (1979) Verapamil therapy: A new approach to the pharmacologic treatment of hypertrophic cardiomyopathy. I. Hemodynamic effects. Circulation 60:1201–1207
9. Singh BN, Ellrodt G, Peter CT (1978) Verapamil: A review of its pharmacological properties and therapeutic use. Drugs 15:169–171
10. Rosen MR, Wit AL, Hoffman BF (1975) Electrophysiology and pharmacology of cardiac arrhythmias. VI. Cardiac effects of verapamil. Am Heart J 89:665–673
11. Epstein SE, Henry WL, Clark CE, Roberts WC, Maron BJ, Ferrans VJ, Redwood DR, Morrow AG (1974) Asymmetric septal hypertrophy. Ann Intern Med 81:650–680
12. Fleckenstein A, Döring HJ, Kammermeier H (1968) Beziehung zwischen den Spiegeln an energiereichen Phosphat und verschiedenen Insuffizienzformen. In: Reindell H, Keul J, Doll E (eds) Herzinsuffizienz Pathophysiologie und Klinik. Internat Symposium, 2.–5. Nov 1967, Hinterzarten. Thieme, Stuttgart, pp 216–226
13. Nayler WG, Szeto J (1972) Effect of verapamil on contractility oxygen utilization, and calcium exchangeability in mammalian heart muscle. Cardiovasc Res 6:120–128
14. Newman RK, Bishop VS, Peterson DF, Leroux EJ, Horwitz LD (1977) Effect of verapamil on left ventricular performance in conscious dogs. J Pharmacol Exp Ther 201:723–730
15. Atterhög JH, Ekelund LG (1975) Hemodynamic effects of intravenous verapamil at rest and during exercise in subjectively healthy middle-aged men. Eur J Clin Pharmacol 8:317–322
16. Seabra-Gomes R, Richards A, Sutton R (1976) Hemodynamic effects of verapamil and practalol in man. Eur J Cardiol 4:79–85
17. Smith HJ, Goldstein RA, Griffith JM, Kent KM, Epstein SE (1976) Regional contractility. Selective depression of ischemic myocardium by verapamil. Circulation 54:629–635
18. Bonow RO, Rosing DR, Bacharach SL, Green MV, Kent KM, Lipson LC, Maron BJ, Leon MB, Epstein SE (1981) Effects of verapamil on left ventricular systolic function and diastolic filling in patients with hypertrophic cardiomyopathy. Circulation 64:787–796

**Long-Term Results of Different
Therapeutic Interventions in
Comparison with Verapamil**

Synopsis

R. HOPF

There is currently scant hope that therapy which will eliminate the basic cause of hypertrophic obstructive cardiomyopathy will appear in the near future. Symptomatic treatment is thought to acutely reduce the outflow tract gradient and, in the long run, perhaps to arrest or reduce the process of myocardial hypertrophy.

Recognized modes of therapy include operative procedures, medication with beta-blocking agents and calcium antagonists, and, in certain cases, pacemaker implantation.

Surgery is only possible in the obstructive type of hypertrophic cardiomyopathy. Since 1961, three procedures have been recommended and are established: myotomy, myectomy (both alone or in combination), and mitral valve replacement. A common objective of these methods is to eliminate the outflow tract gradient and mitral insufficiency.

In most patients, surgery leads to an impressive subjective improvement associated with increased work capacity. The outflow tract gradient is usually reduced and often eliminated; left ventricular filling pressure is lowered in two-thirds of all patients. Echocardiographically, a reduction or disappearance in systolic anterior movement of the mitral valve and an enlarged outflow tract can be demonstrated. By using 2-D echocardiography a reduction of interventricular septal thickness can be seen in nearly all patients. The subsequent development of congestive cardiomyopathy occurs, but seems to be rare. More frequently the late postoperative period is characterized by the reappearance of complaints or the onset of rhythm disturbances in the absence of left ventricular dilatation or recurrence of outflow tract obstruction. This suggests that surgical treatment cannot prevent the progression of the underlying cardiomyopathy.

The question of mortality in operated patients is of special interest. Initially, perioperative mortality was 10–15%, attributable to aortic or mitral insufficiency, low output, or rhythm disturbances. With greater experience mortality could be reduced to about 5%. In the late postoperative period annual mortality is 1.5–3.2%. The mean annual mortality of operatively treated patients, therefore, lies between 3 and 4%, a rate which does not differ significantly from that of untreated patients.

In 1964 propranolol became available as the first beta-blocking agent for routine clinical use. Based on the observation that adrenergic stimulation leads to increased obstruction in hypertrophic cardiomyopathy, beta blockade was expected to reduce the intraventricular gradient. But the results were disappointing. Whereas the augmentation of the obstruction following isoprenaline administration could be attenuated, only a slight reduction in the resting gradient was seen. Following beta blockade, left ventricular filling pressure could be increased as well as decreased. No improvement in left ventricular diastolic function could be observed.

Corresponding to these findings, the clinical results of long-term beta blocker therapy proved disappointing. Initial improvement in about 50% of all patients is usually followed by renewed deterioration. There is some evidence that better results might be achieved with long-term application of very high doses (400 mg propranolol/day). The prognosis does not appear to improve with beta blockade: the mean annual mortality is between 3 and 4%.

The calcium ion has been found to play an important role in hypertrophy and contractility of the myocardium. In 1973 first attempts were made to treat patients with hypertrophic cardiomyopathy with calcium antagonists.

With oral doses of 480–720 mg verapamil/day, 75% of patients improve subjectively, and patients without preexisting complaints remain free of symptoms. In 80% objective improvement can be verified. Clinical improvement is generally associated with a reduction in the left ventricular outflow tract obstruction and filling pressure, although the correlation between the magnitude of gradient reduction and improved exercise capacity is not strong; hence, additional factors other than reduction in gradient probably also contribute to improved symptoms. One such effect may be the improvement verapamil causes in left ventricular diastolic function. Some studies have suggested that left ventricular muscle mass is reduced during long-term verapamil therapy, but other studies have failed to find a significant difference. Thus, whether verapamil leads to a clinically important reduction in hypertrophy or improves prognosis, as preliminary findings suggest, remains to be determined.

Efficacy of Operation for Obstructive Hypertrophic Cardiomyopathy:

A 20-Year Experience with Ventricular Septal Myotomy and Myectomy

BARRY J. MARON, JEAN-PAUL KOCH, STEPHEN E. EPSTEIN, and
ANDREW G. MORROW

Summary

Since 1960, at the National Institutes of Health, ventricular septal myotomy and myectomy has been the mode of treatment for severely symptomatic patients with hypertrophic cardiomyopathy and obstruction to left ventricular outflow who do not respond to medical therapy. Our long-term results of operation for hypertrophic cardiomyopathy are reviewed in 240 patients operated upon through 1979. Postoperatively, most patients (70%) had improved symptomatically with marked reduction in left ventricular outflow gradient at rest. However, 8% of the patients died of causes related to operation. 9% had persistent or recurrent severe functional limitation, and 7% died up to 19 years postoperatively due to underlying cardiomyopathy. Of 17 late postoperative deaths, eight were sudden and nine were due to chronic heart failure. In particular, atrial fibrillation appeared to be a significant contributing factor to poor clinical outcome. Long-lasting clinical improvement occurred in most patients who survived operation for hypertrophic cardiomyopathy. However: (1) 10% of patients deteriorated clinically over the 5-year average follow-up; and (2) there is a continued, small annual postoperative mortality.

Hypertrophic cardiomyopathy is a primary disease of cardiac muscle which may be associated with obstruction to left ventricular outflow. Many patients with hypertrophic cardiomyopathy incur severe symptoms and functional limitation refractory to treatment with propranolol or verapamil.

Operation (septal myotomy and myectomy) for patients with hypertrophic cardiomyopathy and obstruction to left ventricular outflow has been shown to be beneficial in most patients with regard to amelioration of symptoms and relief of the outflow gradient [1–8]. Although previous reports from our institution and from other centers have described the early alterations in functional and hemodynamic state which follow operation [1, 3–8], long-term follow-up data in a large group of operated patients have only recently become available [9]. The following represents a summary of the long-term consequences of operation for hypertrophic cardiomyopathy in a consecutive series of 240 patients who have been followed at the National Heart, Lung, and Blood Institute (NHLBI) for 1–20 years.

Selection of Patients

Between January 1960 and April 1980, 280 patients with hypertrophic cardiomyopathy were operated upon at the NHLBI. The 240 patients who underwent operation between January 1960 and May 1979, and hence had at least a 1-year follow-up, are the subject of this report.

The 240 patients ranged in age from 9 to 76 years (median 44); 130 were men and 110 were women. The clinical condition of each of the 240 patients was determined as of May 1980. The period of postoperative follow-up of the survivors was 1–20 years with a mean follow-up of 5 years.

The vast majority of patients were selected for operation based upon meeting each of the following criteria: (1) severe symptoms of heart disease (New York Heart Association functional class III or IV), despite a therapeutic trial with propranolol or verapamil, or both; (2) marked obstruction to left ventricular outflow (i.e., ≥ 50 mmHg gradient) under basal conditions or with provocative interventions; and (3) absence of intercurrent disease constituting a contraindication to cardiac operation. However, of note, 11 patients were operated upon solely or primarily because of a prior episode of ventricular fibrillation [10], or frequent syncope, and one patient because of a family history of frequent premature sudden death [11].

Operative Procedure to Relieve Obstruction in Hypertrophic Cardiomyopathy: Ventricular Septal Myotomy and Myectomy

A brief description of the operative procedure employed to relieve obstruction in hypertrophic cardiomyopathy is provided [12]. A vertical aortotomy is made and extended obliquely to the aortic anulus in the noncoronary sinus of Valsalva. The normal aortic valve is retracted, and the ridge or bulge of hypertrophic muscle in the interventricular septum is visible below the base of the right coronary valve leaflet. Posteriorly, the anterior mitral leaflet is seen, and is often obviously thickened and opaque. The right coronary leaflet is then retracted with a special cloth-covered retractor, and after the heart has arrested and become flaccid, much of the septum can be rotated anteriorly and into the operative field. A #10 knife blade, attached to an angled handle, is then passed into the septum just below the base of the right coronary leaflet at a point 2–3 mm to the right of the commissure between the left and right coronary leaflets. The blade is inserted through the septum toward the apex for a distance of about 4 cm, and is then withdrawn as its cutting edge incises the septum with a sawing motion directed toward the ventricular lumen and the retractor (Fig. 1). A second myotomy is made in the same manner, parallel to the first one and about 1 cm to the right of it (Fig. 2 A). At the most prominent part of the septum the incisions should be about 1.5 cm in depth, and if necessary the muscle fibers are split by digital pressure to achieve this depth. With a conventional knife a transverse incision is then made at the base of the right coronary leaflet connecting the proximal portions of the myotomies. The bar of muscle which has been isolated can be freed from the surrounding septum for a variable distance by incision of its attachments (Fig. 2 B), and can usually be excised intact (Fig. 3).

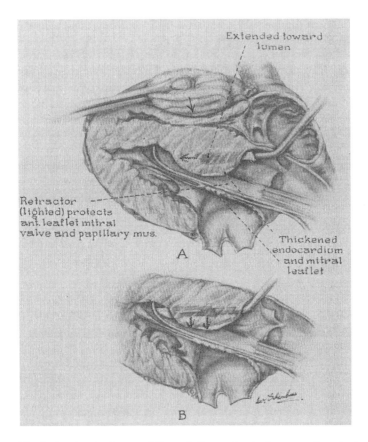

Fig. 1. A retractor is passed through the anulus to the apex; it protects the mitral valve and papillary muscles. The first myotomy is made with an angled knife just to the right of the center of the right coronary leaflet. The blade is inserted into the septum in the long axis of the ventricle for a distance of at least 4 cm. The knife is withdrawn as its edge incises the septum with a sawing motion directed toward the ventricular lumen and the retractor

Results

Postoperative Deaths

Of the 240 patients, 190 have survived to date, 20 died of the consequences of operation, and 30 died late after operation of causes that could not be related to the operative procedure *per se* (Fig. 4). In 13 of these 30 patients, death could *not* be attributed to hypertrophic cardiomyopathy.

The remaining 17 patients died of causes that appeared related to hypertrophic cardiomyopathy, 7 months to 20 years after the operation (mean 4 years). At death, these patients ranged in age from 22 to 64 years (median 49 years), and seven were over 55 years of age. At the time of death three patients were in functional class I, five were in class II, and nine were in classes III or IV. Eleven of the 17 patients had postoperative hemodynamic studies. In each of these patients either no or a small outflow gradient was present under basal conditions.

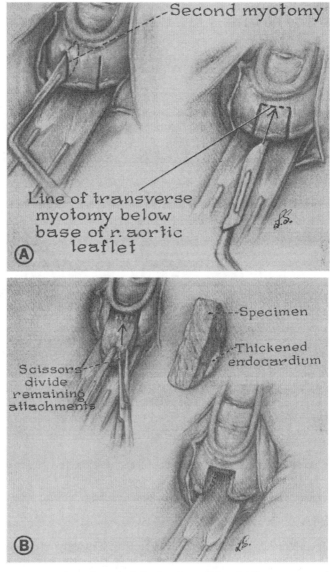

Fig. 2. A A second vertical myotomy is made to the left of and parallel to the first myotomy. A transverse incision is then made, connecting the vertical ones at the base of the right coronary leaflet. The bar of muscle between the vertical myotomies is largely detached from the septum. **B** Remaining attachments of the muscle bar to the septum are divided under direct vision with straight scissors. After completion of the muscle resection, a rectangular channel (1 by 1.5 cm) extends from the valve ring toward the apex for about 4 cm

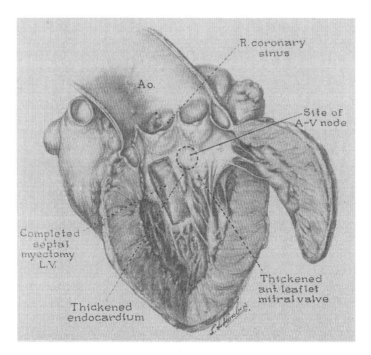

Fig. 3. Semidiagrammatic representation of the left ventricle after completion of the septal myotomy-myectomy. The relations of the channel to the valve leaflets and to the adjacent membranous septum (and conduction tissue) are shown. The apical end of the floor of the channel blends smoothly onto the wall of the distal left ventricle

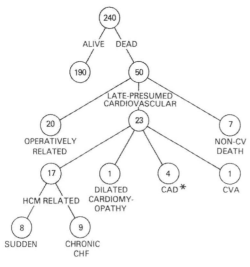

Fig. 4. Flow diagram showing clinical outcome for the 240 patients operated on, 1960–1980, for hypertrophic cardiomyopathy (*HCM*). *CAD*, coronary artery disease; *CHF*, congestive heart failure; *CVA*, cerebrovascular accident; *, Includes 3 patients who died suddenly (one of whom had an acute myocardial infarction) and one other patient who died after coronary artery bypass graft surgery

Eight of the 17 patients died suddenly and unexpectedly, presumably due to an arrhythmia. At the time of death each of these eight patients was engaged in sedentary activity (including one who was asleep). The remaining nine patients died after chronic illnesses characterized by progressive, severe congestive heart failure. The 17 patients who died late and the 190 long-term survivors did not differ with respect to age at operation, sex distribution, or preoperative functional class. The annual mortality rate for late deaths due to cardiomyopathy was 1.5%.

Identification of Potential Contributing Factors to Late Postoperative Death

Of the 17 patients who died late after operation, 14 had potentially deleterious associated cardiovascular or general medical problems that had been identified preoperatively, postoperatively, or both. These abnormalities included clinically significant chronic obstructive pulmonary disease in three patients, obesity in three, systemic hypertension in two, particularly severe, chronic congestive heart failure associated with frank pulmonary edema in six, significant coronary heart disease in three, ventricular fibrillation in two, and chronic alcoholism in one patient. Furthermore, paroxysmal atrial fibrillation appeared to be a significant contributing factor to poor clinical outcome (by virtue of depressing cardiac function, or as an antecedent to a cerebrovascular accident), i.e., preoperative and/or postoperative atrial fibrillation was present in nine (52%) of the 17 patients who died late postoperatively.

Symptomatology

The latest preoperative and the most recent postoperative symptomatic state of the 190 survivors and the 17 patients who died late of hypertrophic cardiomyopathy are summarized in terms of New York Heart Association functional classes (Fig. 5). Of the 185 patients who had functional limitation preoperatively and have survived to

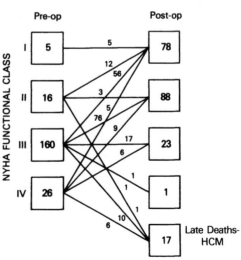

Fig. 5. Preoperative and postoperative functional class and clinical outcome in 207 patients who survived operation. Twelve other patients who died of cardiovascular causes unrelated to hypertrophic cardiomyopathy (*HCM*) have been excluded. NYHA, New York Heart Association

the present, 164 (88%) have perceived (without the need for cardioactive medications) an improvement in their symptomatic state after operation sufficient to be assigned to at least one lower functional class (Fig. 6).

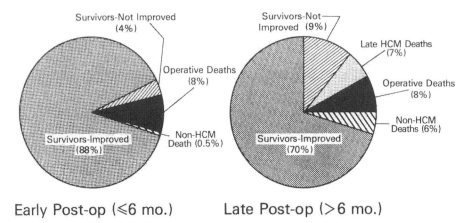

Fig. 6. Short-term and long-term clinical results in patients after operation for hypertrophic cardiomyopathy (*HCM*)

The other 21 patients were not significantly improved when most recently evaluated postoperatively (Fig. 6). However, 15 of these 21 patients did experience transient but significant improvement (i.e., to at least one lower functional class) *early* after operation (Fig. 6). Likewise, 15 of the 17 patients who died late postoperatively of hypertrophic cardiomyopathy also experienced symptomatic improvement early after operation.

Surviving patients and those who died late of hypertrophic cardiomyopathy did not differ with respect to the particular symptom complex present preoperatively. Of the 185 surviving patients who had been symptomatic preoperatively, 146 (79%) had congestive symptoms (dyspnea with exertion, fatigue, orthopnea, or paroxysmal nocturnal dyspnea) and chest pain; syncope had occurred in 111 of these 185 patients. In 31 (17%) of the 185 patients congestive symptoms were present, but not chest pain. Of the eight remaining patients, six had only chest pain and syncope and just two had chest pain alone. Of the 17 patients who died late of hypertrophic cardiomyopathy, 11 had both congestive symptoms and chest pain preoperatively and the remaining six patients had congestive symptoms only; 12 of the 17 patients had syncope preoperatively.

Hemodynamic Data

Preoperative cardiac catheterization was performed in each of the 190 surviving patients and also in the 17 patients who died late of hypertrophic cardiomyopathy;

postoperative catheterization (usually 6 months after operation) was performed in 194 of these 207 patients.

Preoperatively, the peak systolic pressure gradients between the left ventricle and a systemic artery recorded under basal conditions ranged from zero to 210 mmHg, and in 161 of the 207 patients the outflow gradient was >50 mmHg (Fig. 7). The 46 patients with gradients of <50 mmHg under basal conditions each

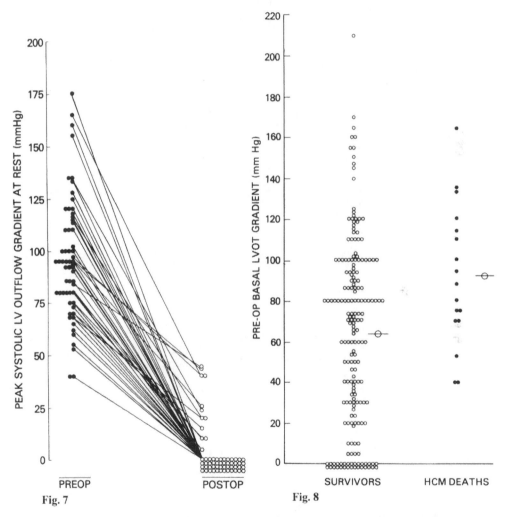

Fig. 7. Peak systolic left ventricular outflow tract pressure gradient measured preoperatively and postoperatively under basal conditions in the initial 60 patients operated upon with basal preoperative gradients ≧ 40 mmHg. It was not possible to plot the data for each of the 240 patients operated upon although the hemodynamic results for the 60 patients shown here are representative of the entire study group

Fig. 8. Comparison of preoperative left ventricular outflow tract (*LVOT*) gradients under basal conditions for survivors and patients who died late postoperatively of hypertrophic cardiomyopathy (*HCM*). ⊖, Mean gradient for each group of patients

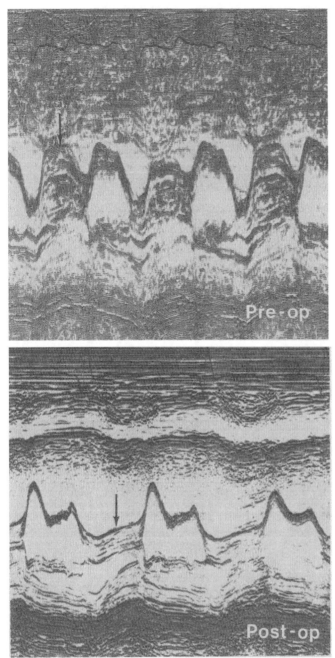

Fig. 9. Echocardiographic demonstration of relief of left ventricular outflow tract obstruction after septal myotomy-myectomy. Marked systolic anterior motion of the anterior mitral leaflet (*arrow*) is present preoperatively and was responsible for substantial obstruction to left ventricular outflow in this 12-year-old boy with hypertrophic cardiomyopathy. Postoperatively, there is no systolic anterior motion of the anterior mitral leaflet (*arrow*) and no left ventricular outflow tract obstruction was measured at catheterization

had gradients of ≧ 50 mmHg produced by provocative maneuvers or interventions. The magnitude of the preoperative left ventricular outflow gradient under basal conditions was significantly greater in the 17 patients who died late of hypertrophic cardiomyopathy (mean 92 ± 8 [SEM] mmHg) than in the 190 survivors (64 ± 3 mmHg; $P<0.02$) (Fig. 8).

Postoperatively, peak systolic pressure gradients between the left ventricle and a systemic artery recorded under basal conditions were less than the preoperative gradient in all but four patients [in whom the gradient increased from 5 to 20 mmHg over the preoperative value]. Postoperatively, no outflow gradient was present under basal conditions in 139 of 194 patients (Figs. 7 and 9). No significant difference was evident between the 190 survivors and 17 patients who died late with regard to the change between the preoperative and postoperative outflow gradient under basal conditions (mean 87 mmHg each) (Fig. 10).

Persistent functional limitation following operation could not be attributed to a poor hemodynamic result. Of the 21 patients in whom marked symptomatology

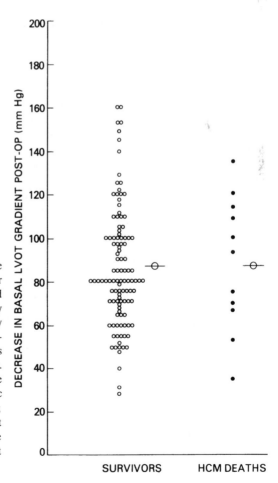

Fig. 10. Change between preoperative and postoperative gradient under basal conditions for survivors and patients who died late postoperatively of hypertrophic cardiomyopathy (*HCM*). Shown only for those patients with preoperative gradients ≧ 50 mmHg under basal conditions. Preoperative hemodynamic data were obtained at the final cardiac catheterization before operation; postoperative data were obtained at the most recent postoperative catheterization. ⊖, mean gradient for each group of patients

Table 1. Electrocardiographic evidence of conduction defects in 107 patients before and after operation for hypertrophic cardiomyopathy

Type of ECG conduction abnormality	No. patients preoperative	No. patients postoperative
None	78 (73%)	4 (4%)
Typical LBBB	2 (2%)	47 (45%)
IVCD	8 (7%)	31 (30%)
Left anterior hemiblock [a]	12 (11%)	11 (11%)
Left axis deviation [b]	7 (7%)	10 (10%)
Complete heart block with functioning pacemaker postop	0	4

IVCD, intraventricular conduction defect; LBBB, left bundle branch block.
[a] Left axis deviation $(>-30°)$, normal QRS duration, small Q_I, R_{III}.
[b] QRS axis $>-30°$, but absence of Q_I and R_{III} and normal QRS duration.

persisted after operation, 17 had no or trivial postoperative left ventricular outflow obstruction under basal conditions (≤ 25 mmHg).

Electrocardiographic Findings

Preoperative and postoperative electrocardiographic data were obtained in the initial 107 patients who underwent septal myotomy-myectomy [9]. Preoperatively, 29 (27%) of the 107 patients showed evidence of conduction abnormalities on the electrocardiogram. Postoperatively, conduction abnormalities were present in 99 (96%) of 103 patients in whom an electrocardiogram without pacemaker artifact was available (Table 1); 47 (45%) of the 103 patients showed typical left bundle branch block.

Discussion

The present study is an analysis of the long-term results of septal myotomy-myectomy in all patients operated upon since 1960, when the first such procedure was performed at the NHLBI, through 1980. Thus, patients have been followed for 1–20 years, with an average follow-up of over 5 years.

We recommend operation, with rare exception, only if symptoms severely impair the quality of life and are not sufficiently improved by the administration of propranolol or verapamil. Operative mortality has consistently been 5–10%. All but 2% of our operative survivors have experienced substantial alleviation of their cardiac symptoms early after operation. In addition, postoperatively 98% of our patients manifested marked reduction or abolition of the left ventricular outflow gradient measured under basal conditions.

However, septal myotomy-myectomy does not always prevent progression of symptoms and does not always prevent fatal events. For example, 15 patients who experienced symptomatic improvement early after operation deteriorated subsequently and are now in functional classes III or IV. In addition, patients continued to die following operation from causes presumably related to their underlying cardiac disease. These deaths have either been sudden and probably due to a ventricular arrhythmia, or have occurred in the setting of chronic and progressive congestive heart failure. Such observations indicate that in patients with hypertrophic cardiomyopathy the cardiomyopathic process is the factor which determines the patient's ultimate course. It is, of course, impossible to determine from these data if the patients who eventually did die would have died earlier had operation not been carried out.

It is important to emphasize that the series of patients described in this report does not represent a selected population, but includes virtually all severely symptomatic patients seen at the NHLBI with hypertrophic cardiomyopathy who were not benefited by propranolol or verapamil therapy. Hence, some patients with associated medical and cardiovascular problems that may have contributed in a deleterious fashion to their subsequent clinical course were operated upon, even through they could not realistically have been expected to derive as long-lasting symptomatic benefit from operation as other patients. In this regard, our data have shown that those patients who died late postoperatively or were severely symptomatic at long-term postoperative evaluation had significantly more associated medical or cardiovascular problems than those patients who survived and were improved postoperatively [9].

Of note, although late cardiac deaths still occurred, the annual rate of such events was relatively small, i.e., 1.5%. Of possible relevance to this statistic is that an annual mortality rate of about 3% has been reported for patients with hypertrophic cardiomyopathy who were not operated upon [13, 14]. The implication of this comparison is that operation does not increase, and may decrease, long-term mortality. However, such a comparison of nonoperated and operated patients is of dubious validity since patients who undergo operation constitute a different subgroup than do the nonoperated patients. Hence, it is impossible to determine definitively whether operation alters the longevity of patients with hypertrophic cardiomyopathy. Such information could only be obtained from a prospective study involving randomization of patients.

Unfortunately, our analysis of preoperative functional status, hemodynamic findings, and conduction abnormalities on the electrocardiogram did not prove to be useful in predicting which patients were at risk of late postoperative death, or which patients would not experience functional improvement. Of note, however, patients who died late of hypertrophic cardiomyopathy had significantly higher preoperative left ventricular outflow gradients (under basal conditions) than did those patients who have survived postoperatively.

In addition, the presence of atrial fibrillation seemed to be a particularly poor prognostic sign. In this regard, 7 of the 17 patients who died from hypertrophic cardiomyopathy late postoperatively experienced multiple episodes of atrial fibrillation. Whether such a rhythm disturbance reflects irreversible left ventricular dysfunction that ultimately causes death, or is itself an etiologically important primary cause of death, remains to be determined. However, it should be pointed out that the presence of atrial fibrillation is not invariably responsible for poor long-term prognosis, since this rhythm occurs in 15% of the long-term survivors [9]. Thus, atrial fibrillation *per se* cannot serve as the sole indication for operation in the absence of severe symptoms.

In conclusion, about 70% of our patients with hypertrophic cardiomyopathy experienced substantial long-term symptomatic benefit from septal myotomy-myectomy. In addition, many of the patients who ultimately died or in whom severe symptoms recurred did experience gratifying initial symptomatic relief that often persisted for years after operation. As a result of these observations we believe that septal myotomy-myectomy is indicated for patients with hypertrophic cardiomyopathy who are severely symptomatic and whose symptoms do not respond satisfactorily to nonoperative treatment.

References

1. Morrow AG, Reitz BA, Epstein SE, Henry WL, Conkle DM, Itscoitz SB, Redwood DR (1975) Operative treatment in hypertrophic subaortic stenosis: Techniques, and the results of pre- and post-operative assessment in 83 patients. Circulation 52:88
2. Barratt-Boyes BG, O'Brien KP (1971) Surgical treatment of idiopathic hypertrophic subaortic stenosis using a combined left ventricular-aortic approach. In: Wolstenholme GEW, O'Connor M (eds) Hypertrophic obstructive cardiomyopathy, Ciba foundation study group No 37. JA Churchill, London, p 150
3. Epstein SE, Henry WL, Clark CE, Roberts WC, Maron BJ, Ferrans VJ, Redwood DR, Morrow AG (1974) Asymmetric septal hypertrophy. Ann Intern Med 81:650
4. Tajik AJ, Giuliani ER, Weidman WM, Brandenburg RO, McGoon DC (1974) Idiopathic hypertrophic subaortic stenosis. Long-term surgical follow-up. Am J Cardiol 34:815
5. Morrow AG, Fogarty TJ, Hannah HJ, Braunwald E (1968) Operative treatment in idiopathic hypertrophic subaortic stenosis. Techniques, and the results of preoperative and postoperative clinical and hemodynamic assessments. Circulation 37:589
6. Agnew TM, Barratt-Boyes BG, Brandt PWT, Roche AHG, Lowe JB, O'Brien KP (1977) Surgical resection in idiopathic hypertrophic subaortic stenosis with a combined approach through aorta and left ventricle. J Thorac Cardiovasc Surg 74:307
7. Bigelow WG, Trimble AS, Auger P, Marquis Y, Wigle ED (1966) The ventriculo-myotomy operation for muscular subaortic stenosis. A reappraisal. J Thorac Cardiovasc Surg 52:514
8. Adelman AG, Wigle ED, Ranganathan N, Webb GD, Kidd BSL, Bigelow WG, Silver MD (1972) The clinical course in muscular subaortic stenosis: A retrospective and prospective study of 60 hemodynamically proved cases. Ann Intern Med 77:515
9. Maron BJ, Merrill WH, Freier PA, Kent KM, Epstein SE, Morrow AG (1978) Long-term clinical course and symptomatic status of patients after operation for hypertrophic subaortic stenosis. Circulation 57:1205
10. Morrow AG, Koch J-P, Maron BJ, Kent KM, Epstein SE (1980) Left ventricular myotomy and myectomy in patients with obstructive hypertrophic cardiomyopathy and previous cardiac arrest. Am J Cardiol 46:313
11. Maron BJ, Lipson LC, Roberts WC, Savage DD, Epstein SE (1978) "Malignant" hypertrophic cardiomyopathy: Identification of a subgroup of families with unusually frequent premature deaths. Am J Cardiol 41:1133
12. Morrow AG (1978) Hypertrophic subaortic stenosis. Operative methods utilized to relieve left ventricular outflow obstruction. J Thorac Cardiovasc Surg 76:423
13. Shah PM, Adelman AG, Wigle ED, Gobel FL, Burchell HB, Hardarson T, Curiel R, De La Calzada C, Oakley CM, Goodwin JF (1975) The natural (and unnatural) history of hypertrophic obstructive cardiomyopathy. Circ Res [Suppl II] 34, 35:II–179
14. Hardarson T, De La Calzada CS, Curiel R, Goodwin JF (1973) Prognosis and mortality of hypertrophic obstructive cardiomyopathy. Lancet 2:1462

Functional Results in Medically and Surgically Treated Patients with Hypertrophic Obstructive Cardiomyopathy *

B. Lösse, H. Kuhn, and F. Loogen

Summary

In 25 patients with hypertrophic obstructive cardiomyopathy (HOCM), the hemodynamic effects of medical (propranolol) and surgical (transaortal septal myectomy) therapy were determined by measuring the following circulatory parameters at rest and during maximal exercise before and after therapy: heart rate, stroke volume, cardiac output, and pulmonary artery pressure. Twelve patients were investigated immediately before and after medical therapy of 1–7 (mean 3) months duration with daily doses of 120–360 (mean 205 ± 70) mg propranolol. Thirteen patients were examined 1 week to 28 months (mean 7.5 months) before and 3 weeks to 35 months (mean 10 months) after operation. Propranolol induced a significant reduction of heart rate and cardiac output, a slight increase in stroke volume (only at rest significant), and a slight further increase in the pathologically elevated exercise pulmonary artery pressure, with the pulmonary vascular resistance remaining unchanged. Although 4 of 12 patients reported some subjective improvement, exercise capacity did not change (72.7 ± 28.4 watts before, 72.9 ± 24.9 watts after propranolol). Myectomy, on the other hand, induced no change in heart rate, a significant increase in stroke volume during exercise, a slight increase in cardiac output during exercise, and a significant fall in the pathologically elevated pulmonary artery pressure by a mean of 3.8 mmHg at rest and 12.7 mmHg during identical exercise. Twelve of the 13 operated patients reported a marked subjective improvement, and the exercise capacity increased from an average of 59.1 ± 16.9 watts to 81.8 ± 22.6 watts. Thus, the clinical and functional result of surgical therapy was significantly better than that of medical therapy and induced, in contrast to medical therapy, a significant hemodynamic improvement and increase in exercise capacity.

Introduction

The most thoroughly investigated therapeutic approaches for the treatment of patients with hypertrophic obstructive cardiomyopathy (HOCM) are medical trials with beta-blocking agents and surgery, consisting of ventricular septal myotomy and myectomy. Long-term effects of both procedures on clinical symptoms and resting hemodynamics are well known [1, 2, 4–7, 11–13, 15, 16, 21–25] as well as acute effects of propranolol during exercise on some parameters of left ventricular function and systemic circulation [4, 5, 8, 24, 26]. However, there are relatively few

---

* Supported in part by a grant of the Deutsche Forschungsgemeinschaft, SFB 30 Kardiologie

252   B. Lösse et al.

published data concerning the long-term hemodynamic effects during exercise [3, 4, 17, 24]. Extending an earlier study [14], we have therefore compared in the following report the effects of both therapeutic procedures on several important circulatory parameters at rest and during exercise. The results will demonstrate the superiority of surgical treatment.

Patients and Methods

The present series is based on a total of 25 patients. One group was medically treated with propranolol, the other was operated upon using the Morrow procedure of ventricular septal myotomy and myectomy [16]. The diagnosis of HOCM had been confirmed in all patients by heart catheterization and left ventricular angiography.

Exercise measurements were performed with patients in supine position on a bicycle ergometer; work load was increased stepwise to a maximum terminated by angina, dyspnea, or exhaustion. Pulmonary artery and, if possible, pulmonary artery wedge pressure were continuously measured as well as oxygen consumption (paramagnetic method, Oxycon, Mijnhardt). Pulmonary artery and systemic arterial oxygen content were discontinuously measured at rest and during each exercise level after reaching a steady state (Lex-O_2-Con, Lexington Instruments). Cardiac output was calculated from oxygen consumption and arteriovenous oxygen content difference, and stroke volume from cardiac output and heart rate.

The medically treated group consisted of 12 patients, six men and six women aged 32 to 50 (mean 40.3 ± 8.5) years. Exercise measurements were performed immediately before and after a therapy of 1–7 (mean 3) months duration with daily doses of 120–360 mg (mean 205 ± 70 mg) propranolol, the dose being adjusted to achieve a heart rate between 50 and 60 beats per minute.

The surgically treated group consisted of 13 patients, ten men and three women aged 24–52 (mean 38.9 ± 9.0) years. All patients had been pretreated with propranolol without satisfactory results. Exercise measurements were performed 1 week to 28 months (mean 7.5 months) before and 3 weeks to 35 months (mean 10 months) after surgery. Propranolol therapy had been discontinued at least 3 days (in most cases several weeks) before the preoperative exercise test in all patients except two, who received a continued dose of 160 and 240 mg propranolol, respectively. At the postoperative exercise test, 6 of the 13 patients were under beta-blocking treatment with 30–120 mg propranolol because of rhythm disturbances or tachycardias observed in the immediate postoperative period.

Results

Both the medically and the surgically treated groups of patients were of comparable age (Table 1). Heart catheterization data demonstrated no significant differences between the two groups, though the subsequently operated patients demonstrated a tendency toward higher values of left ventricular enddiastolic pressure and left ventricular outflow tract gradient. Furthermore, the surgically treated patients initially reached lower maximal exercise levels, which was responsible for the lower maximal heart rates. The reduced cardiac output in the subsequently operated

Table 1. Initial heart catheterization and hemodynamic data in 25 patients with HOCM subsequently treated with propranolol (n = 12) or septal myectomy (n = 13).

			Propranolol (n = 12)	Myectomy (n = 13)	P
Age		[yrs]	40.3 ± 8.5	38.9 ± 9.0	n.s
EDP_{LV}		[mmHg]	16.1 ± 7.5	18.8 ± 7.5	n.s
Syst. ΔP_{LV}	Rest	[mmHg]	40.9 ± 34.6	65.3 ± 39.4	n.s.
	Post-ES	[mmHg]	120.0 ± 41.9	130.5 ± 27.0	n.s.
Max. work capacity		[watts]	72.7 ± 28.4	59.6 ± 16.3	n.s.
HR	Rest	[min^{-1}]	82.9 ± 19.9	73.7 ± 7.9	n.s.
	Exercise	[min^{-1}]	140.9 ± 23.6	118.2 ± 19.0	< 0.025
SVI	Rest	[ml · min^{-1}]	42.3 ± 8.4	43.5 ± 13.3	n.s.
	Exercise	[ml · min^{-1}]	51.3 ± 9.8	44.7 ± 11.0	n.s.
CI	Rest	[l · min^{-1} · m^{-2}]	3.50 ± 1.03	3.19 ± 1.07	n.s.
	Exercise	[l · min^{-1} · m^{-2}]	7.27 ± 2.12	5.26 ± 1.61	< 0.025
$\bar{P}_{PA}$	Rest	[mmHg]	17.7 ± 4.9	19.7 ± 5.4	n.s.
	Exercise	[mmHg]	37.7 ± 11.3	45.8 ± 13.8	n.s.

Note that in the surgically treated group the exercise hemodynamic parameters were measured at a lower maximal work load than in the propranolol group. EDP_{LV}, left ventricular end-diastolic pressure; syst. ΔP_{LV}, systolic left ventricular outflow tract gradient at rest or at postextrasystolic (post-ES) provocation; HR, heart rate; SVI, stroke volume index; CI, cardiac index; $\bar{P}_{PA}$, mean pulmonary artery pressure; P, error probability in Student's t test for unpaired data.

patients was in part referable to the lower heart rates and, during exercise, to the lack of stroke volume increase during exercise. In spite of the lower maximal exercise level and the lower cardiac output, surgically treated patients initially exhibited a more pronounced pathologic increase in pulmonary artery pressure during exercise (Table 1).

All these findings indicate a stronger hemodynamic impairment of the subsequently operated patients. This is also reflected in the initial functional classification (Fig. 1). Three of the medically treated patients initially were in NYHA class II, the remaining nine patients in class III. Of the surgically treated group, initially only one patient was in class II, the majority of ten patients in class

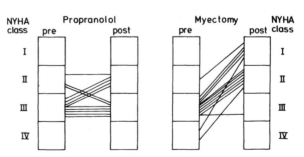

Fig. 1. Clinical classification of 25 patients with hypertrophic obstructive cardiomyopathy before and after medical therapy (propranolol, n = 12) or surgical therapy (myectomy, n = 13)

III, and two patients in class IV. After propranolol, six of the 12 patients remained in the same functional class, four improved by one class, and two deteriorated by one class. The improvement in the four patients consisted of a reduction of palpitations and angina-like symptoms, possibly due in part to the decrease in exercising heart rate. The maximal exercise capacity was on an average not changed in this group (72.7 ± 28.4 watts before propranolol, 72.9 ± 24.9 watts after propranolol). The individual effects of propranolol on maximal exercise capacity are shown in Fig. 2. In contrast, 12 of the 13 operated patients improved, seven of

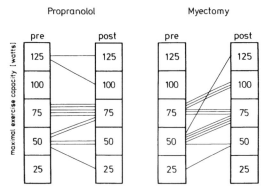

Fig. 2. Individual changes in maximal exercise capacity in 25 patients with hypertrophic obstructive cardiomyopathy after medical (propranolol, n = 12) or surgical therapy (myectomy, n = 13)

them by one class, four by two classes, and one by three classes (Fig. 1). Only one patient remained in the same functional class, and none deteriorated. Three of the operated patients, preoperatively demonstrating outflow tract gradients at rest of 50–125 mmHg in the left ventricle and 15–30 mmHg in the right ventricle, were recatheterized. None of them had a demonstrable gradient in the right or left ventricular outflow tract. Maximal exercise capacity rose in the whole surgically treated group significantly from an average of 59.6 ± 16.3 watts to 81.8 ± 20.8 watts ($P<0.005$). The individual effects of surgical therapy on maximal exercise capacity are shown in Fig. 2.

Heart rate decreased after propranolol significantly (Fig. 3A, Table 2). Probably due to the test conditions in the laboratory, resting heart rate was higher than at control measurements under outpatient conditions. Surgical therapy induced no significant change in heart rate (Fig. 3A, Table 3).

Stroke volume showed a different behaviour in individual patients after both therapeutic procedures (Fig. 3B, Tables 2, 3). As a whole, stroke volume increased at rest in the medically treated patients, whereas the surgically treated patients exhibited an increase during exercise.

As a result of the changes in heart rate and stroke volume, cardiac index fell significantly in the propranolol treated patients (Fig. 3C, Table 2). The changes in the operated patients were more heterogeneous, with no significant changes observed (Fig. 3C, Table 3). It should be noted, however, that six patients received

Functional Results in Medically and Surgically Treated Patients 255

propranolol postoperatively versus two at the preoperative exercise test. Since propranolol decreases cardiac output, it is possible that this drug masked a potential increase in cardiac index subsequent to surgery. Despite the reduction of cardiac index, pulmonary artery pressure exhibited no change at rest during propranolol therapy. During exercise, however, a tendency towards further elevations of the initially pathologically augmented values was observed (Fig. 3 D, Table 2). These

Table 2. Hemodynamic findings ($\bar{x}\pm s$) before and after therapy with propranolol in 12 patients with HOCM

		Propranolol (n = 12)			
		Pre	Post	Change	P
HR	Rest	83.7 ±21.2	62.5 ± 6.9	− 25.3%	< 0.0025
[min⁻¹]	Exercise	138.3 ±23.8	107.9 ±19.4	− 22.0%	< 0.0001
SVI	Rest	40.7 ± 6.9	45.7 ±10.3	+ 12.3%	< 0.05
[ml · m⁻²]	Exercise	50.9 ±10.5	54.7 ±15.2	+ 7.5%	n.s.
CI	Rest	3.50± 1.02	2.91± 0.63	− 16.9%	< 0.005
[l · min⁻¹· m⁻²]	Exercise	7.12± 2.20	5.91± 1.94	− 17.0%	< 0.0005
$\bar{P}_{PA}$	Rest	17.7 ± 4.9	17.8 ± 5.7	+ 0.6%	n.s.
[mmHg]	Exercise	37.3 ±10.2	41.3 ±12.1	+ 10.2%	n.s.
PVR	Rest	104.3 ±45.1	104.4 ±41.6	+ 0.1%	n.s.
[dyn · s · cm⁻⁵]	Exercise	79.0 ±33.4	88.6 ±41.8	+ 12.2%	n.s.

HR, heart rate; SVI, stroke volume index; CI, cardiac index; $\bar{P}_{PA}$, mean pulmonary artery pressure; PVR, pulmonary vascular resistance; P, error probability in the two-tailed Student's t test for paired data. The exercise values were measured at identical exercise levels in the pre- and posttreatment test, averaging 68±26.4 watts.

Table 3. Hemodynamic findings ($\bar{x}\pm s$) before and after septal myectomy in 13 patients with HOCM. Same abbreviations as in Table 2. The exercise values were measured in each patient at identical exercise levels in the pre- and postoperative test, averaging 57.7±15.8 watts

		Myectomy (n = 13)			
		Pre	Post	Change	P
HR	Rest	73.7 ± 7.9	79.6 ±14.7	+ 8.0%	n.s.
[min⁻¹]	Exercise	118.2 ±19.0	113.8 ±21.2	− 3.7%	n.s.
SVI	Rest	43.5 ±13.3	39.9 ± 5.8	− 8.3%	n.s.
[ml · m⁻²]	Exercise	44.7 ±11.0	50.6 ±10.1	+ 13.2%	< 0.025
CI	Rest	3.18± 1.07	3.17± 0.66	− 0.3%	n.s.
[l · min⁻¹· m⁻²]	Exercise	5.26± 1.61	5.73± 1.45	+ 8.9%	n.s.
$\bar{P}_{PA}$	Rest	19.7 ± 5.4	15.9 ± 3.5	− 19.3%	< 0.05
[mmHg]	Exercise	45.9 ±13.8	33.2 ± 6.6	− 27.7%	< 0.05

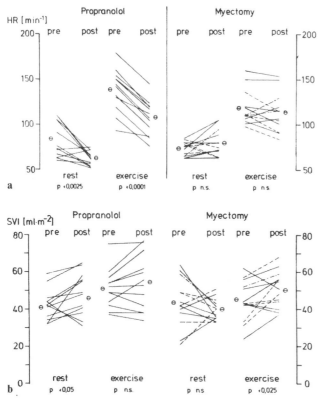

Fig. 3a–d. Hemodynamic data at rest and during exercise at identical levels in the pre- and posttreatment evaluation (68.8 ± 26.4 watts in 12 propranolol treated patients, 57.7 ± 15.8 watts in 13 surgically treated patients). **a** heart rate (HR). **b** stroke volume index (SVI). **c** cardiac index (CI). **d** mean pulmonary artery pressure ($\bar{P}_{PA}$). The *interrupted lines* in the right half of these figures indicate patients who were on propranolol either preoperatively or postoperatively: – – – –, preoperatively no drug, postoperatively propranolol, – · – · –, preoperatively propranolol, postoperatively no drug. Statistical comparisons were performed using the two-tailed Student's t test for paired data

changes, however, were not statistically significant. In addition, no change was observed in pulmonary vascular resistance (derived from cardiac output, pulmonary artery pressure, and pulmonary artery wedge pressure) (Table 2).

In contrast, myectomy induced in most patients a substantial fall of pulmonary artery pressure at rest and, more pronounced, during exercise (Fig. 3D, Table 3). The decrease averaged 3.8 mmHg at rest and 12.7 mmHg at identical exercise levels.

Discussion

The primary effort of all therapy in HOCM should be directed to alleviate the patient's disabling symptoms, to increase their reduced exercise capacity, and to

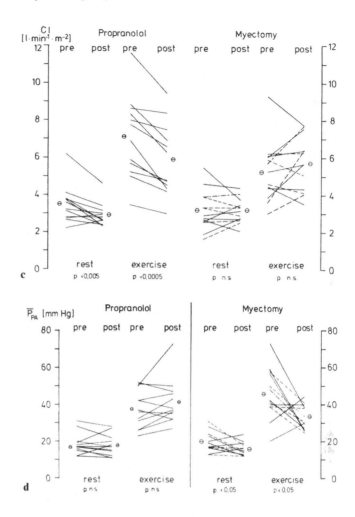

prolong life. The efforts of the present study were directed to assessing the effects of treatment on symptoms, hemodynamics, and exercise capacity. As our findings demonstrate, improved symptoms and increased exercise capacity were unsatisfactorily reached with beta-blocking agents. We found only a small increase in resting stroke volume, and the ability to increase stroke volume during exercise was not improved following treatment. The small increases in stroke volume were, however, not sufficient to compensate for the significant reduction in heart rate. Thus, cardiac output at rest and especially during exercise was significantly reduced. Furthermore, even if left ventricular outflow tract obstruction may have been reduced in some patients, this had no beneficial effect on elevated pulmonary artery pressures. Despite the reduced cardiac output, pulmonary artery pressures exhibited a further rise as compared to pretreatment values. Since pulmonary vascular resistance remained unchanged, this rise was referable to an increase in left ventricular filling pressure, a finding which has been reported in recent studies after long-term treatment with beta-blocking agents [13, 24].

These findings demonstrate that propranolol in general does not improve the pathologic hemodynamic situation in patients with HOCM (i.e., elevation of left ventricular end-diasystolic pressure, and the inability to increase stroke volume during exercise). In fact, further deterioration occurs in that the left ventricular filling pressure increases. Propranolol also impairs the compensatory mechanism of exercise-induced increasing heart rate, which is essential [10] to maintain an adequate cardiac output in these patients. This may explain the relatively low rate of persistent symptomatic improvement (4 of 12 patients), which was consistent with earlier observations in larger series [1, 13, 22]. It further explains why, with definite individual exceptions (Fig. 2), average exercise tolerance of the patients does not increase, a finding also demonstrated by other authors [4, 23]. Only some patients with initial high cardiac output achieved higher exercise levels under propranolol, probably due to subjective symptomatic improvement related to the reduced heart rate (i.e., palpitations). But since heart rate and cardiac output were diminished irrespective of the initial values, patients with initially reduced cardiac output were further compromised and reached lower maximal exercise levels than before treatment.

In contrast to these disappointing results of propranolol treatment, surgical treatment resulted in a significantly better and more pronounced symptomatic improvement and induced a marked rise in exercise tolerance (Fig. 2). The surgical procedure directly reduces or abolishes the obstruction of the left ventricular outflow tract in nearly all patients [1, 2, 7, 11–13, 15–18, 21, 25] by widening the outflow tract. Additionally, an increased left ventricular distensibility may be achieved. Specifically, our findings demonstrate that patients who preoperatively could not increase stroke volume during exercise could achieve such an increase after operation. In conjunction with recent radionuclide angiographic findings, which demonstrated a slightly decreased left ventricular ejection fraction after operation [3], this provides evidence of an augmented left ventricular end-diastolic volume. Since heart rate was not influenced, this increased stroke volume was accompanied by a tendency for cardiac output to rise slightly (this trend may have been more definite were it not for the fact that six patients had been under propranolol treatment at the postoperative exercise test, while only two were on propranolol during the preoperative study). Despite this tendency for cardiac output to increase, pulmonary artery pressures were substantially reduced, indicating a significant fall in left ventricular filling pressures. These changes during maximal exercise are consistent with recent observations of other authors [17]. These favorable hemodynamic effects were accompanied in our series by a marked clinical improvement of one to three functional classes according to the New York Heart Association in 12 of 13 patients, and were documented by a significant increase in exercise tolerance.

The results of this study clearly demonstrate, insofar as clinical symptoms, exercise capacity, and hemodynamics are concerned, that surgical therapy of HOCM is by far superior to medical therapy with beta-blocking agents. Whether the recently introduced medical treatment with the calcium antagonistic drug

Functional Results in Medically and Surgically Treated Patients 259

verapamil [9, 19, 20] is superior to propranolol therapy and equal to surgical therapy, remains to be established in long-term trials directed to changes in clinical symptoms and exercise hemodynamics.

Since the measurements of the present study have been performed an average of 10 months (range 3 weeks to 35 months) after operation, the final persistence of the observed beneficial effects cannot be definitely determined. Earlier studies have demonstrated that the operation-induced reduction of left ventricular outflow tract obstruction and the symptomatic improvement persist in the majority of patients over considerable mean follow-up periods of up to more than 5 years [12, 13, 15, 16, 25], and in individual patients up to 17 years [15]. Therefore, it may be assumed that the hemodynamic improvement will equally persist.

A more extended recommendation of surgical treatment, which seems to be justified from the clinical and hemodynamic data presented in this study, cannot be given unless the surgical risk is taken into account. Whereas earlier studies have reported considerable operative mortality rates [2, 7, 22, 25], increased surgical experience has significantly reduced the risk of death during operation. Most recently published statistics including 30–124 patients have yielded mortality rates of 0–8% [1, 15, 18, 21]. Of our last 51 patients operated upon during 1976 and 1979, who were usually in an advanced stage of the disease, only two patients (4%) have died in the perioperative period.

Considering the significantly better symptomatic and functional results, surgical therapy conceivably might not be confined to only the most severely compromised patients in functional class III and IV. Provided that an experienced surgical team is available, it seems reasonable to consider expanding the indications for surgery to the moderately compromised patients in class II if they do not benefit from medical therapy. However, since the definite effects of operation on survival are unknown, this approach must still be undertaken with great caution.

References

1. Bigelow WG, Trimble AS, Wigle ED, Adelman AG, Felderhof AG (1974) The treatment of muscular subaortic stenosis. J Thorac Cardiovasc Surg 68:384
2. Binet JP, Langlois J, Conso JF, Plache C (1976) Traitement chirurgical de 52 cardiomyopathies obstructives. Arch Mal Coeur 69:777
3. Borer JS, Bacharach SL, Green MV, Kent KM, Rosing DR, Seides SF, Morrow AG, Epstein SE (1979) Effect of septal myotomy and myectomy on left ventricular systolic function at rest and during exercise in patients with IHSS. Circulation [Suppl I] 60:82
4. Edwards RHT, Kristinsson A, Warrell DA, Goodwin JF (1970) Effects of propranolol on response to exercise in hypertrophic obstructive cardiomyopathy. Br Heart J 32:219
5. Flamm MD, Harrison DC, Hancock EW (1968) Muscular subaortic stenosis. Prevention of outflow obstruction with propranolol. Circulation 38:846
6. Frank MJ, Abdulla AM, Canedo MI, Saylors RE (1978) Long-term medical management of hypertrophic obstructive cardiomyopathy. Am J Cardiol 42:993
7. Gerbaux A, Hanania G, Godefroid A, Baragan J, Maouad J, Gay J (1976) Resultats à long terme du traitement chirurgical de la myocardiopathie obstructive par intervention sur le septum interventriculaire. Arch Mal Coeur 69:791
8. Harrison DC, Braunwald E, Glick G, Mason DT, Chidsey CA, Ross J Jr (1964) Effects of beta adrenergic blockade on the circulation, with particular reference to observations in patients with hypertrophic subaortic stenosis. Circulation 29:84

9. Kaltenbach M, Hopf R, Kober G, Bussmann W-D, Keller M, Petersen Y (1979) Treatment of hypertrophic obstructive cardiomyopathy with verapamil. Br Heart J 42:35
10. Kuhn H (1979) Hypertrophische obstruktive Kardiomyopathie. In: Bolte HD (ed) Therapie mit Beta-Rezeptorenblockern. Springer, Berlin Heidelberg New York, p 71
11. Kuhn H, Köhler E, Krelhaus W, Bircks W, Loogen F (1978) Die hypertrophischen Kardiomyopathien – diagnostische und therapeutische Möglichkeiten. Therapiewoche 28:9956
12. Kuhn H, Krelhaus W, Bircks W, Schulte HD, Loogen F (1978) Indication for surgical treatment in patients with hypertrophic obstructive cardiomyopathy. In: Kaltenbach M, Loogen F, Olsen EGJ (eds) Cardiomyopathy and myocardial biopsy. Springer, Berlin Heidelberg New York, p 308
13. Loogen F, Kuhn H, Krelhaus W (1978) Natural history of hypertrophic obstructive cardiomyopathy and the effect of therapy. In: Kaltenbach M, Loogen F, Olsen EGJ (eds) Cardiomyopathy and myocardial biopsy. Springer, Berlin Heidelberg New York, p 286
14. Lösse B, Kuhn H, Krönert H, Rafflenbeul D, Kirschner P, Schulte HD, Loogen F (1980) Hämodynamische Auswirkungen konservativer und operativer Therapie bei hypertrophischer obstruktiver Kardiomyopathie. Z Kardiol 69:470
15. Maron BJ, Merrill WH, Freier PA, Kent KM, Epstein SE, Morrow AG (1978) Long-term clinical course and symptomatic status of patients after operation for hypertrophic subaortic stenosis. Circulation 57:1205
16. Morrow AG, Reitz BA, Epstein SE, Henry WL, Conkle DM, Itscoitz SB, Redwood DR (1975) Operative treatment in hypertrophic subaortic stenosis: Techniques and the results of pre- and postoperative assessments in 83 patients. Circulation 52:88
17. Redwood DR, Goldstein RE, Hirshfeld J, Borer JS, Morganroth J, Morrow AG, Epstein SE (1979) Exercise performance after septal myotomy and myectomy in patients with obstructive hypertrophic cardiomyopathy. Am J Cardiol 44:215
18. Reis RL, Hannah H, Carley JE, Pugh DM (1977) Surgical treatment in idiopathic hypertrophic subaortic stenosis (IHSS): Postoperative results in 30 patients following ventricular septal myotomy and myectomy (Morrow procedure). Circulation [Suppl II] 56:128
19. Rosing DR, Kent KM, Borer JS, Seides SF, Maron BJ, Epstein SE (1979) Verapamil therapy: A new approach to the pharmacologic treatment of hypertrophic cardiomyopathy. I. Hemodynamic effects. Circulation 60:1201
20. Rosing DR, Kent KM, Maron BJ, Epstein SE (1979) Verapamil therapy: A new approach to the pharmacologic treatment of hypertrophic cardiomyopathy. II. Effects on exercise capacity and symptomatic status. Circulation 60:1208
21. Rothlin M, Arbenz U, Krayenbühl HP, Turina J, Senning A (1976) Spätresultate nach Operationen bei muskulärer subvalvulärer Aortenstenose. Z Kardiol 65:501
22. Shah PM, Adelman AG, Wigle ED, Gobel FL, Burchell HB, Hardarson T, Curiel R, De la Calzada C, Oakley CM, Goodwin JF (1974) The natural (and unnatural) history of hypertrophic obstructive cardiomyopathy. Circ Res [Suppl II] 34, 35:179
23. Sowton E (1976) Betarezeptorenblocker bei hypertrophischer Kardiomyopathie. In: Schweizer W (ed) Die Betablocker – Gegenwart und Zukunft. Huber, Bern Stuttgart Wien, p 239
24. Stenson RE, Flamm MD, Harrison DC, Hancock EW (1973) Hypertrophic subaortic stenosis: Clinical and hemodynamic effects of long-term propranolol therapy. Am J Cardiol 31:763
25. Tajik AJ, Giuliani ER, Weidman WH, Brandenburg RO, McGoon DC (1974) Idiopathic hypertrophic subaortic stenosis: Long-term surgical follow-up. Am J Cardiol 34:815
26. Webb-Peploe M (1971) Management of hypertrophic obstructive cardiomyopathy by beta-blockade. In: Wolstenholme GEW, O'Connor M (eds) Hypertrophic obstructive cardiomyopathy, Ciba foundation study group No 37. J & A Churchill, London, p 103

Long-Term Treatment of Hypertrophic Cardiomyopathy with Verapamil or Propranolol. Preliminary Results of a Multicenter Study

G. Kober, R. Hopf, A. Schmidt, M. Kaltenbach, G. Biamino, R. Schröder, P. Bubenheimer, H. Roskamm, P. Hanrath, F. Sonntag, K.-E. v. Olshausen, H. Zebe, W. Kübler, W. Schönung, A. Müller, and M. Schlepper

No clear therapeutic guidelines have as yet emerged in the treatment of obstructive and nonobstructive hypertrophic cardiomyopathy (HCM), a disease entity the etiology of which remains poorly understood.

The long-term administration of beta-adrenergic blocking agents has proven disappointing in a considerable percentage of patients [1]. Surgical intervention represents a therapeutic alternative only in selected, severely symptomatic patients with the obstructive form of hypertrophic cardiomyopathy [2, 3].

In recent years favorable therapeutic results, even in patients who failed to respond to propranolol, have been reported in a nonrandomized study with the long-term administration of the calcium antagonist verapamil [4–6]. Other investigators have recently been able to confirm the effects of verapamil on various pathologic parameters in hypertrophic cardiomyopathy, primarily following acute administration of the drug [7–10]. Long-term clinical results of other groups as well as controlled studies concerning the therapy of hypertrophic cardiomyopathy with calcium antagonists have not yet been published.

The current multicenter study was designed to compare the therapeutic effectiveness of propranolol, which has been used in HCM for a longer period of time, with verapamil in a larger group of patients under controlled conditions. The present manuscript presents the design and preliminary results of this study, which is still in progress.

Methods

The six participating German centers in Bad Krozingen, Bad Nauheim, Berlin, Hamburg, Frankfurt, and Heidelberg agreed upon a uniform protocol for examination, follow-up, and therapy. After confirmation of the diagnosis using noninvasive and invasive techniques, the findings were reported to the central collection point in Frankfurt.

Matched pairs of patients with similar findings, especially with regard to age, complaints, murmurs, electro- and echocardiographic findings, and intraventricular gradients, were formed and therapy with either propranolol or verapamil was assigned.

The first partner of a patient pair was treated with either propranolol or verapamil: Partner 1 of the first pair of patients received verapamil; Partner 1 of the second pair propranolol; Partner 1 of the third pair verapamil again, and so forth. If the first partner of a given pair received verapamil, the second matched partner received propranolol and vice versa.

Therapy was initiated with propranolol 40 mg 3× per day or verapamil 80 mg 3 times per day. One week later the dosage was raised to propranolol 80 mg 3 times per day or verapamil 160 mg 3× per day and, if tolerated well, increased further to propranolol 360 mg per day and verapamil 720 mg per day.

115 patients are currently participating in the study. 33 pairs have been formed; 29 patients are still awaiting the assignment of an appropriate partner. Twenty patients have thus far dropped out of the study for various reasons. To statistically evaluate, say, a possible decline of 0.5 mV in the Sokolow Index during 2 years of therapy, complete follow-up studies on at least 50 patient pairs are required.

The results of such follow-up studies for the 1st and 2nd year following the initiation of therapy are available for only a few patient pairs. For this reason, it is not possible to compare the two forms of therapy in terms of matched groups at this time.

Results

Fig. 1 shows how 70 patients assessed the effect of therapy on a variety of subjective complaints which were present before the onset of treatment. Forty patients belong to the verapamil group and 30 received propranolol. The absolute incidence of any given symptom prior to therapy is represented by the height of the column. The percentage of patients in whom any given symptom improved, remained unchanged, or worsened is shown by the column subdivisions. Prior to therapy, for

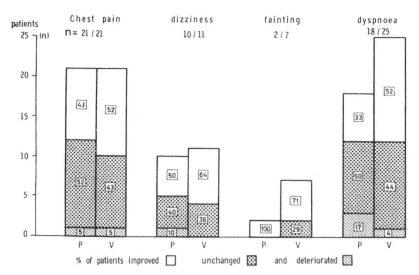

Fig. 1. Changes in four major symptoms in 70 patients with hypertrophic cardiomyopathy treated with propranolol (n=30) or verapamil (n=40). The height of the columns represent the absolute incidence of any given symptom, the column subdivisions the percent change in symptoms

example, 21 of 40 patients (52%) in the verapamil group and 21 of 30 patients (70%) in the propranolol group displayed angina pectoris. During verapamil therapy, angina pectoris improved in 52%, dizziness in 64%, and dyspnea in 52% of the patients.

The response was not quite as good with propranolol: angina pectoris improved in 43%, dizziness in 50%, and dyspnea in 33%. Syncope, a relatively rare symptom, cannot yet be evaluated for the two agents.

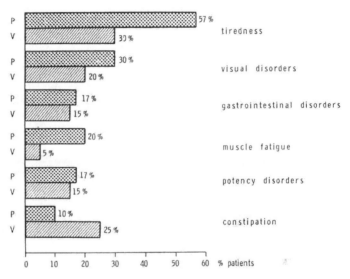

Fig. 2. Side effects of long-term treatment of hypertrophic cardiomyopathy with verapamil (▨, n = 30 = 100%) or propranolol (▨, n = 40 = 100%). Preliminary results of a multicenter study

If the percentages of complaints which worsened are totalled, a figure of 32% is obtained for propranolol and 9% for verapamil. Verapamil thus appears to be superior to propranolol both in terms of providing relief as well as failing to aggrevate existing symptoms.

Fig. 2 shows new symptoms which arose among the 70 treated patients as well as side effects for both drugs. In no case did they force termination of therapy. A relatively high percentage of patients reported general tiredness and visual disturbances, both more often in association with propranolol. The high frequency of visual complaints in the propranolol group seems to be particularly noteworthy in light of changes in the eyes of beagles observed experimentally during the administration of verapamil (Knoll company, personal communication). Only constipation was reported more often in the verapamil group and is probably related to the muscle relaxation effect of calcium antagonists. If the percentage figures for all symptoms are again collected, the results for propranolol (151%) are somewhat worse than for verapamil (110%).

Fig. 3 shows the preliminary course of therapy, which at this point in the study is not based on paired comparisons. The pretreatment values of the parameters

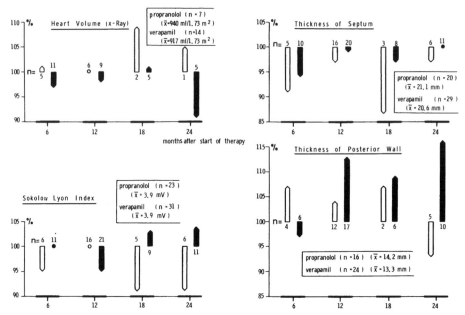

Fig. 3. Percent change in heart volume (X-ray), Sokolow-Lyon Index (ECG), and left ventricular septal and posterior wall thickness (echo) in two different patient groups treated with propranolol (*open arrows*) and verapamil (*closed arrows*). Pretreatment values (in brackets) were assumed to equal 100%. The results shown for 6 to 24 months after start of therapy are based on different patients

being studied (radiographically calculated heart volume, Sokolow-Lyon-Index, echocardiographically measured wall thickness of the interventricular septum, and posterior wall of the left ventricle) were assumed to equal 100%. Mean initial values are given additionally in brackets. The percent change from this initial value is represented by the length of the arrows. Studies of statistical significance were not judged to be meaningful because of the small numbers involved and various follow-up intervals.

Heart volume (upper normal limit for males 800 ml/1.73 m² and for females 700 ml/1.73 m²) showed a tendency to decline during verapamil therapy (mean initial value was 917 ml/1.73 m²), whereas in the propranolol group (mean initial value 940 ml/1.73 m²) no change or even slight increase could be observed.

Based upon a mean initial Sokolow Index of 3.9 mV, propranolol therapy was associated with a 5–10% decline for various follow-up intervals. The initial value of 3.9 mV for the verapamil group remained nearly unchanged.

The mean thickness of the interventricular septum (initial value prior to propranolol 21.1 mm and prior to verapamil 20.6 mm) showed a tendency to decline with both agents. By contrast, the thickness of the left ventricular posterior wall (mean initial values prior to propranolol 14.2 mm and prior to verapamil 13.3 mm) increased.

Table 1 shows the reasons why 20 patients dropped out of the study prematurely. In 12 patients – five received propranolol and seven verapamil –

therapy had to be terminated on noncardiac grounds. In eight instances, treatment was ended on a therapy-related basis: six patients stopped taking propranolol because it was ineffective, caused congestive heart failure, or induced gastrointestinal complaints. One verapamil patient did not continue because of gastrointestinal complaints and another because of dizziness.

Table 1. Reasons for terminating therapy (20 of 115 patients)

Nontherapy related			12
	Propranolol	Verapamil	
	5	7	
Therapy related			8
	Propranolol	Verapamil	
Ineffective	3	–	
Congestive Heart failure	1	–	
Gastrointestinal complaints	2	1	
Dizziness	–	1	

Discussion

In a randomized study of patients with obstructive and nonobstructive hypertrophic cardiomyopathy, the effectiveness of the beta-adrenergic blocking agent, propranolol, was compared with that of the calcium antagonist, verapamil. Because of the novelty of this therapeutic concept as well as the high doses, especially of verapamil, employed, a double-blind study did not appear justifiable. The formation of patient pairs is essentially free of bias, since assignment is made on the basis of previously established data by an investigator who has not seen the patient personally.

The changes in subjective complaints and the appearance of new symptoms and side effects during therapy are important both for the evaluation of different forms of treatment as well as patient compliance.

Both agents were able to ameliorate the subjective complaints of the patients. When the frequency of improvement or deterioration is assessed in percentage terms, verapamil appears to be superior to propranolol, although the numbers are too small to make meaningful, statistically valid statements.

Irritating side effects also occurred more often with propranolol, although in no case did they force discontinuation of the drug. Only in a very small number of patients was an agent withdrawn for reasons directly related to therapy. For this reason, it is not possible to draw any clear distinctions between the two agents.

The preliminary results of follow-up studies in a small number of patients demonstrates some efficacy for both drugs. The findings, however, appear to vary widely according to the time at which the follow-up investigations were made. The rather poor uniformity of objective data might be related to the fact that in general the findings of different patients became available when the various follow-up studies were made. Even at this point of the study, the inability to compare groups based on the patient pairs contributes to the widely varying results.

Summary

Patients with comparable severe hypertrophic cardiomyopathy were randomly assigned a treatment regimen with propranolol, a beta-blocking agent, or verapamil, a calcium antagonist. Preliminary results from nonmatched patient groups suggest that complaints improved more noticably and side effects occurred less often with verapamil than propranolol. Objective parameters indicate a trend toward improvement, although so far no definite differences between the two agents are recognizable.

References

1. Kuhn H, Loogen F (1978) Die Anwendung von Beta-Rezeptorenblockern bei hypertrophischer obstruktiver Kardiomyopathie. Internist (Berlin) 19:527–531
2. Maron BJ, Merrill WH, Freier PA, Kent KM, Epstein SE, Morrow AG (1978) Long-term clinical course and symptomatic status of patients after operation for hypertrophic subaortic stenosis. Circulation 57:1205–1213
3. Epstein SE, Morrow AG, Henry WL, Clark CE (1973) The role of operative treatment in patients with JHSS. Circulation 48:677
4a. Kaltenbach M, Hopf R, Keller M (1976) Calciumantagonistische Therapie bei hypertroph-obstruktiver Kardiomyopathie. Dtsch Med Wschr 101:1284
4b. Kaltenbach M, Hopf R, Kober G, Bussmann WD, Keller M, Petersen Y (1979) Treatment of hypertrophic obstructive cardiomyopathy with verapamil. Br Heart J 42:35–42
5. Hopf R, Keller M, Kaltenbach M (1976) Die Behandlung der hypertrophen obstruktiven Kardiomyopathie mit Verapamil. Verh Dtsch Ges Innern Med 82:1054–1057
6. Kober G, Hopf R, Lemke R, Kaltenbach M (1978) Klinische Studie zur Therapie der hypertrophen obstruktiven Kardiomyopathie mit Calzium-Antagonisten. VI. Kolloquium, Paul Martini Stiftung, Göttingen 137–148
7. Hirzel HO, Troesch W, Jenni R, Krayenbuehl HP (1980) Reduction of septal thickness following verapamil in patients with hypertrophic obstructive cardiomyopathy. VIII Eur Congr Cardiol Paris, 22–26 June 1980, 140
8. Schmidt P, Pavek P, Klein W (1979) Echokardiographische und hämodynamische Untersuchungen zur Beeinflussung der hypertrophischen obstruktiven Kardiomyopathie durch Verapamil. Z Kardiol 68:89–92
9. Rosing DR, Kent KM, Borer JS, Seides ST, Maron BJ, Epstein SE (1979) Verapamil therapy: A new approach to the pharmacologic treatment of hypertrophic cardiomyopathy. I. Hemodynamic Effects. Circulation 60:1201–1207
10. Rosing DR, Kent KM, Maron BJ, Epstein SE (1979) Verapamil therapy: A new approach to the pharmacologic treatment of hypertrophic cardiomyopathy. II. Effects on exercise capacity and symptomatic status. Circulation 60:1208–1213

Effects of Different Calcium Blockers and Implications Regarding Therapy of Hypertrophic Cardiomyopathy

Synopsis

G. KOBER

Our understanding of the calcium ion's cellular mechanisms of action as well as of substances that interfere with calcium metabolism – the so-called calcium antagonists – has grown considerably in recent years. Many questions, however, remain unanswered.

Calcium is of great significance in the function of all bodily cells, especially those comprising cardiac and vascular muscle as well as the specialized conduction system of the heart. More than ten sites of action for calcium ions have already been identified intracellularly and on the cell membrane. The term "calcium antagonists" refers to a group of agents with different molecular structures but which share an experimental ability to inhibit calcium-induced electromechanical coupling in cardiac and vascular muscle.

Individual calcium antagonists, however, have been shown in animal experiments and human studies to possess considerably different modes of action. A wide range of effects has been observed on the heart and peripheral vasculature. Several agents have antiarrhythmic properties. Varying degrees of negative inotropic activity have also been described. These dissimilarities are thought to result from the number of receptor sites occupied on the cell membrane and organelles. Different structures appear to have different levels of sensitivity to different calcium antagonists. This phenomenon may be related to the distribution of cell organelles, the presence of specific calcium receptors, and the characteristics of the cell membrane.

It thus becomes clear that there can be no single prototype for the calcium antagonists. Calcium's broad range of effects is inhibited extremely variably and only more or less specifically. Moreover, these agents also show varying degrees of interference with the transmembrane flux of sodium and potassium. This factor may provide a further explanation for the widely different properties exhibited by individual substances.

Because calcium antagonists induce a considerable spectrum of pharmacological effects, each such agent must be the object of careful clinical trials once animal experiments and studies on isolated organs have been completed. A demonstrated therapeutic effect is initially valid only for the substance and mechanism of action being investigated.

As the following papers illustrate, attempts to identify the similarities and differences among various calcium antagonists have stimulated the design of many imaginative studies in animals and man.

The Antianginal Efficacy of Seven Different Calcium Antagonists

H.-J. BECKER, R. HOPF, G. KOBER, and M. KALTENBACH

Experience with calcium antagonists in the treatment of hypertrophic cardiomyopathy (HCM) has been restricted essentially to verapamil. It is not known whether other agents with calcium antagonistic properties may exert comparable effects. The evaluation of such drugs in patients with HCM is difficult. Comparison of different calcium antagonists, however, is possible in respect to the antianginal activity [1, 3, 4, 6, 13, 16, 18, 21, 22, 23, 24, 25, 26].

We investigated the antianginal activity of seven different calcium antagonists in patients with coronary heart disease. ST-segment changes during exercise were used as parameter of ischemia.

Methods

Only patients with well-documented coronary heart disease were included. No other medication was administered during the study. ST-segment depression was reproducible in preceeding exercise tests. Placebo tests before and after termination of therapy were performed. Exercise tests were performed at the same time of day to exclude diurnal variations [11]. Exercise tests were not symptom limited. Work load and duration of exercise were determined in preceeding tests and maintained throughout the study even if the patients were able to tolerate longer exercise time or higher work loads during therapy.

In different groups of patients with coronary heart disease seven calcium antagonists were tested. ST-segment depression was measured during and after exercise using an arm-assisted step test [14, 15]. For each minute of exercise and recovery ST-segment depression was measured, averaged, and the values for each minute added (Fig. 1). The resulting sum of ST depression was compared to the corresponding value in the placebo tests from the same patient.

Results

Prenylamine, the oldest calcium antagonist, proved ineffective in reducing ischemic ST-segment depression in a dosage of 240 mg po (Table 1, Fig. 2).

Verapamil reduced ischemic ST-segment depression. The improvement was 26% after 160 mg po, 51% after 320 mg po, and 40% after 5 mg iv. While intravenous application did not reduce heart rate during exercise, oral administration of the high dosage led to a reduction in heart rate during exercise by 8% (see Tables 1, 2, Fig. 2).

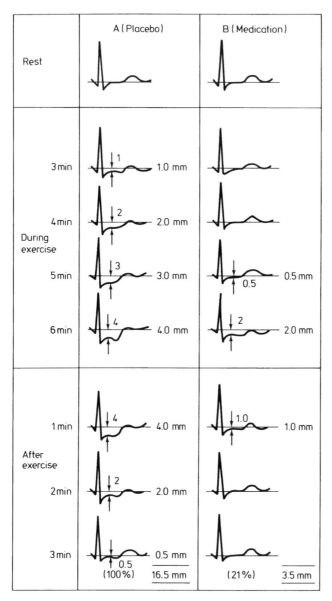

Fig. 1. Behavior of the ST segment in the exercise test in patients with typical ischemic reaction, under *A* (placebo) and under *B* (medication). The measurement of the ST depression is shown schematically. The numerical value given underneath refers to the sum of the ST depression from minute to minute. For the comparison of the results in a given patient, the total ST depression in the control test was always set at 100%

The Antianginal Efficacy of Seven Different Calcium Antagonists

Table 1. Antianginal effect of different calcium antagonists

Drug	Dosage (mg)	Time after application investigated (min)	Improvement of ST depression (mm)		%	n
Prenylamine	240	90	–	–	n.s.	13
Verapamil	160	60	10.7	7.86	26[a]	17
	320	90	10.4	5.1	51[a]	24
	5 i.v.	5	11.2	7.9	30[a]	16
Nifedipine	20	30	17.3	8.9	48[a]	18
	1.0 i.v.	60	14.2	2.9	78[a]	7
	0.1 i.c.	60	14.2	4.8	63[a]	7
Fendiline	300	135	15.9	16.5	n.s.	20
	450	135	15.9	14.3	n.s.	20
Perhexilene maleate	200	120–180	10.9	7.3	33[a]	15
	400	120–180	10.9	6.9	37[a]	15
Etafenone	150	90	8.85	7.6	n.s.	10
	300	90	8.1	5.6	31[a]	5
	450	90	8.1	5.0	38[a]	5
Diltiazem	50	90	10.6	7.6	28[a]	10

n.s., not significant.

[a] Significant ($2\,P < 0.05$–0.001)

Table 2. Heart rate before and after different calcium antagonists

Drug	Dosage (mg)	Heart rate rest		standing		exercise	
		before	after	before	after	before	after
Verapamil	160	70	71	79	80	118	116
	320	71	75	81	84	130	120
	5 i.v.	69	72	79	82	118	114
Nifedipine	20	75	76	–	–	122	122
	1.0 i.v.	66	73	–	–	105	102
	0.1 i.c.	66	65	–	–	105	103
Fendiline	300	76	78	83	84	121	120
	450	76	77	83	85	121	117
Perhexilene	200	67	67	–	76	116	105
maleate	400	64	64	–	68	116	103
Etafenone	150	72	70	82	78	115	114
	300	71	64	81	72	112	110
	450	69	79	79	83	110	117
Diltiazem	60	71	68	81	77	123	120

Nifedipine also had a marked effect on ischemic ST shifts during exercise after 20 mg po. The average improvement was almost 50%. A similar reduction could be achieved after the injection of 1.0 mg iv. Blood pressure showed a marked decrease with both routes of application, whereas heart rate remained unchanged or increased with interindividual variations. Paradoxic reactions with a marked reduction in blood pressure and increase in heart rate leading to a worsening of ischemic ST-segment patterns were occasionally seen. In a separate study [16], the effect of a small

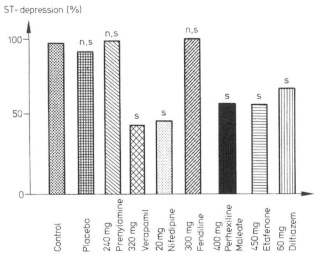

Fig. 2. Antianginal activity of seven different calcium antagonists

dose of nifedipine injected directly into the coronary circulation (0.1 mg into the left coronary artery) was evaluated. A similar reduction of ischemic ST-segment changes was seen as after 20 mg orally. There was no change in heart rate after intracoronary administration.

Fendiline was given to 20 patients with coronary heart disease. No significant improvement in ST-segment depression was seen after 300 mg po. Long-term treatment with 50 mg three times daily over a period of 4 weeks was also ineffective. Even the additional administration of 300 mg (a total dose of 450 mg fendilin) yielded results that did not differ significantly from placebo. Heart rate and blood pressure were not affected.

Perhexilene maleate in a dosage of 200 mg po over a period of 2 weeks diminished ischemic ST-segment depression in 15 patients by 33%. A dose of 400 mg led to an improvement of 37%. Heart rate during exercise was reduced significantly by 10% [6].

Etafenone in a dosage of 150 mg orally given to ten patients with coronary heart disease reduced ischemic ST-segment changes not significantly. Five patients received 300 and 450 mg. At these dosages the improvement of ST-segment depression was 31–38%. Heart rate was not affected significantly. These high dosages led to marked side effects. The five patients complained of dizziness and headache. Therefore these dosages will probably not be tolerated in a long-term treatment.

Diltiazem was given to ten patients in a dosage of 60 mg po. The improvement of ischemic ST-segment depression was 28%. In contrast the reduction of heart rate by diltiazem at rest and during exercise was not significant [19].

Discussion

These results demonstrate that calcium antagonists differ in terms of antianginal potency. These agents display marked structural variations and may have dissimilar mechanisms of action and a variety of effects [17, 30, 31]. Fleckenstein [8] assumes that the different effects are attributable to different doses. Increasing dosages may reveal similar effects in animal experiments but cannot be tested in humans.

Fendiline, which has a chemical structure similar to that of prenylamine, showed no antianginal effect, as did prenylamine.

Other calcium antagonists with divergent chemical structures (diltiazem, etafenone, nifedipine, perhexilene maleate, and verapamil) are potent antianginal drugs.

The antianginal effect of nifedipine, perhexilene maleate, and verapamil is undisputed [1, 3, 4, 6, 9, 12, 13, 16, 18, 19, 22–26, 29]. Similar claims for fendiline has been made by Enenkel [5], Reiterer [27], Schäfer [28], and Streicher [32].

The effect seen by Enenkel [5] and Streicher [32] was small. Enenkel [5] found that ischemic depression improved by 0.5 mm in only 50% of the patients; one-third became worse. Reiterer [27] investigated hemodynamic data with the combination of beta blocker and fendiline and attributed the efficacy of fendiline to a nitroglycerin-like effect.

Diastolic pulmonary artery pressure increased with the combination of oxprenolol and fendiline, however. The addition of nitroglycerin led to a reduction in diastolic pulmonary artery pressure by 6 mmHg. Schäfer [28], who observed favorable effects during fendiline therapy, employed symptom-limited exercise tests.

Bucher [2], in a clinical trial, found etafenone to be effective in comparison with placebo in a dosage of 150 mg three times daily. We found etafenone in a single dose of 150 mg ineffective, whereas higher doses were effective but revealed side effects. The study of Bucher does not appear valid because additional drugs (nitroglycerin, analgeties, and sedatives) were permitted, and only subjective symptoms were assessed.

Conclusion

The calcium antagonist verapamil seems effective in the treatment of angina pectoris and hypertrophic cardiomyopathy. The antianginal properties of other drugs classified as calcium antagonists are not uniform, however. Prenylamine and fendiline, for example, have no antianginal activity, whereas five other agents reduce ST-segment depression during exercise. Side effects vary; whereas nifedipine tends to increase heart rate, verapamil appears to depress sinus node activity and atrioventricular conduction.

The demonstrated differences in the antianginal effect of the various calcium antagonists have implications toward possible use in the treatment of hypertrophic cardiomyopathy. The favorable results achieved with verapamil may not automatically apply to other calcium antagonists.

References

1. Bala Subramanian V, Bowler M, Paramasivon R, Lahiri A, Raftery EB (1980) Verapamil in ischemic heart disease. Experience in 100 patients assessed by objective methods. Calcium antagonism in cardiovasc therapy. Experience with Verapamil. Internat Symp Florence
2. Bucher J, Fischer J, Karobath H, Wenger R (1972) Zweifach klinischer Doppelblindversuch mit der neuen koronarwirksamen Substanz Etafenon und einem Kontrollpräparat. Herz/Kreislauf 4:56–61
3. Becker H-J, Kaltenbach M, Kober G (1975) Comparison of the effects of adalat with other substances on myocardial ischemia under loading conditions. In: Lochner W, Braasch W, Kroneberg G (eds) 2nd Adalat Symposium. Springer, Berlin Heidelberg New York, p 156–163
4. Eklund LG, Atterhög JH, Melin AL (1973) Effect of nifedipin on exercise tolerance in patients with angina pectoris. In: Hashimoto K, Kimura E, Kobayashi T. 1st international Nifedipin (Adalat) Symposium. Tokyo Press, p 144–149
5. Enenkel N, Spiel R (1980) Effekt von Fendilin auf Belastungs-EKG und Belastungshämodynamik bei Koronarkranken. In: Fleckenstein A, Roskamm H (eds) Calcium-Antagonism. Springer, Berlin Heidelberg New York, p 326–330
6. Ferlemann H-J, Krehan L, Kaltenbach M (1979) Wirkung von Perhexilinmaleat auf das Belastungs-EKG von Patienten mit koronarer Herzerkrankung. Z Kardiol 68:826–831
7. Ferlinz J, Easthope JL, Aronow WS (1979) Effects of verapamil on myocardial performance in coronary disease. Circulation 59, No 2:313–319
8. Fleckenstein A (1980) Steuerung der myokardialen Kontraktilität, ATP-Spaltung, Atmungsintensität und Schrittmacherfunktion durch Calcium-Ionen. Wirkungsmechanismus der Calcium-Antagonisten. In: Fleckenstein A, Roskamm H (ed) Springer, Berlin Heidelberg New York, p 1–28
9. Goebel G, Mannes GA, Kafka W, Fleck E, Rudolph W (1977) Behandlung der Angina pectoris mit Perhexillinmaleat. Herz 3:289–297
10. Hagemann K, Lochner W, Niehues B (1975) Studies on the extracardial effects of nifedipine in anesthetized dogs. In: Lochner W, Braasch W, Kroneberg G (eds) 2nd Adalat Symposium. Springer, Berlin Heidelberg New York, p 49–53
11. Henkels V, Blümchen G (1977) Tageszeitliche Schwankungen der Belastungs-Koronarinsuffizienz. Muench. Med Wochenschr [Suppl I] 119:58–63
12. Hopf R, Schmidt H, Kaltenbach M (1978) Kombination von Isosorbiddinitrat mit Nifedipin bei der Behandlung der koronaren Herzkrankheit. Z Kardiol [Suppl V] 67
13. Hosoda S, Kasanuki H, Miyata K, Endo M, Hirosawa K (1973) Results of a clinical investigation of nifedipine in angina pectoris with special reference to its therapeutic efficacy in attacks at rest. In: Hashimoto K, Kimura E, Kobayashi T. 1st International nifedipine symposium. Tokyo Press, p 185–189
14. Kaltenbach M (1974) Die Belastungsuntersuchung von Herzkranken. Böhringer, Mannheim
15. Kaltenbach M, Becker H-J, Kollath J, Spitz P, Kober G (1971) Exercise electrocardiogram and selective coronary arteriography. In: Kaltenbach M, Lichtlen P (eds) Coronary heart disease. Thieme, Stuttgart, p 66–78

The Antianginal Efficacy of Seven Different Calcium Antagonists

16. Kaltenbach M, Schulz W, Kober G (1979) Effects of nifedipine after intravenous and intracoronary administration. Am J Cardiol 44:832–838
17. Kaufmann R (1977) Differenzierung verschiedener Kalziumantagonisten. Muench Wochenschr [Suppl I] 119:6–11
18. Kelly DT, Freedmann SB, Richmond DR (1980) Coronary spasm at rest and during exercise and response to treatment with verapamil. Calcium antagonism in cardiovascular therapy. Experience with verapamil. Intern Symposium Florence
19. Kober G, Berlad T, Hopf R, Kaltenbach M (1981) Die Wirkung von Diltiazem und Nifedipin auf ST-Senkung und Herzfrequenz im Belastungs-EKG bei Patienten mit koronarer Herzerkrankung. Z Kardiol 70:59–65
20. Lichtlen P (1975) Coronary and left ventricular dynamics under nifedipine in comparison to nitrates, beta blocking agents and dipyridamol. In: Lochner W, Braasch W, Kroneberg G (eds) 2nd International Adalat Symposium. Springer, Berlin Heidelberg New York, 212–224
21. Lichtlen PR, Engel H-J, Wolf R, Amende J (1980) The effect of calcium antagonistic drug nifedipine on coronary and left ventricular dynamics in patients with coronary heart disease. In: Fleckenstein A, Roskamm H (eds) Calcium Antagonismus. Springer, Berlin Heidelberg New York, p 270–281
22. Mabuchi G, Kishida H, Suzuki K (1973) Clinical effect of nifedipine on variant form of angina pectoris. In: Hashimoto K, Kimura E, Kabayashi T. 1st International nifedipine symposium. Tokyo press, 177–184
23. Parodi O, L'Abbate A, Simonetti I, Severi S, Marzullo P, Trivella MG, Maseri A (1980) Verapamil in the treatment of vasospastic angina pectoris. Calcium antagonism in cardiovascular therapy. Experience with verapamil. International Symposium Florence
24. Ponti CD, Vincenz M (1980) Acute and chronic effects of verapamil exercise induced angina. Calcium antagonism in cardiovascular therapy. Experience with verapamil. International Symposium Florence
25. Raftos J (1980) Verapamil in the long-term treatment of angina pectoris. Calcium antagonism in cardiovascular therapy. Experience with verapamil. International Symposium Florence
26. Reiterer W (1976) Belastbarkeit Koronargefäßkranker unter Perhexilin. Herz/Kreislauf 8, Nr 3:132–139
27. Reiterer W (1980) Der Einfluß von Fendilin als Monotherapie und in Kombination mit einem Beta-Rezeptorenblocker auf die Belastungshämodynamik. In: Fleckenstein A, Roskamm H (eds) Calcium-Antagonismus. Springer, Berlin Heidelberg New York, p 305–313
28. Schäfer N, Belz GG, Stauch M, Schneider B (1980) Fendilin und Isosorbiddinitrat bei koronarer Herzkrankheit. Dtsch Med Wochenschr 105:1253–1258
29. Schnellbacher K, Kalusche D, Roskamm H (1980) Hämodynamik während belastungs-induzierter Angina pectoris von Fendilin und Nifedipin. In: Fleckenstein A, Roskamm H (eds) Calcium-Antagonismus. Springer, Berlin Heidelberg New York, p 314–317
30. Scholz H (1980) Physiologische und pharmakologische Grundlage der Therapie mit sog. Calcium-Antagonisten. Dtsch Ärzteblatt 7:381–387
31. Spies HF, Schulz W, Werner H, Appel E, Becker H-J, Kaltenbach M (1980) Einfluß von Calcium-Antagonisten Verapamil, Nifedipin, Fendilin auf Blutdruck und Herzfrequenz. In: Fleckenstein A, Roskamm H (eds) Calcium-Antagonismus. Springer, Berlin Heidelberg New York, p 252–257
32. Streicher KA, Guckenbiel W, Olbermann W (1976) Einfluß von Fendilinhydrochlorid (Sensit) im Belastungstest bei Patienten mit koronarer Herzerkrankung. Med Welt 27:1395–1397

Differentiation of Calcium-Antagonistic Drugs with Respect to Their Myocardial Effects

R. Kaufmann, R. Bayer, R. Rodenkirchen, and R. Mannhold

Calcium ions trigger and control numerous elementary cell functions. They play a pivotal role in excitation-contraction coupling of all types of muscle, in stimulus secretion coupling of glands and neurotransmission, in the control of enzyme activities, in the control of membrane excitability, in the formation of membrane to membrane contacts, in lymphocyte transformation and activation, in blood clotting, or in microtubulus assembly, to mention only a few.

Among the drugs interfering with Ca-controlled cellular activities, the so-called Ca antagonists have attracted particular attention. According to a definition given first by Fleckenstein [1], Ca antagonists are said to inhibit the inflow of Ca across the excited cellular membrane, thus, for instance, reducing contractile activation and energy requirements in cardiac cells. Following these pioneering studies numerous drugs were subsequently included in the group of Ca antagonists simply by analog conclusion. However, closer exploration of their pharmacodynamics more and more revealed dissimilar modes and sites of action rather than a strict common principle such that the term "Ca antagonist" became somewhat vague. The main items in this regard may be summarized as follows:

1. Ca antagonists are structurally unrelated. For instance, verapamil has some structural similarities with papaverine, nifedipine with the coenzyme NADH, whereas diltiazem is clearly related to well-known tranquilizers (Fig. 1)
2. Ca antagonists interfere with different cellular sites, each controlling Ca movements. Thus, the effects exerted are qualitatively different [2, 3, 4]. In addition, organ-specific actions must be taken into account [5]
3. Amongst "Ca antagonists" there are also agents subsequently found *not* to inhibit transmembrane Ca influx but to act intracellularly [6]

Therefore, in the light of current thinking one may tentatively coin a new definition: *"Ca antagonists are a very heterogeneous group of agents with dissimilar pharmacodynamic and pharmacokinetic properties acting at different sites. Their only common denominator is a reduction of Ca ions needed to maintain or induce specific cellular activities."*

The central role of Ca ions in controlling a large variety of body functions implies that Ca antagonists may affect the performances of many different organs. Only some of the established or suspected effects are of therapeutic benefit so far. These are, for instance, tocolysis; the spasmolytic action in stomach, ureter, and esophagus; depression of myocardial contractile and pacemaker activities; and, most important, relaxation of vascular smooth muscle. On the other hand, beneficial effects have been reported without a clear-cut understanding of why and how Ca antagonists exert their therapeutic action. This applies in particular to the actual topic of cardiomyopathia where, with our lack of insight into etiologic or

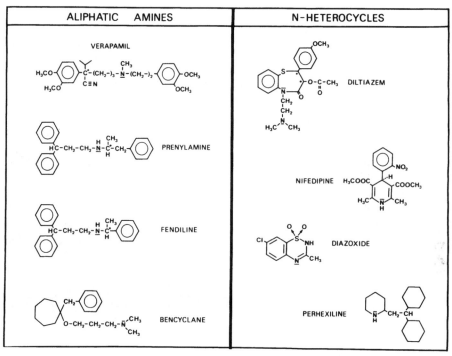

Fig. 1. Chemical structure of established and suspected Ca antagonists

pathogenetic determinants, we can only refer to a black box model to assess therapeutic drug effects. Since we are dealing with heart muscle in general, we will focus our attention on Ca antagonistic effects exerted directly in heart muscle tissues, especially in ventricular working myocardium.

It is well known that all Ca antagonists reduce myocardial contractile force but with different potency. If, however, working conditions of isolated papillary muscles are changed in a way that heart does in body, qualitative differences of actions also appear. For instance, the normal heart responds to a sudden increase in frequency with an increase in contraction amplitudes. This effect develops in a staircase-like manner, the well-known Bowditch phenomenon. The steady state contractions reached at each stimulation frequency define the amplitude frequency relationship (AFR).

In verapamil-treated cardiac muscles this picture drastically changes: Each increase in beat rate is now followed by a negative staircase. Thus, the AFR is inversed. That means that the negative inotropic potency of verapamil is not only dose- but also frequency-dependent to a large extent. At a given dose its effect increases with increasing heart rate. In contrast, prenylamine leaves the staircase phenomena and AFR nearly unaffected. In this case depression of contractility is *not* dependent on heart rate. On the other side perhexiline strongly reduces contractility at low stimulation frequencies whereas, at the more physiologic frequency of 60 beats/min (temperature 32°C), its action is rather weak. Consequently perhexiline tends to steepen the AFR.

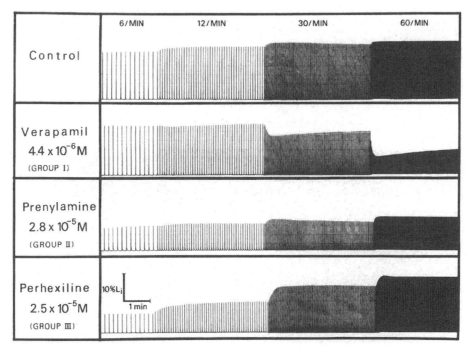

Fig. 2. Original recordings of amplitude-frequency pattern in isotonically contracting cat papillary muscles, stimulated with stepwise increasing frequencies from 6 to 60/min. Effects of verapamil, prenylamine, and perhexiline as compared to a representative control registration

Thus, in heart muscle, one may subdivide Ca antagonists into three groups according to the above patterns of inotropic actions (Fig. 2):

I) Compounds inverting the AFR such as verapamil, fendiline, and diltiazem
II) Negative inotropic drugs which do not change the shape of the AFR such as prenylamine and nifedipine
III) Drugs accentuating the AFR such as perhexiline, diazoxide, and bencyclane

It would be interesting to know whether this classification is relevant as to the efficacy of Ca antagonists in the therapy of hypertrophic cardiomyopathy.

Among group I and II we find the "classical" Ca antagonists verapamil, prenylamine, and nifedipine where, by means of voltage clamp investigations direct evidence as to their inhibitory action on transmembrane Ca^{2+}-inward current through the so-called slow channel exists [4, 7, 8, 9]. Figures 3 and 4 give examples of such evidence and, at the same time, also demonstrate that, for instance, nifedipine and (−)-verapamil act rather differently on slow channel conductivity. Isolated cat papillary muscles were first stimulated at a rate of 6/min and an action potential was recorded (labeled 6 in the upper panel of Figs. 3 and 4). Then voltage clamp conditions were switched on to measure the slow inward current (labeled 6 in the lower panel). Cycle frequency was then increased to 60/min and the slow

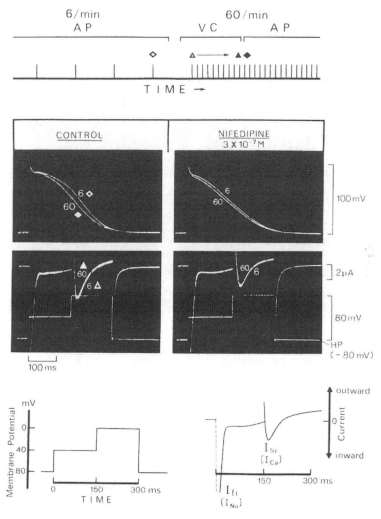

Fig. 3. Voltage clamp experiments to test the influence of the repetition rate on the slow Ca^{2+}-inward current and AP configuration under control conditions and after the addition of nifedipine. In the upper panel the protocol is given; the preparations were first stimulated with a frequency of 6/min and an action potential was recorded (labeled ◇). Thereafter stimulation rate was increased and at the same moment voltage clamp conditions were switched on to record the slow inward current for ten subsequent cycles (labeled 6 △—60 ▲). Then voltage clamp conditions were switched off and the first of the following action potentials recorded (labeled 60 ◆).

The middle panel shows original recordings of the membrane potential and the superimposed current traces.

The lower panel shows schematically the method to separate the slow inward current from the fast inward current. A first depolarizing clamp step from the holding potential (–80 mV) to –40 mV activated the fast inward current (I$_{fi}$, first downward deflection of the current trace) which within a few milliseconds was inactivated. After 150 ms the membrane was further depolarized to zero potential eliciting the slow inward current (I$_{si}$, second downward deflection). After 150 ms the clamp cycle was terminated by repolarizing the membrane back to –80 mV

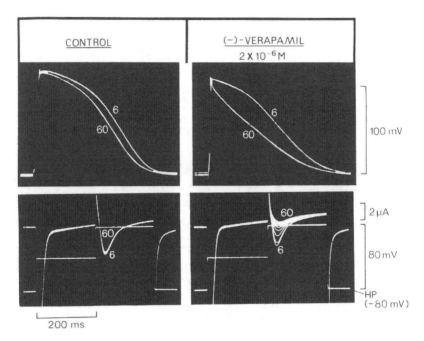

Fig. 4. Voltage clamp experiments to test the influence of (–)-verapamil on slow Ca^{2+}-inward current. Same experimental protocol as in Fig. 3

inward current recorded for 10 consecutive cycles. At the end of this period another action potential was recorded (labeled 60) for comparison. Figure 3 shows that the extent to which nifedipine depresses the plateau of the action potential and reduces the slow inward current does not depend on cycle frequency whereas under the same experimental conditions (–)-verapamil (the Ca antagonistic active isomer of verapamil [2]) is almost ineffective at 6/min but fully abolishes slow inward current at 60/min (with a corresponding strong depression of the plateau phase). These voltage clamp findings are in agreement with the above mentioned patterns of negative inotropic actions of both drugs.

In the case of diltiazem and fendiline an inhibition of the slow Ca^{2+}-inward current has not been proven by the voltage clamp technique so far, but the depression of the plateau phase of monophasic action potential and the mode of their negative inotropic action (i.e., inversion of the AFR) led us to suggest that diltiazem and fendiline may also reduce Ca supply by direct interference with the slow inward channel. A further common denominator of these drugs (groups I and II) is the fact that their negative inotropic potencies inversely correlate with their lipophilicity (Table 1) [10].

Although the group I and II drugs are classified as "specific" slow (Ca) channel inhibitors, one must, nevertheless, be aware that these drugs act via different and drug specific sites of action. Recent structure-activity investigations revealed that Ca antagonists need rather specific, but in each case quite different, molecular requirements of optimal drug-receptor interaction. For instance, the negative inotropic action of verapamil depends mainly on electronic and steric properties of

Differentiation of Calcium-Antagonistic Drugs 281

the substituent, whereas in the case of nifedipine steric and/or lipophilic parameters are of major importance [11, 12].

If one extends contractile pattern analysis to parameters such as amplitude-interval relationship, postextrasystolic potentiation, or paired stimulation pattern, dissimilar pharmacodynamic patterns of the compounds also emerge.

For the drugs steepening the AFR (group III such as perhexiline, bencyclane, diazoxide; see also Fig. 2) there is no experimental evidence for a specific slow (Ca) channel inhibition. Instead, their effects on cellular Ca metabolism appear to be rather nonspecific and may not even be always the main basis of their therapeutic action. Since they all have been introduced after the concept of Ca antagonism as a therapeutic principle, they were labeled as Ca antagonists for convenience rather than for their demonstrated pharmacodynamic properties. In like manner, a large variety of older well established drugs such as antiarrhythmics (e.g., aprindine, diphenylhydantoin), barbiturates (e.g., phenobarbital), and tranquilizers (e.g., flurazepam), which all have more or less pronounced negative inotropic side effects of the group III type, could have been named Ca antagonists. Contrary to the specific Ca antagonist (groups I and II), all these compounds not only need high concentrations for half maximal effects, but their negative inotropic potency positively correlates with the drug's lipophilicity [10]. We therefore suggest that the Ca antagonistic property of these drugs is nonspecific. They may alter membrane functions by hydrophobic interactions with membrane lipoproteins. This mode of

Table 1. Negative inotropic potencies (cat papillary muscles, stimulation rate 60/min, 32° C) of (established and suspected) Ca antagonists as related to their relative lipophilicity. Note that only in specific slow channel inhibitors the negative inotropic potency increases when lipophilicity decreases. As minor changes in molecular structure of specific Ca antagonists do not change the typical inotropic pattern (verapamil → D 600, nifedipine → nimodipine → niludipine) it is supposed that the altered inotropic potency is due to changes in the drug's affinity to its site of action

Type of Ca antagonist		Generic name	Neg. inotrop. potency Verapamil = 1	Lipophilicity Verapamil = 1
Specific slow Ca-channel inhibitors acting at specific sites ((1–5)	1 {	Verapamil	1.00	1.00
		D 600	2.82	1.06
	2	Prenylamine	0.18	1.55
	3	Fendiline	0.07	2.61
	4 {	Nifedipine	6.86	0.64
		Nimodipine	2.69	2.64
		Niludipine	1.35	4.58
	5	Diltiazem	0.36	1.27
Unspecific compounds acting by hydrophobic interactions		Perhexiline	0.11	2.70
		Bencyclane	0.06	2.15
		Aprindine	0.04	1.46
		Flurazepam	0.02	1.00
		DPH	0.02	0.03
		Diazoxide	0.01	− 0.55
		Phenobarbital	0.002	− 0.52

282 R. Kaufmann et al.

Table 2. Established and suspected effects of (established and suspected) Ca antagonists on cardiac transmembrane currents

Substance	Na^+-inward current	Ca^{2+}-inward current	K^+-outward current
Verapamil	Inhibition (AP)	Inhibition (vc, AP, ni)	Presumable inhibition (AP)
Prenylamine	Inhibition (AP)	Inhibition (vc, AP, ni)	Presumable inhibition (vc, AP)
Nifedipine	No effect (AP)	Inhibition (vc, AP, ni)	Presumable Increase (vc, AP)
Fendiline	Inhibition (AP)	Inhibition ? (AP, ni)	$\varnothing$
Diltiazem	Inhibition (AP)	Inhibition ? (AP, ni)	Presumable inhibition (AP)
Bencyclane	Inhibition (AP)	Inhibition ??? (ni)	$\varnothing$
Perhexiline	Inhibition (AP)	Inhibition ??? (ni)	$\varnothing$
Diazoxide	$\varnothing$	Inhibition ??? (ni)	$\varnothing$

vc, as evidenced by voltage clamp experiments; AP, as evidenced by alterations of monophasic action potentials; ni, as evidenced by negative inotropic effect; $\varnothing$, experimental data controversal or not available.

action has already been postulated to explain the negative inotropic side effects of certain β-receptor blockers [13, 14].

With respect to cardiac electrophysiology it is important to notice that most – if not all – of the Ca antagonists also interfere with sodium and/or potassium conductivity of the cardiac membrane. Table 2 compiles the relevant data from our and other laboratories [3, 4, 7, 8, 9, 15, 16, 17].

Perhaps with the only exception of nifedipine, all drugs listed in Table 2 inhibit to a certain extent the fast (or slow) Na-inward current. A particularly interesting example is the racemic ($\pm$)-verapamil in which the "Na-antagonistic" property was found to be merely related to the ($+$)-enantiomer whereas the ($-$)-enantiomer represents the Ca-antagonistic principle [18, 19]. Further verapamil, prenylamine, and diltiazem tend to prolong the transmembrane action potential by an inhibition of the late K-outward current. In contrast, nifedipine shortens cardiac action potential. This and voltage clamp experiments suggest that nifedipine increases the late K-outward current.

Hence, one must accept the idea that the action of Ca antagonists (either specific or nonspecific) is not restricted to interference with transmembrane Ca movements. Additional side effects on Na^+ and K^+ current may be rather important and eventually the key to understand why some Ca antagonists have antiarrhythmic properties and others not.

We are far away from fully understanding the action of Ca antagonists, but current evidence points to the following conclusions:
1. From our investigations on isolated cardiac preparations it is obvious that a specific Ca antagonistic action can only be attributed to a rather small group of drugs.

Differentiation of Calcium-Antagonistic Drugs

2. Within this group a large variety of different but drug-specific actions can be detected. This indicates that Ca antagonists act via rather defined cellular sites, each probably representing specific drug receptors.
3. The action of even the specific Ca antagonists is not always restricted to inhibition of the slow Ca^{2+}-inward current. More or less pronounced additional actions involve changes of cardiac sodium and/or potassium conductance.
4. It is not readily apparent which of the findings in isolated preparations is clinically relevant. However, there is growing evidence that the potency and the pharmacodynamic pattern exerted by Ca antagonists also differ widely in patients. For instance, the dissimilarities in antianginal and antiarrhythmic action and the quite unique efficacy of verapamil in the therapy of hypertrophic cardiomyopathy can only be understood if one accepts the idea of drug specific actions within the group of Ca antagonists. Therefore we feel that the differentiation based on investigations of the molecular mode of action of Ca antagonists is more than of academic interest.

It is hoped that the evidence presented will trigger further clinical studies to elucidate the actions of Ca antagonists.

References

1. Fleckenstein A, Kammermeier H, Döring HJ, Freund HJ, Grün G, Kienle A (1967) Zum Wirkungsmechanismus neuartiger Koronardilatatoren mit gleichzeitig Sauerstoff-einsparenden Myokard-Effekten, Prenylamin und Iproveratril. Z Kreislaufforsch 56:716–744, 839–858
2. Bayer R, Hennekes R, Kaufmann R, Mannhold R (1975) Inotropic and electrophysiological actions of verapamil and D 600 in mammalian myocardium. I. Pattern of inotropic effects of the racemic compounds. Naunyn Schmiedebergs Arch Pharmacol 290:49–68
3. Bayer R, Rodenkirchen R, Kaufmann R, Lee J, Hennekes R (1977) The effects of Nifedipine on contraction and monophasic action potential of isolated cat myocardium. Naunyn Schmiedebergs Arch Pharmacol 301:29–37
4. Bayer R, Ehara T (1978) Comparative studies on calcium-antagonists. In: Van Zwieten PH, Schönbaum E (eds) The action of drugs on Ca-metabolism, Progress in pharmacol vol 2, Nr 1. Fischer, Stuttgart New York, pp 31–37
5. Grün G, Fleckenstein A (1972) Die elektromechanische Entkoppelung der glatten Gefäßmuskulatur als Grundprinzip der Coronardilatation durch 4-(Nitrophenyl)-2,6-dimethyl-1,4-dihydropyridine-3,5-dicarbonsäure-dimethylester (BAY a 1040, Nifedipine). Arzneim Forsch 22:334–344
6. Rahwan RG, Faust MM, Witiak DT (1977) Pharmacological evaluation of new calcium antagonist: 2-substituted 3-methylamine-5,6-methylene-diozyindenes. J Pharmacol Exp Ther 201:126–137
7. Haas HG, Kern R, Benninger C, Einwächter HM (1975) Effects of Prenylamine on cardiac membrane currents and contractility. J Pharmacol Exp Ther 192:688–701
8. Ehara T, Kaufmann R (1978) The voltage- and time-dependent effects of (–)-Verapamil on the slow inward current in isolated cat ventricular myocardium. J Pharmacol Exp Ther 207:49–55
9. Kohlhardt M, Fleckenstein A (1977) Inhibition of the slow inward current by Nifedipine in mammalian ventricular myocardium. Naunyn Schmiedebergs Arch Pharmacol 298:267–272

10. Rodenkirchen R, Mannhold R, Bayer R, Steiner R (1978) Correlations between negative inotropic potency and lipophilicity of Ca antagonists (Abstr). In: 7th International Congress of Pharmacology, Paris. Pergamon Press, Oxford New York, p 488
11. Mannhold R, Steiner R, Haas W, Kaufmann R (1978) Investigations on the structure-activity relationships of Verapamil. Naunyn Schmiedebergs Arch Pharmacol 302:217–226
12. Rodenkirchen R, Bayer R, Steiner R, Bossert F, Meyer H, Möller E (1979) Structure-activity studies on Nifedipine in isolated cardiac muscle. Naunyn Schmiedebergs Arch Pharmacol 310:69–78
13. Hellenbrecht D, Lemmer B, Wiethold G, Grobecker H (1973) Measurement of hydrophobicity, surface activity, local anaesthesia and myocardial conduction velocity as quantitative parameters of the non-specific membrane affinity of nine β-adrenergic blocking agents. Naunyn Schmiedebergs Arch Pharmacol 277:211–226
14. Rauls DO, Baker JK (1979) Relationship of non-specific antiarrhythmic and negative inotropic activity with physicochemical parameters of propranolol analogues. J Med Chem 22:81–86
15. Nakajima H, Hoshiyama M, Yamashita K, Kiyomoto A (1975) Effect of Diltiazem on electrical and mechanical activity of isolated cardiac ventricle muscle of guinea pig. Jap J Pharmacol 25:383–392
16. Fleckenstein A, Fleckenstein-Grün G, Byon YK, Courret G (1977) Fundamentale Herz- und Gefäßwirkungen des Ca-antagonistischen Koronartherapeutikums Fendilin (Sensit[R]). Arzneim Forsch 27:562–571
17. TenEick RE, Singer DH (1973) Effects of Perhexiline on the electrophysiologic activity of mammalian heart. Postgrad Med J [Suppl]:32–42
18. Bayer R, Kaufmann R, Mannhold R (1975) Inotropic and electrophysiological actions of verapamil and D 600 in mammalian myocardium. II. Pattern of inotropic effects of the optical isomers. Naunyn Schmiedebergs Arch Pharmacol 290:69–80
19. Bayer R, Kalusche D, Kaufmann R, Mannhold R (1975) Inotropic and electro-physiological actions of verapamil and D 600 in mammalian myocardium. III. Effects of the optical isomers on transmembrane actions potentials. Naunyn Schmiedebergs Arch Pharmacol 290:81–97

The Concept of Calcium Antagonist Therapy in Cardiac Hypertrophy

Different Calcium Antagonists with Respect to Therapeutic Efficacy in Hypertrophic Cardiomyopathy. Combined Therapy with Calcium Antagonists and Other Drugs?

M. KALTENBACH, G. KOBER, and R. HOPF

Verapamil seems to offer an effective treatment of hypertrophic cardiomyopathy superior to beta blockade (3). Two important questions which may lead to further steps in the treatment of this disease should be answered:
1. What may be the therapeutical efficacy of other calcium antagonists instead of verapamil (e.g., nifedipine)?
2. Can we expect an increased therapeutic efficacy from the combination of calcium antagonists with beta blockers or other drugs?

Verapamil Versus Nifedipine

From pharmacological and experimental data it seems that nifedipine has calcium antagonistic properties comparable to verapamil. In clinical experience verapamil, however, has antiarrhythmic properties which nifedipine lacks [2–4].

Thus, from a theoretical point of view nifedipine could be used instead of verapamil provided the goal of treatment is related to calcium ion inhibition rather than to the prevention of arrhythmias. It has been postulated, however, that there are differencies among calcium antagonists concerning the more central (heart muscle) effect of substances like verapamil or more peripheral (vascular smooth muscle) effects of drugs like nifedipine. The question whether verapamil and nifedipine have similar actions in an intact organism as compared to isolated preparations is also unanswered. As shown by Becker et al. (see this volume p. 270) nifedipine as well as verapamil demonstrate clear antianginal activities. This is in contrast to several other calcium antagonists, which have no antianginal actions despite similar favorable pharmacological properties in animal experiments. The clinically relevant similarities between nifedipine and verapamil, as well as their differencies, can therefore only be derived from studies performed in humans. In many clinical experimental studies performed over the last 10 years in our institution, the following results were obtained:

Antianginal Effect

Both verapamil and nifedipine reveal antianginal properties as documented by the influence on exercise-induced ST depression in patients with angina pectoris. The studies were performed with different doses and different forms of application:

		Antianginal effect
Verapamil orally	160–320 mg	+
Verapamil i.v.	5– 10 mg	+
Nifedipine orally	10– 20 mg	+
Nifedipine i.v.	1.0 mg	+
Nifedipine i.c.	0.1 mg (infused into the left coronary artery)	+

Negative Inotropic Effect

Contractility remains uninfluenced if verapamil is given intravenously over a short period of time. If verapamil, however, is slowly infused or given orally contractility is depressed. Apparently the negative inotropic effect of the substance is counteracted by increased sympathetic tone if the drug is injected over a short period of time and therefore creates pronounced hypotension:

	Contractility	Heart rate
Verapamil 10 mg i.v. injected in 2 min	unchanged	↑
Verapamil 10 mg i.v. infused in 10 min	↓	(↓)
Verapamil 160 mg orally	↓	(↓)
Verapamil 1.5 mg in coronary artery	↓	(↓)

After nifedipine administered orally or intravenously, no change in contractility occurred. After infusion into the left coronary artery, however, depressed contractility was evident (4):

	Contractility	Heart rate
Nifedipine 20 mg orally	unchanged	↑
Nifedipine 1.0 mg i.v.	unchanged	↑
Nifedipine 0.1 mg i.c. (infused into left coronary artery)	↓	unchanged

From these data it seems uncertain whether oral nifedipine will achieve the same beneficial effects in hypertrophic cardiomyopathy as verapamil, if the therapeutic influence on hypertrophic cardiomyopathy is related to the negative inotropic effect upon the myocardium. The effect may be similar, however, if the main beneficial influence is related to improved myocardial relaxation due to an alteration in Ca^{++} availability not reflected in an alteration of myocardial contractility.

Calcium Antagonists *and* Beta Blockers

The next question that arises in respect to therapy of HCM is whether a combination of calcium antagonists with beta blockers could have therapeutical efficacy. It has been shown that the antianginal activity of nifedipine and beta blockers may be additive [1]. It has also been demonstrated that a combination of

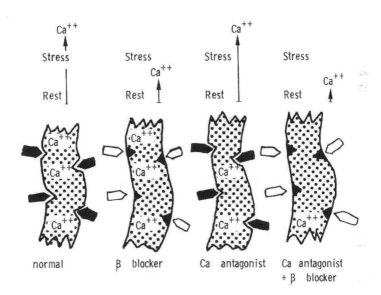

Fig. 1. Calcium ion availability within the cardiac muscle cell. With beta blockade no marked reduction at rest is achieved while the increase during stress may be reduced. With a calcium antagonist a reduction occurs at rest while the increase during stress may be the same. Combination of a calcium antagonist with beta blockade may reduce calcium ion availability at rest as well as during stress

calcium antagonists with beta blockers can be applied without particular complications.

The effects at the cellular level carried by beta blockers, calcium antagonists, and the combination of calcium antagonists with beta blockers may be different if one assumes the actions as shown in Fig. 1. The reduced calcium ion availability associated with the combination of calcium antagonists and beta blockers may, during stress, result in a situation that is considerably different from that achieved with verapamil or beta blockade alone. It seems not impossible therefore that combined therapy might provide another form of treatment in patients with hypertrophic cardiomyopathy.

Competitive Inhibition of Ca Ions by Increased K or Mg Concentration

Finally, we must consider the concept, derived from the experiments of Fleckenstein in isolated heart muscle preparations and of Lossnitzer in the Syrian hamster, that increased concentrations of K or Mg ions competitively inhibit calcium ions. If the concentration of these ions can be effectively increased in humans, the beneficial effects seen in experiments can possibly be utilized in patients. To determine whether this approach will provide, alone or in combination with calcium antagonists, another form of treating patients with cardiac hypertrophy, a clinical trial has been started in our institution.

Conclusions

Based on the results obtained in patients with hypertrophic cardiomyopathy and with angina pectoris due to coronary disease as well as on the experimental findings obtained in intact animals and in isolated muscle preparations, the following conclusions can be drawn at present:
1. Verapamil treatment may offer an effective approach to medical therapy of hypertrophic cardiomyopathy and perhaps of hypertrophy of other origin.
2. It seems possible that the therapeutic efficacy of calcium antagonists is enhanced by the addition of beta blockers.
3. Competitive inhibition of myocardium calcium ions by increased concentration of K and Mg ions might provide another therapeutic principle, which either alone or in combination with calcium antagonists, can possibly be applied to humans.

References

1. De Ponti C, Galli MA, Mauri F, Salvadé P, Carù B (1978) Effects of association of calcium antagonists with nitroderivatives or β-blocking drugs in effort angina. In: Kaltenbach M, Lichtlen P, Balcon R, Bussmann WD (eds) Coronary heart disease. Thieme, Stuttgart, pp 316–323
2. Fleckenstein A (1980) Steuerung der myocardialen Kontraktilität, ATP-Spaltung, Atmungsintensität und Schrittmacher-Funktion durch Calcium-Ionen – Wirkungs-mechanismus der Calcium-Antagonisten. In: Fleckenstein A, Roskamm H (eds) Calcium-Antagonismus. Springer, Berlin Heidelberg New York, pp 1–28
3. Kaltenbach M, Hopf R, Keller M (1976) Calciumantagonistische Therapie bei hypertroph-obstruktiver Kardiomyopathie. Dtsch Med Wochenschr 101:1284
4. Kaltenbach M, Schulz W, Kober G (1979) Effects of nifedipine after intravenous and intracoronary administration. Am J Cardiol 44:832–837
5. Lossnitzer K, Mohr W, Konrad A, Guggenmoos R (1979) Heredity cardiomyopathy in the syrian golden hamster: Influence of verapamil as calcium antagonist. In: Kaltenbach M, Loogen F, Olsen EGJ (eds) Cardiomyopathy and myocardial biopsy. Springer, Berlin Heidelberg New York, pp 27–37

Clinical Pharmacology of Verapamil in Hypertrophic Cardiomyopathy

Synopsis

R. G. McAllister, Jr.

Although verapamil has been clinically evaluated and used for over a decade, the pharmacokinetics and pharmacodynamics of the drug are only now being defined. In part, at least, this may be attributed to difficulties encountered in early efforts to measure verapamil in plasma. However, it is also clear that an appreciation of the need for definitive studies of a drug's kinetic characteristics and for plasma level effect correlations has but recently spread to the community of clinicians who use new pharmacologic agents. Formerly the exclusive province of clinical pharmacologists, the terms "half-life", "drug-protein binding", "distribution volume", and "first-pass effect" have all begun to enter the vocabulary of the bedside physician.

This has occurred at a propitious time in the evolution of new drugs for use in cardiovascular disorders. Verapamil and the other slow-channel blocking agents are potent drugs with enormous therapeutic potential, and their beneficial effects have already been demonstrated in patients with ischemic heart disease, supraventricular tachyarrhythmias, hypertension, and cardiomyopathic conditions in which the diastolic relaxation processes are impaired (the "hypertrophic" variants). The potential for toxicity, however, is as real as that for therapeutic benefit since these drugs antagonize an essential biochemical process – the transmembrane flux of calcium. It is essential, therefore, that the kinetic properties of such compounds be known prior to widespread patient use, that questions regarding drug metabolism and elimination in various patient age groups and in different disease states be clearly answered. In other words, the "therapeutic window" for verapamil and similar drugs, a range of plasma concentrations where desired drug effects occur but toxicity is minimal or absent, must be defined in a variety of patients. For the slow-channel calcium antagonists to be most safely and effectively used in clinical practice, the clinically relevant pharmacology of these drugs must be more intensively studied.

The contributions in this section are oriented toward this approach. The fact that more questions are raised than answers given reflects the present state of the art.

Pharmacokinetics, Bioavailability, and ECG Response of Verapamil in Man

MICHEL EICHELBAUM and ANDREW SOMOGYI

Although verapamil has been widely used in the treatment of various cardio-vascular disorders for the past 20 years, knowledge of its physiological disposition in man has been rather scant. This paucity of knowledge in verapamil's pharmacokinetic, bioavailability, and metabolism has been due to the lack of convenient, specific, and sensitive methods for the measurement of verapamil in biological fluids. With the quite recent development of analytical methods such as mass fragmentography, gas chromatography with nitrogen-FID, and liquid chromatography with fluorescence detection, it is now possible to quantify with high specificity and sensitivity verapamil in biological fluids [1–4].

In an initial study from this laboratory, on the physiological disposition of verapamil both after intravenous and oral administration of 14 C-verapamil, we used a specific and sensitive mass fragmentographic method [4]. It was shown that the absorption of verapamil was complete but that bioavailability was low and systemic clearance high, indicative of a drug with a high first-pass effect [5]. In this initial study large interindividual variations in first-pass metabolism were noted, hence raising the possibility that conventional techniques for bioavailability assessment (giving the drug on two separate occasions) might lead to false values of kinetic parameters after oral dosing.

Intravenous Pharmacokinetics and Absolute Bioavailability

A new method for studying drug pharmacokinetics was employed for verapamil. This method, using stable labeled techniques, involved giving verapamil both by the intravenous and oral route simultaneously, so that time-dependent changes in clearance are avoided. Thus the two experiments which are normally required for the assessment of absolute bioavailability are carried out in a single experiment [6].

Six volunteers were studied and following intravenous administration, the plasma concentration time curve could best be described by either a mono- or biexponential equation in accordance with a one or two compartment-open model.

Figure 1 shows the plasma concentration time profile in two of the subjects, one requiring a monoexponential, the other a biexponential equation, indicating that verapamil distributes rapidly and achieves an equilibrium with body tissues in a short period of time and hence its pharmacological responses should be quickly elicited. Table 1 lists the various pharmacokinetic parameters for verapamil. The volume of distribution was extensive and ranged from 4.5 to 9.9 l/kg, thus indicating extensive tissue binding. Total plasma clearance ranged from 0.98 to 1.45 liters/min and approached that of normal liver blood flow (1.5 liters/min). Since

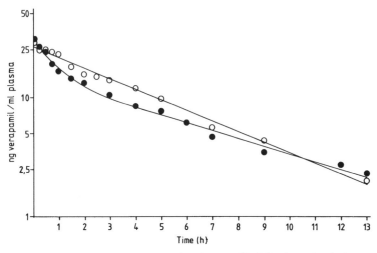

Fig. 1. Verapamil plasma concentration-time profile following a 5-min intravenous infusion of 10 mg verapamil. One subject (○) required a monoexponential equation to describe the data whereas another subject (●) required a biexponential equation [6]

less than 4% of the dose is recovered unchanged in urine [7], it can be deduced that the systemic clearance of verapamil is most likely liver blood flow dependent. The terminal half-life was on average 3.7 h.

By using the total blood clearance of verapamil as reflecting hepatic clearance, the extraction ratio was approximately 0.74. Thus the absolute bioavailability would be 0.26 (one minus extraction ratio). This predicted value (26%) is in excellent agreement with the observed mean value of 22% (Table 1). From these data it is evident that verapamil is a drug whose systemic clearance is liver blood flow dependent, thus resulting in extensive first-pass metabolism. The site of first-pass metabolism is the liver, for in a recent study [8] involving a patient examined before and after construction of a mesocaval shunt, it was found that the bioavailability was increased to 82% from a preshunt value of 38%.

A comparison of the pharmacokinetic parameters between male and female subjects indicated that sex might influence verapamil disposition, for females had larger volumes of distribution, higher total plasma clearance values, and longer terminal half-lifes. These were not statistically significant owing to the small number of subjects in each group.

In our earlier study the protein binding of verapamil was on average 90%, indicating that the clearance of verapamil is binding insensitive so that both the free and bound drug can be taken up by the liver.

Relative Bioavailability

While it is generally assumed that the bioavailability or clearance of drugs administered orally should remain constant, this assumption does not hold for

Table 1. Pharmacokinetic parameters of verapamil following the simultaneous administration of 10 mg verapamil i.v. and 80 mg d_3-verapamil orally [6]

Subject	IV			oral			
	$t_{1/2\beta}$ (h)	Cl_p (liters/min)	V_β (liters/kg)	$t_{1/2\beta}$ (h)	Cl_o (liters/min)	t_{max} (min)	F(%)
1	4.72	1.454	9.91	4.13	7.05	60	20.6
2	5.32	1.084	9.97	4.92	8.96	30	12.1
3	3.17	1.453	4.86	2.94	8.38	60	17.3
4	3.89	0.979	7.01	4.35	3.04	90	32.2
5	2.76	1.288	4.46	2.36	6.63	180	19.4
6	3.41	1.288	4.53	3.69	4.24	60	30.4
Mean	3.69[a]	1.258	6.76	3.51[a]	6.38	60[b]	22.0
±S.D.	–	0.194	2.64	–	2.32	–	7.79

Pharmacokinetic parameters: $t_{1/2\beta}$, elimination half-life; Cl_p, total plasma clearance; V_β, apparent volume of distribution; Cl_o, apparent oral clearance; t_{max}, time of maximum plasma level; F, bioavailability.

[a] Harmonic mean
[b] Median

highly cleared drugs subject to substantial first-pass metabolism. Besides, large intra- and interindividual variations in bioavailability and clearance were noted (Table 1), thus resulting in substantial alterations in bioavailability within the same subject when verapamil was administered orally on two separate occasions. This conclusion was drawn from the results obtained in a study in which the relative bioavailability of the commercial tablet formulation was compared with a solution of verapamil using stable labeled techniques in the same six subjects as the absolute

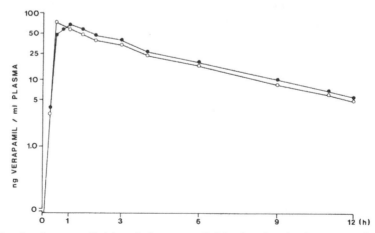

Fig. 2. Plasma levels of verapamil (●) and d_3-verapamil (○) after the simultaneous oral administration of 80 mg verapamil as tablet (●) and as solution (○) [9]

bioavailability study [9]. The inference was made that substantial changes in first-pass metabolism in the same subject occur, because the bioavailability of the tablet was as high as 190% relative to the solution when the areas under the curves were compared for the solution in the absolute bioavailability study to the tablet in the relative bioavailability study. When the tablet and solution were compared on the same day there were no statistically significant differences in the maximum plasma concentration, time of maximum plasma concentration, half-life, and oral clearance. The relative bioavailability of the tablet compared to the solution was 108.07%, with 95% confidence interval, lying between 89.1 and 127.1% (Table 2, Fig. 2). Thus it can be concluded that the tablet is fully available relative to the

Table 2. Pharmacokinetic data and relative bioavailability of verapamil tablet (T) compared with an oral solution of d_3-verapamil (S) in six subjects [9]

Parameter	T		S
c_{max} (ng/ml)	63.6 ± 14.8 [a]		68.8 ± 29.5
t_{max} (h)	2.0 ± 0.9		1.5 ± 0.9
$t_{1/2\beta}$ (h)	3.40 [b]		3.56 [b]
Cl_o (liters/min)	4.36 ± 1.22		4.67 ± 1.10
F (%)		108.07 ± 8.97	

Pharmacokinetic parameters: c_{max}, maximum plasma concentration; t_{max}, time of c_{max}; $t_{1/2\beta}$, elimination half-life; Cl_o, apparent oral clearance; F, relative bioavailability of tablet to solution.
[a] Mean ± S.D.
[b] Harmonic mean

optimally available solution. This statement could not be elicited if the tablet and solution were given on separate occasions; hence the advantage of the stable labeled technique. The slightly higher relative bioavailability of the tablet is probably due to it containing slightly more than the stated content [9].

Chronic Administration

In five subjects from the previous two studies, chronic dosing with verapamil was initiated as 80 mg four times daily. On four occasions over a period of 3 weeks, the morning dose was substituted with a solution of deuterated verapamil and the pharmacokinetics measured at steady state without necessitating withdrawal of verapamil.

Pronounced inter- and intraindividual variations in the area underneath the curve (oral clearance) were noted. The mean oral clearance values between occasions ranged from 3.23 to 4.16 liters/min with coefficients of variation ranging from 26 to 85%. The between subject mean oral clearance ranged from 2.19 to 6.1 liters/min with coefficients of variation of 12–50%. Within the same subject the oral clearance varied more than threefold. As well, the morning trough level ranged from 25 to 31 ng/ml between days, and from 10 to 46 ng/ml between subjects with large variations in the same subject. There was no evidence of a saturation of first-pass metabolism, since the half-life and volume of distribution remained the same. Fig. 3 shows the plasma levels of verapamil during chronic treatment in one subject. Because of the large inter- and intraindividual variations observed, a true "steady-state" situation is never fully achieved. Hence, a low trough value on one occasion can also result in a high value on another occasion without implying that the subject or patient is a poor absorber of verapamil (Eichelbaum et al., manuscript in preparation).

Hence, it is felt that the monitoring of plasma levels of verapamil can lead to false and potentially adverse conclusions concerning a patient's handling of verapamil, and therefore, good clinical assessment ought to prevail over plasma level monitoring.

ECG – Response

Whereas our knowledge of the pharmacokinetics and bioavailability of verapamil has improved substantially and is now nearly complete, the question of whether the pharmacokinetics, that is plasma levels, are related to pharmacodynamics has not been studied in detail in man. So far, neither therapeutic nor toxic verapamil plasma levels have been established.

In a recent study we investigated the effects of verapamil on PR interval in relation to verapamil plasma levels following single intravenous and oral administration, and during chronic treatment [10].

A close relationship between verapamil plasma concentration and effect on PR interval could be established both after intravenous and oral administration and during chronic oral treatment. After intravenous administration, a linear

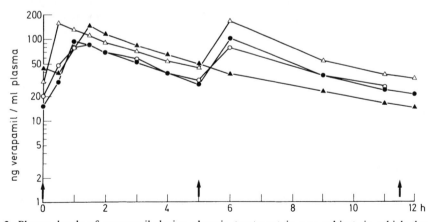

Fig. 3. Plasma levels of verapamil during chronic treatment in one subject, in which the morning tablet dose was substituted with d_3-verapamil on days 2 (○), 8 (●), and 16 (△); on day 21 (▲) chronic dosing was discontinued. The *arrow* on the ordinate indicates the time of drug administration

relationship between verapamil plasma concentration and $\triangle$ PR (y = x(0.74) + 1.8) with a small between subject variation in the slope of the regression (% coefficient of variation 18.7, range 0.71–1.10) was observed. The slope of the oral plasma concentration-response regression (y = x (0.33) –3.0) was statistically significantly ($P<0.05$) less than the slope of the intravenous plasma level response regression. Interindividual variation in the slope was most pronounced (range 0.13–0.47). On average two to three times higher verapamil plasma levels were required after oral administration in order to produce the same increase in $\triangle$ PR as after intravenous administration. In contrast to the single oral dose study, during chronic administration, a hysteresis effect was observed in two subjects. The presence of hysteresis indicates that the pharmacodynamic effect lags behind the plasma concentration (for details see [11]). As after single administration, a relationship between verapamil plasma level and effect on PR interval could be established. However, within the same subject, day to day variations in the steepness of the slope were observed and in one subject the slope approached that of the intravenous plasma level-effect slope. Since, after oral administration of d,1-verapamil, on average three times higher verapamil concentrations are required in order to elicit the same increase in $\triangle$ PR as compared to intravenous administration, the most plausible explanation for this phenomenon seems to be that verapamil undergoes stereoselective presystemic elimination.

The different slopes of the concentration-response curve indicate that the more active 1-isomer is preferentially metabolized during hepatic first-pass metabolism [10].

In support of our assumption is the finding that in patients with liver cirrhosis and/or mesocaval shunt, where bioavailability of verapamil after oral administration is almost complete, the steepness of the concentration-response curve is nearly identical to the intravenous curve [12].

In conclusion, verapamil is a drug whose blood clearance is liver blood flow dependent resulting in low bioavailability per se. The commercial tablet is fully available relative to an optimally available solution. During chronic treatment, the kinetics remain the same but pronounced inter- and intraindividual variations in first-pass metabolism occur. Plasma levels are related to changes in the PR interval, though following oral administration the slope is approximately one-third of that after intravenous administration, suggesting stereoselective presystemic elimination.

References

1. Harapat SR, Kates RE (1980) High performance liquid chromatographic analysis of verapamil II. Simultaneous quantitation of verapamil and its active metabolite, nor-verapamil. J Chromatogr 181:484–489
2. Hege HG (1979) Gas chromatographic determination of verapamil in plasma and urine. Arzneim Forsch 29:1681–1684
3. Jaouni TM, Leon MB, Rosing DR, Fales HM (1980) Analysis of verapamil in plasma by liquid chromatography. J Chromatogr 182:473–477
4. Spiegelhalder B, Eichelbaum M (1977) Determination of verapamil in human plasma by mass fragmentography using stable labelled verapamil as internal standard. Arzneim Forsch 27:94–97

5. Schomerus M, Spiegelhalder B, Stieren B, Eichelbaum M (1976) Physiological disposition of verapamil in man. Cardiovasc Res 10:605–612
6. Eichelbaum M, Somogyi A, Von Unruh GE, Dengler HJ (1981) Simultaneous determination of the I.V. and oral pharmacokinetic parameters of d,l-verapamil using stable labelled verapamil. Eur J Clin Pharmacol 19:133–137
7. Eichelbaum M, Ende M, Remberg G, Schomerus M, Dengler HJ (1979) The metabolism of DL-^{14}C verapamil in man. Drug Metab Dispos 7:145–148
8. Eichelbaum M, Albrecht M, Kliems K, Somogyi A (1980) Influence of mesocaval shunt surgery on verapamil kinetics, bioavailability and response. Br J Clin Pharmacol 10:527–529
9. Eichelbaum M, Dengler HJ, Somogyi A, Von Unruh GE (1981) Superiority of stable labelled techniques in the bioavailability assessment of drugs undergoing extensive first-pass elimination. Studies on the relative bioavailability of verapamil tables. Eur J Clin Pharmacol 19:127–131
10. Eichelbaum M, Birkel P, Grube E, Gütgemann U, Somogyi A (1980) Effects of verapamil on P-R intervals in relation to verapamil plasma levels following single I.V. and oral administration and during chronic treatment. Klin Wochenschr 58:919–925
11. Galeazzi RL, Benet LZ, Sheiner LB (1976) Relationship between the pharmacokinetics and pharmacodynamics of procainamide. Clin Pharmacol Ther 20:278–289
12. Somogyi A, Albrecht M, Kliems G, Schäfer K, Eichelbaum M (1981) Pharmacokinetics, bioavailability and ECG response of verapamil in patients with liver cirrhosis. Br J Clin Pharmacol 12:51–60

Verapamil Plasma Concentrations and Indices of Heart Size in Hypertrophic Obstructive Cardiomyopathy – Evidence for the Existence of a Therapeutic Range

BARRY G. WOODCOCK, RÜDIGER HOPF, and ROLAND KIRSTEN

Summary

1. The question of a relationship between plasma verapamil concentration and pharmacological response in hypertrophic obstructive cardiomyopathy (HOCM) patients was investigated using Sokolow-Lyon index (SLI) and heart volume (HV) measurements.
2. Twenty-six patients were treated with maintenance doses of verapamil (usually 3×160 mg Isoptin daily) and plasma level measurements were done using a gas/chromatographic method specific for verapamil. Considerable interpatient variation in plasma verapamil concentration was present attributable to variability in hepatic first-pass extraction and systemic clearance.
3. Approximately 50% of patients showed 10% decrease in SLI and 40% a 10% decrease in HV. Concentrations of verapamil were usually higher in these patients and in the case of SLI a good correlation was observed between the change in ECG and plasma verapamil level $r = 0.6245$, $P < 0.01$.
4. In HOCM patients plasma concentrations of verapamil in the range 100 to 400 ng/ml (pre-dose concentration 100 ng/ml) will produce clinically important changes in HV and SLI in most patients and these concentrations are suggested as a provisional therapeutic range.
5. In order to ensure that plasma verapamil concentrations in HOCM patients are in the therapeutic range it is necessary to measure plasma verapamil levels.

Verapamil has value in the treatment of several types of cardiovascular disease. For treatment of hypertrophic obstructive cardiomyopathy (HOCM), the oral dose of verapamil (360–480 mg daily) is large in comparison to the intravenous dose (5–10 mg) recommended for producing significant hemodynamic changes, such as a fall in systemic vascular resistance [1]. The need for high oral doses of verapamil has also been reported for the treatment of arrhythmias, where 10–20 times the recommended intravenous dose had to be given in order to observe anti-arrhythmic effects [2]. This difference in the required oral and intravenous dose seems to be due to a first pass effect involving the liver. A first pass effect for verapamil is apparent from early disposition studies with ^{14}C-verapamil in dogs and rats [3] and has been confirmed in man [4].

In the case of HOCM, owing to the chronic nature of the disease and its treatment, a period of as long as a year may be required before it can be decided that a change in dosage is necessary. By this time, however, the pathology may have progressed to an irreversible stage and considerable losses in time and money will have been incurred. Clearly, if such a thing as a therapeutic range exists, the price worth paying for such knowledge would be very high.

Ideally we should like to establish a therapeutic verapamil plasma concentration at the beginning of treatment. With verapamil, as in the case of many other drugs, however, we are unable to rely on our experience using a particular dosage regime to achieve this. The amount of verapamil in blood is not only related to the dose and dosage frequency, but also to physiological and biochemical factors, in particular hepatic hemodynamics and hepatic drug metabolism, the importance of which, in individual patients, cannot easily be assessed from normal clinical tests.

The area under the blood concentration-time curve of verapamil is a function of two extraction processes. These are (1) hepatic first-pass extraction, and (2) systemic clearance.

The first of these determines how much drug enters the systemic circulation, while the second determines how long it stays there. Data on the first-pass extraction of verapamil in HOCM patients, as reflected in measurements of bioavailability, are not available. According to previous studies [5, 6], we can forecast a bioavailability of about 15%, but interpatient variation cannot be predicted on the basis of normal clinical and biochemical parameters. In Fig. 1 it can be seen that having entered the circulation there is a linear correlation between verapamil clearance and hepatic blood flow. The data in Fig. 1 include two HOCM patients, H_1 and H_2; two intensive-care patients with polytrauma, I_1 and I_2; three patients with liver disease L_1, L_2, L_4; and two healthy subjects, N_1 and N_2. The slope is equivalent to the verapamil systemic extraction, estimated at about 0.9. Thus it is obvious that a major proportion of the verapamil is metabolized during the first-pass following an oral dose and this is followed by a rapid systemic elimination process. Not surprisingly this leads to difficulties in relating verapamil dose to verapamil concentration in blood.

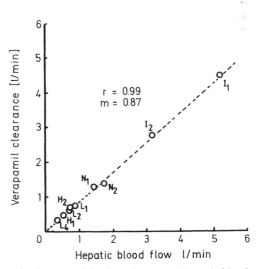

Fig. 1. Correlation between verapamil systemic clearance (blood) and apparent hepatic blood flow. Apparent hepatic blood flow is calculated using standard procedures based on area measurements of the plasma concentration – time curves obtained after oral and intravenous verapamil doses. [5]

300   Barry G. Woodcock et al.

What is the relationship between plasma concentration and response?
This question is in reality three questions in one.
1. What responses?
2. What concentration (or when?)?
3. What relationships?

In this report these questions are provided with answers, and evidence is given to support the view that in HOCM patients a relationship exists between indices of heart size and the plasma concentration of verapamil.

Methods

A group of 26 patients were diagnosed as having HOCM by right and left heart catheterization and echocardiogram and a full clinical report on the antihypertrophic efficacy of verapamil in 22 of the patients has already been published [7]. All patients had normal liver function and were fully compensated without need for additional medication. Approximately 30% of the patients had received a β blocker which was discontinued 1 week prior to commencement of verapamil investigations because of disappointing clinical response. None of the patients had received previous treatment with verapamil.

All patients received maintenance doses of verapamil (see Tables 1, 2) administered three times daily as equal divided doses (Isoptin, Knoll AG). No dosage change had occurred in any patient within the 6-month period prior to measurement of plasma concentrations. The mean duration of verapamil treatment was 2.67 ± 1.09 (S. D.) years, with a range of 1–5 years.

Verapamil levels in plasma were determined in duplicate by gas chromatography with a nitrogen detector after double extraction with heptane. The method is based on that of Hege [8] and has been improved to provide easier and more rapid assays [9].

Sokolow-Lyon Index (SLI) and heart volume (HV) were used as indices of heart size. SLI was obtained from the ECG (lead 6) with a measurement error of 0.25 giving a 5% error for an SLI of 5 (R. Hopf, G. Kober and M. Kaltenbach, personal communication). Heart volume was measured by X-ray with the patient in the supine position [10]. Initial heart volumes for the group were 916 ± 186 ml/1.73 m^2 body surface area. The minimum observation period was 1 year during which two sets of heart size measurements were made. Changes in SLI and HV are expressed as a percentage of the pre-verapamil treatment value, each patient serving as his own control.

Results and Discussion

In 23 HOCM patients a 10% decrease in SLI in 40% of patients (Fig. 2) and a 10% decrease in HV in 50% of patients (Fig. 3) was observed. The individual changes for both parameters in all subjects are listed in Tables 1 and 2.

Plasma concentrations of verapamil in HOCM patients on maintenance therapy are given in Fig. 4. The data on 22 patients refer to a dose of 160 mg t.i.d. Minimum predose verapamil concentrations averaged 75 ng/ml. Time to peak is reported to be about 1 h [4]. The large standard deviation (vertical bars) indicates a high interpatient variation. In Fig. 5 this variability is shown more clearly. Each pair of columns is a single patient on 160 mg Isoptin t.i.d. The bold bars are the predose concentrations or minimum values and the thinner columns are the 1-h peak concentrations. Patients with low predose concentrations usually have low postdose concentrations, pointing to a high first pass effect and losses at the absorption stage may be responsible for the tenfold variation in verapamil plasma concentrations. In Figs. 2 and 3, 40–50% of HOCM patients exhibited a good therapeutic response, defined in this case as a greater than 10% change in HV or SLI. If a correlation exists between response and verapamil plasma concentration

Table 1. Percentage change in Sokolow-Lyon Index with respect to pretreatment values. Verapamil daily doses are usually taken as three equal divided doses. BDC's are morning predose plasma concentrations after on overnight fast. ADC's are plasma concentrations taken 1 h after a test dose of 160 mg verapamil

Patient number	% change in Sokolow Index	Verapamil dose (mg/day)	BDC <25 (ng/ml)	BDC<25 ADC<100 (ng/ml)	BDC >100 (ng/ml)	ADC >300 (ng/ml)
2	− 58	480			●	●
21	− 38	480			●	
11	− 37	480	●	●		
19	− 34	480			●	●
32	− 32	480			●	●
22	− 26	480			●	●
15	− 25	480			●	
27	− 22	480				
28	− 18	480				●
9	− 17	480			●	●
30	− 17	480			●	●
14	− 14	240				
8	− 14	240	●			
20	− 9	480			●	
6	− 8	240	●	●		
17	− 4	320				
29	+ 10	480	●			●
1	+ 11	480	●	●		
16	+ 11	480				
13	+ 13	480	●			
31	+ 16	320	●	●		
18	+ 17	320	●	●		

BDC, before dose plasma concentration; ADC, after dose plasma concentration (1 h of drug administration).

Table 2. Percentage change in heart volume with respect to pretreatment values

Patient number	% change in heart volume	Verapamil dose (mg) per day	BDC <25 (ng/ml)	BDC<25 ADC<100 (ng/ml)	BDC >100 (ng/ml)	ADC >300 (ng/ml)
28	− 29	480				●
26	− 28	480				
22	− 26	480			●	●
17	− 22	320			●	●
19	− 22	480			●	●
16	− 18	480				
27	− 16	480				
13	− 16	480	●			
14	− 15	240				
9	− 14	480			●	●
29	− 13	480	●			●
1	− 10	480	●	●		
6	− 6	240	●	●		
21	− 4	480			●	
15	− 4	480			●	
30	− 2	480			●	●
20	− 2	480			●	
11	− 1	480	●	●		
18	+ 2	320	●	●		
31	+ 2	320	●	●		
8	+ 3	240	●			
2	+ 9	480			●	●
32	+28	480			●	●

BDC, before dose plasma concentration;   ADC, after dose plasma concentration (1 h of drug administration).

then we might expect a satisfactory therapeutic response to be associated with a minimum plasma verapamil concentration of circa 100 ng/ml, since 40–50% of the patients in Fig. 5 have verapamil plasma concentrations above this value.

Tables 1 and 2 show HOCM patients ranked according to percentage change in SLI and HV with the verapamil concentration range marked. It is obvious from Table 1 that patients did less well, judged by changes in SLI, when the verapamil concentration before dose (BDC) was <100 ng/ml and most patients who did well, defined as 10% decrease in SLI, had BDC's > 100 ng/ml and 1-h post-dose concentrations >300 ng/ml. A similar picture is apparent with respect to HV (Table 2).

Sokolow index was well correlated with the predose verapamil concentration, $r=0.6245$, $P<0.01$ (Fig. 6). Taking the threshold as 10% decrease, the efficacy limit is at 100 ng/ml or thereabouts. This threshold is similar to that in the preliminary findings of Follath et al. [11], who observed that after oral doses the verapamil concentration producing an approximately 10% reduction of heart rate in four

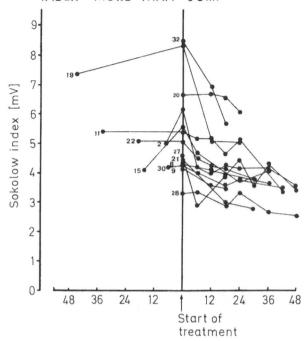

Fig. 2. Sokolow-Lyon index in the precordial electrocardiogram before and during verapamil treatment. All patients in the figure have shown a reduction in Sokolow-Lyon index of at least 10%

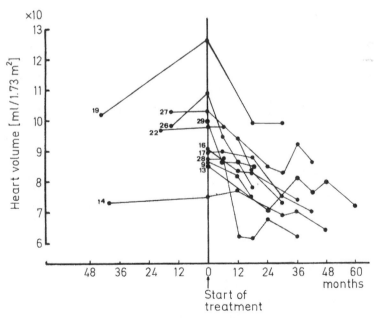

Fig. 3. Heart volume before and during treatment with verapamil. All patients in the figure have shown a reduction in heart volume of at least 10%. Patients are identified with numbers according to Table 2

patients with atrial fibrillation (initial ventricular rate for group 140/min) was approximately 100 ng/ml (Fig.. 7). Dominic et al. [12] also reported a relationship between the decrease in ventricular rate and verapamil concentration, but the response depended on the severity of disease. In a group of less severely ill subjects a decrease of approximately 40% in ventricular rate was achieved at a mean verapamil concentration for the group of 52 ± 7 ng/ml. In a group of patients with concomitant congestive heart failure the reduction in ventricular rate was only 28 ± 11, i.e., about 20%, with a verapamil level of 95 ± 16 ng/ml. This latter group corresponds to those patients examined by Follath et al. [11], since 10 of the 12 subjects in the Follath et al. study were receiving cardiac glycoside medication. Thus in atrial fibrillation, depending on the severity of the disease, minimum verapamil concentrations producing a satisfactory response can be as high as 100 ng/ml.

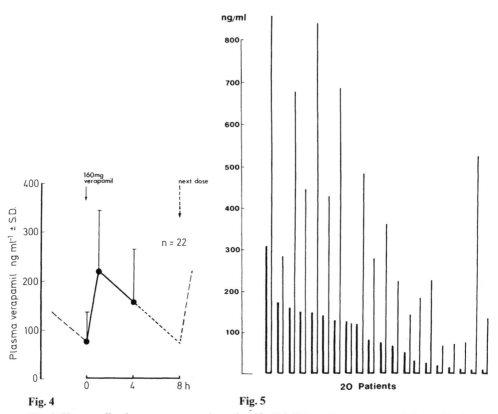

Fig. 4. Fig. 5

Fig. 4. Verapamil plasma concentrations in 22 HOCM patients measured immediately predose and 1 and 4 h after a dose of 160 mg verapamil during maintenance therapy with 480 mg orally given as three equal divided doses

Fig. 5. Plasma verapamil concentrations in 20 patients with hypertrophic obstructive cardiomyopathy. Predose (*bold bars*) and 1 h after test dose of 160 mg orally (*thin bars*). Measurements were made after an overnight fast. Patients were receiving maintenance therapy with 480 mg verapamil given as three equally divided doses daily. Patients are ranked in order of their predose verapamil concentration

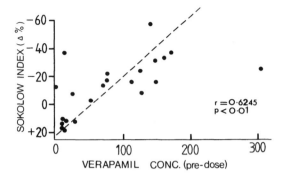

Fig. 6. Correlation between verapamil plasma concentrations and percentage reduction in Sokolow-Lyon index in HOCM patients

The relationship between verapamil plasma concentration and increase in PQ interval has been studied by Koike et al. [13]. Increase in PQ interval was 75% of maximal with verapamil concentrations of 25 ng/ml and near maximal changes were obtained with verapamil plasma concentration of 100 ng/ml, indicating an extremely shallow dose response curve. Thus PQ interval changes may be observed at lower verapamil concentrations than required for a significant change in SLI, HV, or ventricular rate.

Decrease in peripheral vascular resistance (among other cardiovascular responses such as decrease in mean arterial pressure and increase in left ventricular end diastolic pressure) following an intravenous dose of 10 mg verapamil are

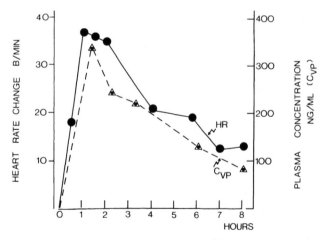

Fig. 7. Plasma verapamil and heart rate reduction following a dose of 120 mg oral verapamil in a patient with atrial fibrillation. In a further three patients receiving the same dose orally the verapamil plasma concentrations 1 h after the dose were 60, 120, and 200 ng/ml and 3 h after the dose 25, 80, and 100 ng/ml respectively. The mean duration of action defined as a decrease of >20 beats/min in heart rate in a comparable group of eight patients following 120 mg verapamil orally was 170 ± 80 min. Data from Follath et al. [11] and unpublished work

exceedingly transient [1] and within a period of 10 min after the administration of verapamil these pharmacological responses can no longer be observed. The plasma verapamil concentration is above 100 ng/ml approximately 5–10 minutes after 10 mg verapamil given intravenously. This suggests that the peripheral vascular effects of verapamil are produced only by high concentrations in comparison to those required to produce a significant change in the PQ interval (B. G. Woodcock and R. Hopf, unpublished work and [13]).

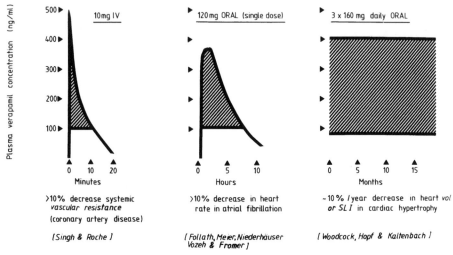

Fig. 8. Schematic illustration of the relationships between cardiavascular effects and plasma concentration of verapamil

The relationships between verapamil plasma concentration and cardiovascular effects of verapamil are compared diagrammatically in Fig. 8. The shaded areas represent concentration regions where a significant pharmacological response occurs. In the left of the diagram is shown the plasma concentration – time curve after 10 mg verapamil i.v. and the shaded area indicates a corresponding reduction in vascular resistance of at least 10% according to Singh and Roche [1]. Singh and Roche did not actually measure verapamil concentrations in their subjects, however, and these have been obtained from other studies (B. G. Woodcock and R. Hopf, unpublished work and [13]). The results show that within 10–15 min after 10 mg verapamil intravenously the plasma concentration is below 100 ng/ml. The results shown in the middle curve have already been discussed above. The shaded area represents the concentration range associated with a change in heart rate of at least 10% after an oral dose of 120 mg verapamil. It should be noted that the time scale for atrial fibrillation patients is in hours in contrast to minutes for changes in vascular resistance after the i.v. dose. In Fig. 8, extreme right, the time scale is in months and the upper line is the plasma level reached in most patients on a maintenance dose of 3×160 mg verapamil daily. The shaded area is that range of concentration giving approximately 10% decrease in SLI per year and is based on the data shown in Fig. 6. In contrast to the data shown in the rest of Fig. 8, SLI responses refer to chronic treatment. It cannot be claimed from these preliminary data that 400 ng/ml verapamil is the upper limit of the therapeutic range in HOCM patients. However, a concentration as high as this is not infrequently seen in HOCM patients as a peak level and is well tolerated.

In conclusion, plasma concentrations vary over a tenfold range on the same dose of verapamil given orally in HOCM patients who are taking their medication regularly [14]. This variability is probably the result of differences in first pass effect influencing absorption and differences in liver blood flow affecting systemic verapamil clearance. When the SLI is used as an index of therapeutic efficacy a reduction of 10% can be achieved in most patients within about 1 year when the plasma verapamil concentration stays above 100 ng/ml. The reduction in muscle mass, as indicated by the SLI, is more regularly seen than a decrease in heart volume. This limit of 100 ng/ml corresponds also to the lower limit above which significant changes in ventricular rate can be anticipated in congestive cardiac failure patients with atrial fibrillation. This concentration also approximates that required for significant changes in cardiovascular parameters such as peripheral vascular resistance and left ventricular end diastolic pressure, although the comparison of these latter transient cardiovascular actions with plasma verapamil concentration has been made using different subjects. Of the 20 HOCM patients in Fig. 5, as many as 50% of the group appear to have had subtherapeutic steady state concentrations of verapamil and an increase in the dose can be recommended so as to bring the verapamil concentration within the range 100–400 ng/ml taking 100 ng/ml as the predose trough concentration. Dosage adjustment like this cannot be made without knowledge of the patients individual verapamil concentrations. Thus verapamil blood levels, as in the case of other antiarrhythmic drugs such as digoxin, lidocaine, and disopyramide, should be monitored, especially so in HOCM patients.

References

1. Singh BN, Roche AHG (1977) Effects of intravenous verapamil on hemodynamics in patients with heart disease. Am Heart J 94:593–599
2. Krikler D (1974) Verapamil in cardiology. Eur J Cardiol 2:3–10
3. McIlhenny HM (1971) Metabolism of ^{14}C-verapamil. J Med Chem 14:1178–1184
4. Schomerus M, Spiegelhalder B, Stieren B, Eichelbaum M (1976) Physiological disposition of verapamil in man. Cardiovasc Res 10:605–612
5. Woodcock BG, Rietbrock I, Vöhringer HF, Rietbrock N (1981) Verapamil disposition on liver disease and intensive-care patients: Kinetics, clearance and apparent blood flow relationships. Clin Pharmacol Ther 29:27–34
6. Woodcock BG, Vöhringer HF (1980) Evaluation of the first pass effect of verapamil in patients. In: Rietbrock N, Woodcock BG, Neuhaus G (eds) Methods in clinical pharmacology. Vieweg, Braunschweig Wiesbaden, pp 218–228
7. Kaltenbach M, Hopf R, Kober G, Bussmann W-D, Keller M, Petersen Y (1979) Treatment of hypertrophic obstructive cardiomyopathy. Br Heart J 42:35–42
8. Hege HG (1979) Gaschromatographic determination of verapamil in plasma and urine. Arzneim Forsch 29:1681–1684

9. Nelson K, Woodcock BG, Kirsten R (1979) Improvement of the quantitative determination of verapamil in human plasma. Int J Clin Pharmacol Biopharm 17:375–379
10. Hopf R, Hopf M, Kober G, Lentz R, Riemann HA, Kaltenbach M (1978) Importance of heart volume determination and electrocardiography in early diagnosis of cardiomyopathy. In: Kaltenbach M, Loogen F, Olsen EGF (eds) Cardiomyopathy and myocardial biopsy. Springer, Berlin Heidelberg New York, pp 227–236
11. Follath F, Meier P, Niederhäuser U, Vozeh S, Fromer M (1978) Pharmacodynamic comparison of oral and intravenous verapamil in atrial fibrillation. Abstract No 1525, 8th World Congress of Cardiology, Tokyo
12. Dominic J, McAllister RG, Kuo C-S, Reddy CP, Surawicz B (1974) Verapamil plasma levels and ventricular rate response in patients with atrial fibrillation and flutter. Clin Pharmacol Ther 26:710–714
13. Koike Y, Shimamura K, Shudo I, Saito H (1979) Pharmacokinetics of verapamil in man. Res Commun Chem Pathol Pharmacol 24:37–47
14. Woodcock BG, Hopf R, Kaltenbach M (1980) Verapamil and norverapamil plasma concentrations during long-term therapy in patients with hypertrophic obstructive cardiomyopathy. J Cardiovasc Pharmacol 2:17–23

Plasma Verapamil Levels in Patients with Hypertrophic Cardiomyopathy: Interpatient Variability and Clinical Usefulness

MARTIN B. LEON, DOUGLAS R. ROSING, and STEPHEN E. EPSTEIN

Summary

Plasma verapamil levels were measured under various clinical conditions using a high-pressure liquid chromatography assay to determine their importance in guiding therapy in patients with hypertrophic cardiomyopathy. In 80 patients on chronic oral verapamil therapy, there was marked variability between patients in plasma verapamil levels for each dosage. In contrast, variability in peak and trough plasma verapamil levels for a given patientnwas relatively small (verapamil peak/trough ratio for 23 patients = 1.66 ± 0.07). Plasma verapamil levels in 27 clinical responders, with improvement in NYHA functional class and >15% increase in exercise capacity, were not different from 15 nonresponders (responders = 153 ± 11, vs nonresponders = 175 ± 18 ng/ml (NS)). In 24 patients with serious electrophysiologic or hemodynamic side effects from verapamil, plasma verapamil levels ranged from 30 to 540 ng/ml (mean plasma verapamil level = 201 ± 23 ng/ml) and there was significant overlap in plasma verapamil levels compared with responders and nonresponders. Thus, in patients with hypertrophic cardiomyopathy on verapamil therapy (1) there is marked interpatient variability in plasma verapamil levels, which may be due to differences in first-pass hepatic metabolism and (2) there is considerable overlap of plasma verapamil levels in responders, nonresponders, and patients with serious side effects. Plasma verapamil levels therefore may be of limited usefulness in predicting therapeutic or toxic effects from oral verapamil therapy in patients with hypertrophic cardiomyopathy.

Introduction

Verapamil has been shown to be an effective alternative to beta-adrenergic blocking drugs in the treatment of hypertrophic cardiomyopathy [1–3] (Rosing et al.[1]). However, our experience over the past 3 years using chronic oral verapamil at the National Institutes of Health has shown that only some patients with hypertrophic cardiomyopathy are benefitted by this form of therapy, while others have no improvement in symptoms or manifest deleterious cardiac side effects. Thus far, no pretreatment clinical predictors for therapeutic responsiveness or toxicity have been identified, leading to speculation that aspects of drug pharmacology may be playing

---

1 R. Rosing et al., A new approach to the pharmacologic treatmeno of hypertrophic obstructive cardiomyopathy with verapamil, unpublished work

an important role in determining clinical efficacy. Therefore, to answer such questions, we used a sensitive high-pressure liquid chromatography assay to measure total plasma verapamil concentrations in a large group of patients with hypertrophic cardiomyopathy in a wide range of clinical situations. The major purposes of the present investigation were (1) to examine the variability of plasma verapamil levels between patients while on chronic oral therapy and (2) to assess the clinical utility of plasma verapamil levels in predicting physiologic, therapeutic, and toxic drug effects.

Methods

Patient Groups and Study Protocols

The subject group consisted of 80 patients with previously diagnosed hypertrophic cardiomyopathy admitted to the Cardiology Service of the National Heart, Lung, and Blood Institute between 1 June 1978 and 31 May 1980. All patients had referrable cardiac symptoms (including chest pain, shortness of breath, and presyncope or syncope) and the vast majority were considered either functional class 3 or 4 according to NYHA classification. All patients had previously been given a trial of beta-adrenergic blocking drugs and now were admitted with the intention of beginning oral verapamil as a therapeutic alternative. Ages ranged from 15 to 80 years (mean 48 ± 1 years), 51% of patients were men and 49% were women. Left and right heart cardiac catheterization during hospital admission were performed in 70% of patients. Evidence of left ventricular outflow tract obstruction at rest or during provocative maneuvers was present in 80% of all patients by either cardiac catheterization or echocardiography [4].

Patients were subdivided into smaller groups to ascertain the impact of plasma drug level assessments on the clinical pharmacology and physiologic effects of verapamil therapy. Group 1 consists of 80 patients begun on oral verapamil therapy as inpatients on the various dosage regimens used in clinical practice; 80 mg T.I.D., 80 mg Q.I.D., 120 mg T.I.D., 120 mg Q.I.D., and 160 mg Q.I.D. All inpatient plasma drug levels were obtained after a minimum of 48 h on a given dose and, in 47 of the patients (58%), plasma levels were also obtained at the time of outpatient clinic evaluation while on chronic oral verapamil therapy. Most plasma levels were obtained without attention to the timing of drug administration and were measured just prior to upright treadmill exercise testing for both inpatients and outpatients in an attempt to correlate changes in exercise capacity with plasma drug concentrations. Group 2A comprises peak (1½ h after a dose) and trough (before the next dose) plasma level data in 12 outpatients with hypertrophic cardiomyopathy on chronic oral therapy taking from 240 mg to 480 mg/day in three or four divided doses. For comparison, group 2B includes peak and trough plasma levels in 11 inpatients with coronary artery disease participating in a different study [5] and treated with oral verapamil at two different dosages (80 mg Q.I.D., and 120 mg Q.I.D.), each for 48 h duration. Group 3 encompasses 27 patients defined as clinical responders (3 A) and 15 patients considered to be clinical nonresponders (3 B). Inclusion into either of these groups required that patients have no significant

Plasma Verapamil Levels in Patients with Hypertrophic Cardiomyopathy 311

inpatient hemodynamic or electrophysiologic side effects on the verapamil dose prescribed at discharge and that they be on chronic oral therapy for at least 3 months. Clinical responders fulfilled two criteria: (1) increase in exercise duration of 15% or greater on standard upright treadmill exercise testing and (2) improvement in outpatient symptomatic status of at least one NYHA functional class. In contrast, nonresponders all had less than a 15% increase in exercise duration and no improvement in functional class. Both inpatient plasma levels (after 48 h drug therapy) and outpatient plasma levels were obtained at the time of exercise testing. Group 4 consists of 24 patients experiencing verapamil-related side effects. These included electrophysiologic abnormalities (AV dissociation or AV-nodal Wenkebach) deleterious hemodynamic consequences (congestive heart failure or symptomatic hypotension), and verapamil-quinidine interactions. Blood was available for analysis at the time of side effects for inpatients and within 2 weeks of a documented complication in outpatients.

Many patients are included in multiple of the afore-mentioned groups as determined by individual diagnostic workups and clinical course.

Assay Techniques

Venous blood was injected into heparinized glass tubes and plasma was immediately sequestered after centrifugation and frozen for future chemical analysis. A highly sensitive, reproducible high-pressure liquid chromatography assay developed in our laboratory [6] and utilizing a commercially available column with fluorometric detection was employed for determination of total verapamil concentration in plasma. Similar assay extraction techniques with either HPLC or gas chromatography have been used by other investigators [7–9] and sensitivity for measurement of plasma verapamil levels is in the 1–2 ng/ml range. Plasma assays were always done in duplicate and in cases where greater than 10% variation in duplicate samples existed the assay was repeated. Mean results of the duplicate samples were reported as the final plasma verapamil level.

Statistical Analysis

Data are expressed as mean $\pm$ SEM unless otherwise stipulated. Statistical analyses were done using standard 2-tailed tests for paired and unpaired data as well as linear regression analyses where appropriate.

Results

Inpatient Plasma Level Variability

In the 80 patients from group 1, 166 plasma verapamil concentrations were measured and mean plasma levels for both inpatients and outpatients showed progressive increments with increasing daily oral verapamil dosage (Table 1, Fig. 1).

Table 1. Verapamil levels in patients with hypertrophic cardiomyopathy on chronic oral therapy

Dose	Mean (ng/ml)	P value	Range (ng/ml)	±2 SD (ng/ml)	n
80 mg TID (240 mg)					
Inpatient	104	} <.05	60–143	74	5
Outpatient	63		32– 82	42	5
Total	84		32–143	72	10
80 mg QID (320 mg)					
Inpatient	127	} ns ⌐ns	15–540	238	24
Outpatient	101		42–202	92	11
Total	119		15–540	202	35
120 mg TID (360 mg)					
Inpatient	173	} ns <.025	30–450	168	30
Outpatient	147		20–322	178	18
Total	163		20–450	172	48
120 mg QID (480 mg)					
Inpatient	167	} ns ⌐ns	72–368	148	34
Outpatient	185		50–596	262	29
Total	174		50–596	208	63
160 mg QID (640 mg)					
Inpatient	292	} ns <.01	–	–	1
Outpatient	254		145–395	180	0
Total	256		145–395	170	10

Further, except at the lowest dose (240 mg/day), there was no difference between inpatient and outpatient plasma levels at each dosage, implying that with chronic oral therapy neither drug compliance nor drug accumulation influenced outpatient plasma level results (Table 1, Fig. 1). Although mean plasma levels generally corresponded with oral dosage changes, there is considerable overlap of individual blood level data in patients taking different dosages and marked interpatient variability at each dosage level (Fig. 2). The ratio of highest to lowest verapamil level for inpatients and outpatients at each total daily dosage varied from 2.7 to 36.0 and averaged 15.6 for all five dosages. Plasma drug level variability between patients was not improved when total daily dosage was corrected for differences in body weight. For all group 1 patients, there was poor correlation between oral dosage in milligram/kilogram/day and plasma verapamil concentrations ($r = 0.296$). Examining more closely the subgroup of patients with verapamil levels below 100 ng/ml ($n = 14$), compared with the remainder of group 1 patients, there were no differences in cardiac output (measured in 11 of 14 patients at the time of catheterization), incidence of clinical congestive heart failure, hepatic function, renal function, or ratio of verapamil dose to body weight. However, although group 1 patients were equally divided among men and women, 12 of 14 patients with verapamil levels less than 100 ng/ml (86%) were women.

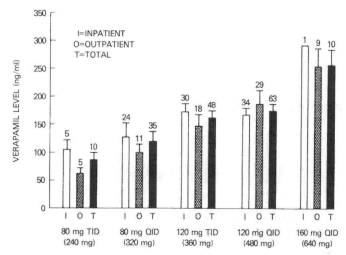

Fig. 1. Mean (+SEM) plasma verapamil levels for inpatients and outpatients with hypertrophic cardiomyopathy on chronic oral therapy. (Numbers above mean bars represent number of samples at each dosage level)

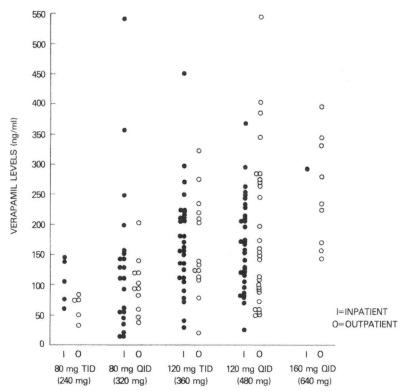

Fig. 2. Individual plasma verapamil level data for inpatients and outpatients with hypertrophic cardiomyopathy on chronic oral therapy

Peak and Trough Plasma Verapamil Levels

Peak plasma verapamil levels correlated well with trough levels in both patients with hypertrophic cardiomyopathy (group 2 A; $r=0.618$, $P<0.05$) and patients with coronary artery disease (group 2 B; $r=0.889$, $P<0.001$ for 320 mg/day and $r=0.897$, $P<0.001$ for 480 mg/day). The average plasma drug level peak to trough ratio for group 2 A was 1.70 (range 1.01–2.42) and for group 2 B was 1.59 (range 1.30–2.72) (Fig. 3). The above data indicate that although differences in verapamil

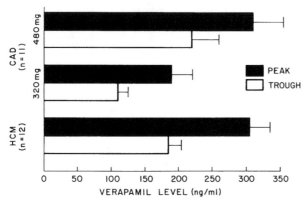

Fig. 3. Mean ($\pm$ SEM) peak and trough plasma verapamil levels in patients with coronary artery disease (at two different dosages, 320 mg/day and 480 mg/day) and in patients with hypertrophic cardiomyopathy

concentrations on a given dose are diminished somewhat when sampling time is considered, additional explanations are required to reconcile the extreme interpatient variability demonstrated in group 1 patients.

Clinical Responders and Nonresponders

In 42 patients with hypertrophic cardiomyopathy begun on oral verapamil therapy as inpatients and continued as outpatients individuals were defined as either clinical responders (group 3 A) or clinical nonresponders (group 3 B, see Methods). The two groups manifested no significant differences in plasma verapamil levels at the time of exercise testing (group 3 A = 153 ± 11 vs group 3 B = 175 ± 18 ng/ml, ns) (Fig. 4). When changes in exercise capacity were examined independently, there was a poor correlation between percent change in exercise duration (compared with inpatient baseline exercise on no medication) and plasma verapamil concentrations for both responders ($r=0.151$) and nonresponders ($r=0.127$).

There were also no changes between inpatient and outpatient plasma levels for both responders and nonresponders (Fig. 4). However, in those individuals where plasma level data are available on a given dose as both inpatients and outpatients (n = 14 in group 3 A and n = 5 in group 3 B), there was a tendency for nonresponders to show a greater decrease in plasma verapamil concentration from inpatient to

Plasma Verapamil Levels in Patients with Hypertrophic Cardiomyopathy 315

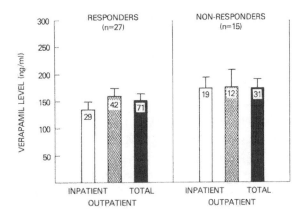

Fig. 4. Mean (±SEM) plasma verapamil levels for inpatients and outpatients in responders and nonresponders. (Numbers within mean bars represent number of samples for each subgroup)

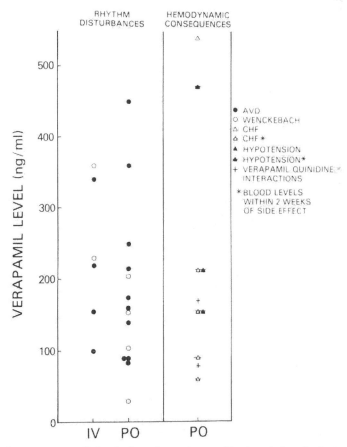

Fig. 5. Individual plasma verapamil level data in patients with drug-induced electrophysiologic and hemodynamic side effects

outpatient values than responders (mean = –85 vs –5 ng/ml, P = 0.05). This suggests that at least in some patients, either poor drug compliance or changing drug metabolism may influence outpatient verapamil levels and clinical responsiveness. No other clinical, hemodynamic, or pharmacologic parameters were useful in predicting therapeutic benefit from chronic oral verapamil therapy.

Patients with Side Effects

The 24 patients in group 4 experienced a variety of verapamil-related side effects including AV dissociation in 14, AV-nodal Wenkebach in six, congestive heart failure in five, symptomatic hypotension in three, and verapamil-quinidine interactions in two others (consisting of marked postural hypotension in one and both hypotension and congestive heart failure in another) (Fig. 5). Plasma verapamil levels were statistically indistinguishable in patients with either rhythm

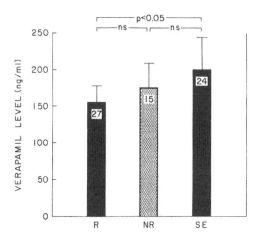

Fig. 6. Mean (±SEM) plasma verapamil levels in responders (R), nonresponders (NR), and patients with side effects (SE). (Numbers within mean bars respresent number of samples for each subgroup)

disturbances (mean = 196 ± 24 ng/ml, range 30–450 ng/ml) or hemodynamic consequences (mean = 213 ± 49 ng/ml, range 52–540 ng/ml). Furthermore, comparing responders, nonresponders, and all patients with side effects, although there was a significant difference between responders and patients with side effects (mean = 201 ± 23 ng/ml, $P<0.05$), there is considerable overlap in individual plasma level data amongst all of these patient groups (Fig. 6).

Discussion

The use of calcium channel blocking agents like verapamil constitutes the first major pharmacologic advance in the treatment of hypertrophic cardiomyopathy since the introduction of propranolol therapy more than a decade ago [10]. Despite almost complete oral absorption of verapamil in humans, drug bioavailability averages only 10–20% of an administered dose, resulting from extensive first-pass hepatic metabolism [11]. The rapid emergence of plasma metabolites and their slow elimination relative to the parent compound [12] has led to speculation that physiologically active metabolic by-products may play an important role in the clinical effects seen with verapamil therapy. However, animal investigations demonstrated that of all major circulating verapamil metabolites, only norverapamil (N-demethylverapamil) possesses significant hemodynamic effects (about 1/5 as potent as verapamil) [13]. Furthermore, studies in patients with hypertrophic cardiomyopathy on long-term oral verapamil therapy have shown no significant accumulation of norverapamil and good correlation between plasma verapamil and norverapamil concentration [14]. Thus, it would seem that measurement of plasma verapamil levels should be an accurate reflection of physiologic drug effects and could prove useful in guiding patient therapy.

In the present study patients given standard oral dosages of verapamil manifested considerable variability in plasma verapamil levels for both inpatients and outpatients at any given dosage and marked overlap of individual plasma level data in patients receiving different dosages (Table 1, Fig. 1, 2). Although plasma level sampling times were usually coupled with exercise testing and therefore were not standardized relative to dosing intervals, peak and trough plasma level differences were not great enough to account for the profound interpatient variabilities revealed (Fig. 3). These observations corroborate the findings of Woodcock et al. who demonstrated a 25-fold difference in trough and a 13-fold difference in peak plasma verapamil concentrations in 20 patients with hypertrophic cardiomyopathy given the same oral dosages [14]. An adequate explanation for the wide interpatient variability of verapamil levels remains somewhat unclear. Patient drug compliance appears to be of minor importance as there are similar degrees of variability and insignificant differences in plasma levels for inpatients and outpatients. Further, dosages correctioned for body weight did little to improve the correlation between dosage (in mg/kg/day) and verapamil concentrations. Oral absorption of verapamil is almost complete and would not be expected to vary greatly from patient to patient. Individual differences in protein binding should also have minimal influences on plasma drug concentrations due to the fact that drugs with predominant first-pass presystemic metabolism generally have rates of hepatic elimination which are not dependent upon protein binding characteristics [15]. Thus, if all the above facts are excluded as possible causes of verapamil level variability one is left with the likelihood that drug metabolism, which is dominated by rapid hepatic biotransformation, is largely responsible for differing plasma verapamil concentrations.

Variability in first-pass hepatic metabolism among patients usually results from either alterations in hepatic blood flow or individual differences in the activity of degradative enzyme processes [16]. Although cardiac output was not measured at the time of oral dosing, in those patients with higher verapamil levels (greater than 1 standard deviation above mean for a given dosage), there was no increased incidence of clinical congestive heart failure and cardiac output measured at the time of cardiac catheterization was no different in this subgroup compared with patients having lower verapamil levels. However, since hepatic clearance of drugs with high hepatic extraction ratios is extremely sensitive to changes in liver blood flow and verapamil may cause profound alterations in cardiovascular hemodynamics, we cannot exclude this as contributing factor in plasma level variability.

Genetic factors and environmental influences can alter the status of hepatic enzymes systems responsible for the metabolism of verapamil. For example, patients with augmented hepatic N-dealkylation enzyme pathways forming circulating plasma verapamil metabolies with minimal hemodynamic activity would have exaggerated first-pass effects resulting in both lower verapamil concentrations and diminished therapeutic efficacy at any oral dosage. Interestingly, in the present study, the vast majority of those individuals with low plasma verapamil levels were women. In the absence of other differentiating clinical features, it seems possible that gender-specific alterations in the capacity of hepatic enzyme systems may be responsible for some of the observed interpatient variability in plasma levels during verapamil therapy. Finally, there is good evidence to suggest that therapy with other drugs having significant first-pass hepatic metabolism, such as propranolol, also results in poor correlation between oral doses and plasma drug concentrations [17, 18].

Several investigators have demonstrated a good correlation between plasma verapamil levels and negative dromotropic actions in dogs using intravenous verapamil [19–21] and in humans with both intravenous and oral verapamil preparations [22, 23]. Thus far, there are only preliminary data addressing the relationship between hemodynamic events and plasma verapamil concentrations [20] and no evidence to indicate that the use of plasma verapamil levels in humans on chronic oral therapy is useful in predicting therapeutic or toxic drug effects. We attempted to answer such questions by comparing plasma drug concentrations in three discrete groups of patients with hypertrophic cardiomyopathy on chronic oral verapamil therapy; clinical responders, clinical nonresponders, and patients with either hemodynamic or electrophysiologic drug-induced side effects. The criteria used to separate responders from nonresponders included objective exercise test performance coupled with blinded assessments of overall symptomatic status and were generally the same criteria used to decide whether individual patients should continue verapamil therapy. No statistical differences were found in plasma verapamil levels between responders and nonresponders in both inpatient and outpatient subgroups (Fig. 4). In some patients, outpatient drug compliance may be a significant factor as there were changes in inpatient versus outpatient plasma drug concentrations corresponding to changes in clinical responsiveness. However, no other distinguishing clinical or pharmacologic features served to separate these two groups.

Patients with verapamil related side effects comprised a heterogenous group manifesting either hemodynamic instability or evidence of pathologic prolongation of AV nodal conduction (Fig. 5). Examination of this group of patients with side effects reveals a wide range in plasma verapamil levels (from 30–540 ng/ml) and no differences between patients with either hemodynamic or electrophysiologic complications. Importantly, there is marked overlap of individual plasma drug level data in responders, nonresponders, and patients with various side effects (Fig. 6).

Based upon these data, it would be difficult to assign a therapeutic range which might predict subsequent success or failure in patients with hypertrophic cardiomyopathy started on oral verapamil therapy. For example, if 100 ng/ml were considered the lower limit of a therapeutic range, then 37% of plasma verapamil levels in responders would be below this limit and 71% of plasma drug levels in nonresponders would be above 100 ng/ml. Likewise, it is problematic to define a toxic plasma verapamil concentration above which most patients manifest drug-related complications. Only 16% of plasma drug levels in patients with serious cardiac side effects were greater than 350 ng/ml. It bears noting that although there are minimal group differences in plasma verapamil levels, no attempts were made to establish individual patient dose-response relationships. It is indeed possible that for a given patient, changes in plasma drug levels would be more closely associated with physiologic and toxic drug effects.

That plasma verapamil levels would correlate poorly with end-organ drug-induced effects is not entirely unexpected and several explanations are plausible. First, it remains uncertain as to whether measurement of total plasma verapamil concentrations is an accurate reflection of circulating drug activity. Although animal studies indicated that most important plasma verapamil metabolites have minimal hemodynamic and electrophysiologic effects [13], such evidence is lacking in humans. Further, commercially available oral verapamil is a racemic mixture of (–) and (+) optical isomers and there is mounting data that only the (–) optical isomer possesses significant calcium channel blocking properties [24]. Thus, depending on the isomeric balance of a given verapamil preparation and differential hepatic metabolism of the optical isomers, total plasma verapamil levels may be a poor index of (–) verapamil concentrations and corresponding pharmacologic activity. Also, localized changes in myocardial blood flow could result in differences in regional myocardial drug availability [25], rendering measurement of plasma verapamil levels an insensitive indicator of cardiac drug effects. Finally, insight is only now being gained regarding the specific mechanisms whereby calcium channel blockers are beneficial in patients with hypertrophic cardiomyopathy and other cardiac disorders. It appears that verapamil's inhibiting effects on transmembrane calcium influx are modulated by multiple ambient influences (including local catecholamine, cyclic-AMP, and phosphodiesterase inhibitor concentrations) [26]. Therefore, if patient drug effects are heavily dependent upon an individual's resting "calcium influx tone", measurement of plasma blood levels would be an imprecise reflection of actual pharmacologic activity. That this may be of clinical importance has been shown in patients with atrial fibrillation and congestive heart failure [22]. Such patients require significantly higher plasma verapamil levels for the same degree of ventricular slowing. This is presumably due to elevated resting catecholamine levels causing augmentation of calcium influx, thereby counteracting the effects of verapamil [22].

In conclusion, the present investigation demonstrates that in patients with hypertrophic cardiomyopathy on oral verapamil therapy: (1) there is marked interpatient variability in plasma verapamil levels for a given dose, which may be due to differences in first-pass hepatic metabolism; and (2) considerable overlap in plasma verapamil levels in patients who are clinical responders, clinical nonresponders, and those with drug-related side effects render the routine measurement of plasma verapamil levels of limited clinical utility in predicting therapeutic or toxic effects.

References

1. Kaltenbach M, Hopf R, Keller M (1976) Calciumantagonistische Therapie bei hypertroph-obstruktiver Kardiomyopathie. Dtsch Med Wochenschr 101:1284
2. Rosing DR, Kent KM, Maron BJ, Epstein SE (1979) Verapamil therapy: A new approach to the pharmacologic treatment of hypertrophic cardiomyopathy. II. Effects on exercise capacity and symptomatic status. Circulation 60:1208
3. Kaltenbach M, Hopf R, Kober G, Bussman WD, Keller M, Peterson DY (1979) Treatment of hypertrophic obstructive cardiomyopathy with verapamil. Br Heart J 42:35
4. Henry WL, Clark CE, Griffith JM, Epstein SE (1975) Mechanism of left ventricular outflow obstruction in patients with obstructive asymmetric septal hypertrophy (idiopathic hypertrophic subaortic stenosis). Am J Cardiol 35:337
5. Leon MB, Rosing DR, Bonow RD, Lipson LC, Epstein SE (to be published) Clinical efficacy of verapamil alone and combined with propranolol in treating patients with chronic stable angina pectoris. Am J Cardiol
6. Jaouni TM, Leon MB, Rosing DR, Fales HM (1980) Analysis of verapamil in plasma by liquid chromatography. J Chrom 182:473
7. Harapat SR, Kates RE (1979) Rapid high-pressure liquid chromatographic analysis of verapamil in blood and plasma. J Chromatogr 170:385
8. McAllister RG, Tan TG, Bourne DA (1979) GLC assay of verapamil in plasma: Identification of fluorescent metabolies after oral drug administration. J Pharmacol Sci 68:574
9. Hege HG (1979) Gas chromatographic determination of verapamil in plasma and urine. Arzneim Forsch 29, 11:1681
10. Cohen LS, Braunwald E (1967) Amelioration of angina pectoris in idiopathic hypertrophic subaortic stenosis with beta-adrenergic blockade. Circulation 35:847
11. Schomerus M, Spiegelhalder B, Stieren B, Eichelbaum M (1976) Physiological disposition of verapamil in man. Cardiovasc Res 10:1
12. Eichelbaum M, Ende M, Renberg G, Schomerus M, Dengler HJ (1979) The metabolism of DL-^{14}C verapamil in man. Drug Metab Dispos 7:154
13. Neugebauer G (1978) Comparative cardiovascular actions of verapamil and its major metabolies in the anaesthetised dog. Cardiovasc Res 12:247
14. Woodcock BG, Hopf R, Kaltenbach M (1980) Verapamil and norverapamil plasma concentrations during long-term therapy in patients with hypertrophic obstructive cardiomyopathy. J Cardiovasc Pharmacol 2:17
15. Blaschke TF (1977) Protein binding and kinetics of drugs in liver diseases. Clin Pharmacokinet 2:32
16. Wilkinson GR (1976) Pharmacokinetics in disease states modifying body perfusion. In: Benet LZ (ed) The effect of disease states on drug pharmacokinetics. American Pharmaceutical Association, Washington DC, p 13
17. Zacest R, Koch-Weser J (1972) The relation of propranolol plasma level to β-blockade during oral therapy. Pharmacology 7:178
18. Chidsey CA, Morselli P, Bianchetti E, Morganti A, Leonchi G, Zanchetti A (1975) Studies of the absorption and removal of propranolol in hypertensive patients during therapy. Circulation 52:313
19. McAllister RG, Bourne DWA, Dittert LW (1977) The pharmacology of verapamil. I. Eleminiation kinetics in dogs and correlation of plasma levels with effects on the electrocardiogram. J Pharmacol Exp Ther 202:38
20. Mangiardi LM, Hariman RJ, McAllister RG, Bhargava V, Surawicz B, Shabetai R (1978) Electrophysiologic and hemodynamic effects of verapamil. Correlation with plasma drug concentrations. Circulation 57:366

21. Keefe DL, Harapat SR, Kates RE (1981) Relationship between pharmacodynamics and myocardial concentration of verapamil (Abstr) Am J Cardiol 47:406
22. Dominic J, McAllister RG, Kuo CS, Reddy CP, Surawicz B (1979) Verapamil plasma levels and ventricular rate response in patients with atrial fibrillation and flutter. Clin Pharmacol Ther 26:710
23. Schwartz JB, Keefe DL, Peters F, Kates R, Harrison DC (1981) Concentrations dependent heart rate suppression with verapamil (Abstr) Am J Cardiol 47:406
24. Bayer R, Hennekes R, Kaufman R, Mannhold R (1975) Inotropic and electrophysiologic actions of verapamil and D-600 in mammalian myocardium: I. Pattern of inotropic effects of the racemic compounds. Naunyn Schmiedebergs Arch Pharmacol 290:49
25. Zito RA, Cardio VJ, Holford T, Zaret BL (1981) Regional myocardial kinetics of lidocaine in experimental infarction: modulation by regional flow. Am J Cardiol 47:265
26. Antman FM, Stone PH, Muller JE, Braunwald E (1980) Calcium channel blocking agents in the treatment of cardiovascular disorders. Part 1: Basic and clinical electrophysiologic effects. Ann Intern Med 93:875

Correlation of Verapamil Plasma Levels with Electrocardiographic and Hemodynamic Effects*

R. G. McAllister, Jr.

Introduction

As further clinical indications for verapamil become apparent, the need to define drug plasma concentrations at which specific pharmacologic effects predictably occur grows increasingly important. The activity of verapamil as an antagonist of calcium-dependent processes provides the basis for a wide range of therapeutic effects, and at the same time allows prediction of the toxicity which must result when the drug is present in excess. High plasma verapamil levels can interfere sufficiently with excitation-contraction coupling [1] to produce profound depression of myocardial pump function [2]. In the same fashion, antagonism of calcium-dependent impulse conduction across the atrioventricular (AV) node can be intense enough to produce complete heart block [2]. Since these manifestations of drug toxicity are potentially lethal, the establishment of plasma concentration ranges at which therapeutic, but not toxic, effects can reasonably be anticipated will allow more consistently effective use of verapamil in patient management.

An additional factor serving as a stimulus for studies seeking to define verapamil plasma level-effect correlations is the observation by Schomerus et al. [3] that orally administered verapamil is subject to extensive first-pass hepatic extraction and metabolism. This results in low bioavailability (10–20% of administered dose) and a wide variation between subjects in plasma drug concentrations produced by fixed oral doses. Similar kinetic patterns have been described for other cardioactive drugs, particularly propranolol [4], and experience has confirmed the predictions that, in such circumstances, the oral dose required to produce therapeutic effects cannot be reliably anticipated. Since avoidance of toxicity is imperative when deleterious effects may be life threatening, as is the case for verapamil, plasma drug level monitoring will be an important aid in rational drug therapy.

Assay Methodology

Verapamil is a papaverine derivative which is extensively metabolized in animals [5] and man [6]. The major metabolites appear to have no significant pharmacologic activity except for the N-demethylated form (nor-verapamil), which has about 20% of the effect of the parent drug as a coronary arterial vasodilator in dogs [7]. Plasma concentrations of verapamil have been measured by a variety of methods, including

---

* Supported in part by a grant from the Knoll Pharmaceutical Company (Whippany, N. J., USA) and by funds from the Veterans Administration.

spectrophotofluorometry [8], gas chromatography, mass spectrometry [9], high-pressure liquid chromatography (HPLC) [10, 11], gas chromatography (GC) using flame-ionization detection [12], and GC with a nitrogen-specific detector [13, 14]. The mass fragmentographic method reported by Spiegelhalder and Eichelbaum [9] is the most sensitive method used, but is laborious and the equipment is unavailable in many laboratories. Spectrophotofluorometry is perhaps the simplest of the various assay methods; it appears to be adequately sensitive (20 ng/ml) and reproducible for clinical studies of verapamil levels after intravenous drug administration [15, 16]. It has, however, the disadvantage of detecting fluorescent metabolites present in plasma after verapamil is given orally and thus is insufficiently specific for studies during oral verapamil use [12].

The HPLC techniques used by Harapat and Kates [10, 17], with various modifications [11] appear to be both sensitive (1–5 ng/ml) and reproducible. In addition, separation between unchanged verapamil and the metabolites appearing after oral drug ingestion can be achieved [11, 17]. Use of a nitrogen-specific detector has improved verapamil assay methodology with GC; Hege reported a sensitivity at 4 ng/ml and linearity in a concentration range between 5–60 mg/ml, but interference with the verapamil peak by norverapamil is apparent at high

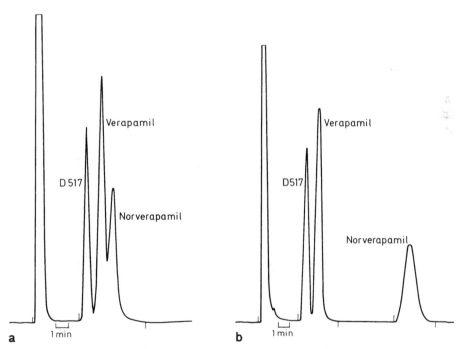

Fig. 1. a Chromatogram of an extract of plasma to which had been added verapamil (50 ng/ml) and norverapamil (50 ng/ml), with D517 as internal standard. Assay conditions are shown in Fig. 2. Note the overlap between verapamil and norverapamil peaks. **b** Effect of addition of acetic anhydride (50 ml) to the same plasma extract shown in Fig. 1 b. The norverapamil peak is widely separated from that of the unchanged drug, allowing quantitation of both compounds

concentrations of the latter [13]. We have seen similar problems in our GC technique (Fig. 1 A), but can achieve distinct separation between parent drug and metabolite by utilizing the addition of acetic anhydride (a technique reported for HPLC use by Jaouni et al. [11]) to react with the demethylated derivative (Fig. 1 B). This modification retains the sensitivity of the GC method and allows a reproducibility in measurement of both verapamil and norverapamil which compares favorably with HPLC techniques (Fig. 2) [17a].

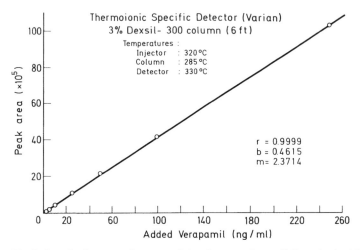

Fig. 2. Standard curve of verapamil in plasma using a GC method with a nitrogen-specific (thermoionic) detector. Extraction techniques were those previously used [12] and acetic anhydride was added prior to injection (see Fig. 1b). Six samples were measured at each point shown and the resulting peak areas integrated electronically

These comments are necessary because the validity of plasma verapamil measurements depends upon the assay techniques used. It is difficult, for example, to assess data on drug plasma levels measured with spectrophotofluorometry after oral drug administration [16], when it has been previously shown that fluorescent metabolites generated during the first pass interfere with the reliability of this particular assay method [12]. Therefore, the interpretation of studies seeking to correlate verapamil's effects with corresponding plasma drug concentrations will depend, in part, on the assay methodology.

In Vitro Studies

Only a few in vitro studies with verapamil have used variable drug concentrations to characterize the observed effects. Rosen et al. varied verapamil concentrations from 10^{-5} m to 2×10^{-7} m (i.e., 4546–91 ng/ml) in determination of the electrophysiologic effects of the drug upon canine Purkinje fiber bundles [18]: at concentrations below 2×10^{-6} M (i.e., 909 ng/ml), the drug had no effect on the

Purkinje fiber action potential but suppressed automaticity induced by low potassium perfusates or ouabain. Hordof et al. found that verapamil concentrations between 100–1000 ng/ml depressed only the action potential plateau of normal human right atrial fibers, but lower concentrations markedly depressed action potentials in fibers from dilated atria [19]. In addition, slow response automaticity was depressed at the lowest drug concentration studied. Imanishi et al. used depolarized ventricular myocardium from guinea pigs pretreated with verapamil to evaluate the effects of the drug on rhythmic automatic depolarizations (RAD) resulting from inactivation of the fast sodium current [20]. At the time of killing, plasma drug levels varied from 100–1850 ng/ml, and the effects on decrease in rate and overshoot of RAD were directly related to the corresponding plasma drug concentrations. A retrospective analysis of these studies reveals that they were accurate in predicting the concentration – effect correlations subsequently derived from in vivo investigations.

In Vivo Studies: Animals

A number of different in vivo models have been used to determine the effects of verapamil. Healthy, anesthetized mongrel dogs tolerated intravenous doses of verapamil up to about 3.5 mg/kg before the onset of electrophysiologic toxicity (i.e., second or third degree heart block) or hypotension [21]. In studies using conscious dogs, the effects of verapamil were shown to be related not only to the amount of drug given but also to the speed of intravenous administration; rates in excess of 3 mg/min resulted in a high incidence of transient heart block [22]. The effects of verapamil on AV conduction, measured as the P-R interval of the surface electrocardiograms (EKG), were shown to be linearly related to corresponding plasma drug levels in these animals; in addition, the P-R interval change versus drug level relationship was similar during periods of rapidly increasing drug plasma concentrations and when plasma levels were falling [15]. Plasma verapamil levels in these studies were measured by spectrophotofluorometry, a method which appears to be valid for studies using single intravenous doses of drug, in contrast to studies where verapamil is given orally and fluorescent metabolites appear rapidly [12].

Using anesthetized, open-chest dogs, Mangiardi et al. studied the effects of various plasma concentrations of verapamil on both electrophysiologic and hemodynamic parameters [2]. The drug was given intravenously in a fashion designed to produce and maintain relatively stable plasma drug levels for 20 min, and the experimental results analyzed for groups of animals in which verapamil levels were low (25–152 ng/ml), intermediate (200–377 ng/ml), or high (400–2000 ng/ml). The drug slowed the sinoatrial pacemaker only at concentrations above 152 ng/ml, and sinus arrest was seen only in the presence of high verapamil levels; significant prolongation of corrected sinus recovery time did not occur at any level of verapamil. A direct relationship between plasma verapamil levels and prolongation of A-H interval was found, with high degrees of heart block occurring during spontaneous rhythm only in the group in which higher plasma drug levels were produced. When atrial pacing was used, heart block appeared earlier, at plasma drug levels of 200 ng/ml, indicating the rate-dependent nature of verapamil's actions on AV nodal impulse conduction. Significant depression of myocardial contractility did not occur at low levels of verapamil (i.e., <152 ng/ml), but increased progressively as plasma concentrations increased. The effects of verapamil in this experimental model are shown in Fig. 3, where the preferential effects of the drug on electrophysiologic parameters are clearly apparent. The higher slope and lower intercept of the plasma level-effect relationship for A-H interval prolongation, as compared with that for decrease in myocardial contractility (expressed as left ventricular dp/dt), indicate that significant effects on AV conduction can be achieved at plasma verapamil levels producing insignificant hemodynamic effects.

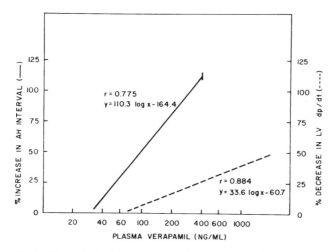

Fig. 3. The relationship between plasma verapamil concentrations and electrophysiologic effects (expressed as % increase in A-H interval) and hemodynamic effects (% decrease in left ventricular dp/dt), from the studies of Mangiardi et al. in anesthetized instrumented dogs [2]. The differing slopes and intercepts indicate that significant degrees of A-H prolongation will occur at plasma drug levels at which insignificant depression of LV dp/dt occurs

Using the same instrumented, anesthetized dog model, Hariman et al. studied the action of $CaCl_2$ on the electrophysiologic and hemodynamic effects of verapamil across a wide range of plasma drug levels (70–2042 ng/ml) [22]. Relatively small amounts of $CaCl_2$ were required to reverse the negative isotropic effects, regardless of plasma concentration of the drug; the vasodilator activity of verapamil, however, was unaffected by $CaCl_2$ administration. In addition, doses of $CaCl_2$ sufficient to reverse the depressant effects on myocardial contractility (15 mg/kg over 5 min) had no effect on verapamil-induced prolongation of A-H interval and slowing of sinus rate. These studies, therefore, demonstrated distinct differences in the susceptibility of verapamil's effects on myocardial, vascular, and electrophysiologic sites to reversal by $CaCl_2$.

Perkins reported that calcium gluconate administration promptly reversed both hypotension and intermittent AV block in a patient who took 3200 mg of verapamil orally; the verapamil concentration was 4000 ng/ml, but the assay used to measure the drug was not defined [23]. In a similar case in which plasma levels were not measured, complete heart block and hypotension occurred in a 14-year-old girl after ingestion of 2400 mg of verapamil; intravenous calcium gluconate produced an increase in the ventricular rate but not resolution of the AV block [24].

In Vivo Studies: Human Subjects

In 1976, Schomerus et al. [3] used mass fragmentography to analyze the pharmacokinetics of verapamil after 10 mg given intravenously over 45 min in three elderly subjects, and after an 80 mg oral dose in an additional three. No pharmacodynamic correlations were reported and the levels of unchanged verapamil in plasma were below 100 ng/ml. Koike et al. used spectrophotofluorometry to study verapamil plasma levels in six normal Japanese subjects (ages 21–68 years) given 10 mg verapamil intravenously over 3–5 min, with electrocardiographic recordings made when blood samples were taken [16]. Prolongation of the P-R interval was found to be linearly related to verapamil plasma concentrations between 25–300 ng/ml. In one of the six volunteers Wenckebach type AV block occurred at a level of 127 ng/ml, disappearing when the drug concentration fell below 63 ng/ml.

We have carried out a similar study in eight young healthy men (ages 24–28 years), to whom 0.2 mg/kg verapamil was given intravenously over 3–5 min [25]. Verapamil concentrations in plasma were measured by GC, using a nitrogen-specific detector, as described earlier in this report (see Figs. 1, 2). The P-R interval on the surface EKG increased in all subjects after verapamil was given, with the maximum interval change for the study group (52 ± 19 ms) corresponding to the peak verapamil level in plasma (270 ± 21 ng/ml). In each individual subject, plasma levels of verapamil were directly related to the degree of P-R interval prolongation; between-subject comparisons, however, were not meaningful because of the variation in effects produced at specific plasma verapamil concentrations. At a drug level of 162 ng/ml, for instance, Wenckebach block occurred transiently in one subject, while similar drug levels in another subject produced a P-R interval increase of only 15 ms. Plasma concentrations below 30 ng/ml had no effect on the P-R interval. A mean decrease in T-wave amplitude of $35 \pm 11\%$ from control was observed just after the drug was given, but rapidly resolved. A slight increase in heart rate (mean $= 13.5 \pm 3.0$ beats/min) and a fall in systolic arterial pressure (mean $= 10.4 \pm 4.4$ mmHg) occurred at peak plasma drug concentrations, with a return to control values within 30–60 min.

A similar between-subject variation in the effects of verapamil on AV conduction was reported by Dominic et al. [26], who studied the action of the drug in patients with atrial fibrillation and flutter. Patients who were clinically stable responded to intravenous verapamil (mean dose $= 0.066 \pm 0.099$ mg/kg) with an average decrease in ventricular rate of 60 beats/min; the corresponding plasma verapamil level was 52 ± 7 ng/ml. In patients with similar dysrhythmias but clinical evidence of cardiac failure, however, a dose threefold as large was required to produce a fall in ventricular rate of only 28 ± 11 beats/min, with a mean verapamil level of 95 ± 16 ng/ml. The marked difference in response between the two groups was attributed to the increased endogenous sympathetic tone in the patients with cardiac failure in which increased levels of norepinephrine [27] would be expected to antagonize the actions of verapamil [28].

The importance of sympathetic activity as a modifier of verapamil effects on the AV junction was recently emphasized by Urthaler and James [29], who found that concentrations of verapamil not toxic to the normal heart readily produced high-grade block after elimination of adrenergic influences in the AV junction by prior administration of propranolol or reserpine. This study provides an explanation for the clinical observation that usual clinical doses of verapamil may be lethal in patients also given antiadrenergic drugs [30–32]. The variability in endogenous sympathetic activity present in different individuals, whether healthy or sick, implies a similar degree of variation in the responses to verapamil seen in different subjects at the same plasma drug concentrations.

Stable patients with sustained supraventricular tachyarrhythmias appear to respond well to rather modest intravenous doses of verapamil (i.e., 10 mg or less), while those who are acutely ill may require considerably larger doses (20 mg) [33]. In a group of 20 patients with reentrant SVT, Sung et al. [34] found that the verapamil plasma concentrations required for conversion to sinus rhythm ranged from $72-195$ ng/ml (mean $= 123 \pm 40$ ng/ml). This range of drug plasma concentrations is generally achieved with administration of $0.1-0.2$ mg/kg over a brief period. A similar group of patients receiving a lower dose had a mean verapamil level of 27 ± 21 ng/ml, and none converted to sinus rhythm.

Few data are currently available on the relationship between verapamil plasma concentrations and myocardial depressant effects in humans. Several studies in catheterization laboratories are now in progress, however, which should help to define the correlations needed.

An additional area which requires further study concerns the relationship between plasma verapamil level and effect after oral drug administration. The difficulties produced by the rapid generation of metabolites after oral verapamil were reviewed earlier, and assay methodology is clearly much more critical in studies seeking to correlate responses to plasma drug level after oral therapy. Because of the intense first-pass extraction of verapamil and its rather low bioavailability [3], plasma levels of the drug will vary widely between individuals receiving the same dose. Plasma level monitoring would seem, therefore, to be potentially useful as a guide to clinical therapy. However, the therapeutic and toxic ranges for verapamil levels after oral drug use have not yet been defined. Again, studies are at present underway in normal subjects to determine oral pharmacokinetics and pharmacodynamics, but the results are not yet available.

A few observations are, however, available in patients. Woodcock et al. used a GC method to measure verapamil levels in patients with hypertrophic cardiomyopathy who were receiving chronic oral therapy [14]. As expected, they found considerable (25-fold) variation among patients taking a similar oral dose. Drug levels in some patients were clearly in a range associated with toxicity after intravenous administration (i.e., above 350 ng/ml), but no evidence of deleterious drug effects were reported. Unpublished observations from our laboratory (six patients) also suggest that patients will tolerate verapamil levels following oral drug therapy that are higher than those required to produce similar effects with intravenous drug. An explanation for this is not yet available, but current speculation centers on the racemic nature of verapamil and the demonstration that (–) verapamil is more potent as a vasodilator, myocardial depressant, and negative dromotropic agent than the (+) form [35]. Since current assay procedures measure both isomers, selective extraction of the (–) isomer by the liver after oral therapy would result in a preponderance of the less potent (+) form in the circulation, and higher levels of drug would be required for desired effects than after intravenous drug use.

Summary

The effects of verapamil after intravenous administration are closely related to corresponding plasma drug levels, both in animal experiments as well as in healthy subjects and patients. In the absence of prior treatment with antiadrenergic drugs, patients generally tolerate plasma levels up to 200–300 ng/ml without significant hemodynamic effects but with progressive impairment in AV conduction. Levels above 300 ng/ml have not been well studied in humans but are associated with myocardial depressant effects in dogs. The variability between subjects in the effects on AV conduction at similar drug plasma levels is probably due to differences in endogenous sympathetic activity. Intravenous calcium administration is effective in reversing the negative inotropic effects of verapamil regardless of drug plasma concentration but the electrophysiologic effects are less readily affected.

Too little information is available to define plasma level-effect correlations after oral verapamil use, but preliminary observations suggest that patients may require higher plasma drug concentrations for equivalent effects than needed after intravenous drug.

Finally, evaluation of assay methodology is critical to interpretation of studies seeking to correlate plasma drug levels with effects. The rapid production of fluorescent metabolites after oral drug requires assay techniques capable of separating the parent drug from less active derivatives, while simpler methods appear to suffice for studies with intravenous verapamil administration.

References

1. Haeusler G (1972) Differential effect of verapamil on excitation-contraction coupling in smooth muscle and on excitation-secretion coupling in adrenergic nerve terminals. J Pharmacol Exp Ther 189:672–682
2. Mangiardi LM, Hariman RJ, McAllister RG Jr, Bhargava V, Surawicz B, Shabetai R (1978) Electrophysiologic and hemodynamic effects of verapamil. Correlation with plasma drug concentrations. Circulation 57:366–372
3. Schomerus M, Spiegelhalder B, Stieren B, Eichelbaum M (1976) Physiological disposition of verapamil in man. Cardiovasc Res 10:605–612
4. Nies AS, Shand DG (1975) Clinical pharmacology of propranolol. Circulation 52:6–12
5. McIlhenny HM (1971) Metabolism of (^{14}C) verapamil. J Med Chem 14:1178–1184

6. Eichelbaum M, Ende M, Remberg G, Dengler HJ (1979) The metabolism of DL-(^{14}C) verapamil in man. Drug Metab Dispos 7:145–148
7. Neugebauer G (1978) Comparative cardiovascular actions of verapamil and its major metabolites in the anesthetized dog. Cardiovasc Res 12:247–254
8. McAllister RG Jr, Howell SM (1976) Fluorometric assay of verapamil in biological fluids and tissues. J Pharm Sci 65:431–432
9. Spiegelhalder B, Eichelbaum M (1977) Determination of verapamil in human plasma by mass fragmentography using stable isotope-labelled verapamil as internal standard. Arzneim Forsch 27:94–97
10. Harapat SR, Kates RE (1979) Rapid high-pressure liquid chromatographic analysis of verapamil in blood and plasma. J Chromatogr 170:385–390
11. Jaouni TM, Leon MB, Rosing D, Fales HM (1980) Analysis of verapamil in plasma by liquid chromatography. J Chromatogr 182:473–477
12. McAllister RG Jr, Tan TG, Bourne DWA (1979) GLC assay of verapamil in plasma: Identification of fluorescent metabolites after oral drug administration. J Pharm Sci 68:574–577
13. Hege HG (1979) Gas chromatographic determination of verapamil in plasma and urine. Arzneim Forsch 29:1681–1684
14. Woodcock BG, Hopf R, Kaltenbach M (1980) Verapamil and norverapamil plasma concentrations during long-term therapy in patients with hypertrophic obstructive cardiomyopathy. J Cardiovasc Pharmacol 2:17–23
15. McAllister RG Jr, Bourne DWA, Dittert LW (1977) The pharmacology of verapamil. I. Elimination kinetics in dogs and correlation of plasma levels with effect on the electrocardiogram. J Pharmacol Exp Ther 202:38–44
16. Koike Y, Shimamura K, Shudo I, Saito H (1979) Pharmacokinetics of verapamil in man. Res Comm Chem Pathol Pharmacol 24:37–47
17. Harapat SR, Kates RE (1980) High-performance liquid chromatographic analysis of verapamil. II. Simultaneous quantitation of verapamil and its active metabolite, norverapamil. J Chromatogr 181:484–489
17a. Todd, GD, Bourne DWA, McAllister RG Jr (1980) Measurement of verapamil concentrations in plasma by gas chromatography and high-pressure liquid chromatography. Ther Drug Mon 2:411–416
18. Rosen MR, Ilvento JP, Gelband H, Merker C (1974) Effects of verapamil on electrophysiologic properties of canine cardiac Purkinje fibers. J Pharmacol Exp Ther 189:414–422
19. Hordof AJ, Edie R, Malm JR, Hoffman BF, Rosen MR (1976) Electrophysiologic properties and response to pharmacologic agents of fibers from diseased human atria. Circulation 54:774–779
20. Imanishi S, McAllister RG Jr, Surawicz B (1978) The effects of verapamil and lidocaine on the automatic depolarizations in guinea-pig ventricular myocardium. J Pharmacol Exp Ther 207:294–303
21. Reimer KA, Lowe JE, Jennings RB (1977) Effect of the calcium antagonist verapamil on necrosis following temporary coronary artery occlusion in dogs. Circulation 55:581–587
22. Hariman RJ, Mangiardi LM, McAllister RG Jr, Surawicz B, Shabetai R, Kishida H (1979) Reversal of the cardiovascular effects of verapamil by calcium and sodium: Differences between electrophysiologic and hemodynamic responses. Circulation 59:797–804
23. Perkins CM (1978) Serious verapamil poisoning: Treatment with intravenous calcium gluconate. Br Med J 2:1127
24. Da Silva OA, De Melo RA, Filho JPJ (1979) Verapamil acute self-poisoning. Clin Toxicol 14:361–367

25. Dominic JA, Bourne DWA, Tan TG, Kirsten EB, McAllister RG Jr (1981) The pharmacology of verapamil. III. Pharmacokinetics in normal subjects after intravenous drug administration. J Cardiovasc Pharmacol 3:25–38
26. Dominic JA, McAllister RG Jr, Kuo CS, Reddy CP, Surawicz B (1979) Verapamil plasma levels and ventricular rate response in patients with atrial fibrillation and flutter. Clin Pharmacol Ther 26:710–714
27. Thomas JA, Marks BH (1978) Plasma norepinephrine in congestive heart failure. Am J Cardiol 41:233–245
28. Zipes DP, Fischer JC (1974) Effects of agents which inhibit the slow channel on sinus node automaticity and atrioventricular conduction in the dog. Circ Res 34:184–192
29. Urthaler F, James TN (1979) Experimental studies on the pathogenesis of asystole after verapamil in the dog. Am J Cardiol 44:651–656
30. Benaim ME (1972) Asystole after verapamil. Br Med J 2:169
31. Krikler D (1974) Verapamil in cardiology. Eur J Cardiol 2:3–10
32. Witchitz S, Haiat R, Tarrade T, Chiche P (1975) Accidents cardiovasculaires au cours des traitements par le verapamil. A propos de 6 observations. Nouv Presse Med 4:337–341
33. Hagemeijer F (1978) Verapamil in the management of supraventricular tachyarrhythmias occurring after a recent myocardial infarction. Circulation 57:751–755
34. Sung RJ, Elser B, McAllister RG Jr (1980) Intravenous verapamil for termination of re-entrant supraventricular tachycardias. Intracardiac studies correlated with plasma verapamil concentrations. Ann Intern Med 93:682–689
35. Satoh, Yanagisawa T, Taira N (1980) Coronary vasodilator and cardiac effects of optical isomers of verapamil in the dog. J Cardiovasc Pharmacol 2:309–318

Subject Index

Arrhythmia
  ambulatory ECG-monitoring 12, 14, 171
  and septal thickness 12
  and sudden death (see sudden death)
Asymmetrical septal hypertrophy 23

Bowditch-phenomenon 277

Calcium-antagonisme 115, 268
Calcium-antagonists
  amplitude-frequence-relationship 277
  antianginal effects 269
  cardio-protective effects 106, 107, 118, 119
  and contractility 277
  hemodynamic effects 138
  myocardial effects 276
  negative inotropic effects 278
  pharmacological differentiation 276
  slow inward current 278, 280
  sodium- and potassium conductivity 282
Calcium-overload 115
Calcium-uptake 119
Cardiothoracic ratio 216
Congestive cardiomyopathy
  histologic findings 59

Diltiazem 273
  effect on ST-segment depression 273

Echocardiography 5, 18, 19, 20, 23, 25, 27,
  148, 171, 189, 195, 219
  comparison of m-mode and two-dimen-
    sional echo in HCM 27
  m-mode 19, 23, 164, 171, 189, 207
  two-dimensional 20, 25
Etaphenone 272
  effect on ST-segment-depression 272
  side effects 272
Exercise-testing 188, 192

Fendiline 272
  antianginal activity 272
  effect on ST-segment-depression 272

Heart volume 179, 181
  (see also HOCM)
Hypertrophic cardiomyopathy
  and arrhythmia 12
  clinical characterization 5
  diastolic ventricular function 14
  Echocardiography 11, 25, 164, 207, 218
    comparison of m-mode and two-dimen-
      sional 27
    m-mode 5, 19, 23, 164, 189, 207
    two-dimensional 5, 20, 25
  filling pressure 14
  functional limitation 31
  hemodynamic findings 9
  histologic findings 7, 46
  left atrial diameter 183, 208
  mortality 8
  muscle-cell disorganization 38
    and clinical findings 38
  natural history 8
  outflow-tract obstruction 33
  quantitative histologic findings 46
  septal thickness 10, 207, 214
  Sokolow-Lion-Index 218
  symptoms 31, 166, 190
  terminology 5
  types of ventricular hypertrophy 25, 33
  ventricular compliance 14
  ventricular function 14
  verapamil treatment 163, 177
    (see also HOCM)
Hypertrophic   cardiomyopathy   in   animals 73
  clinical findings 75
  cross-anatomic findings 79, 80
  ECG 75
  histologic findings 82, 84
  sudden death 75
Hypertrophic non-obstructive cardiomyopathy 161
  clinical course 216
  enddiastolic ventricular diameter 214

Subject Index

left atrial diameter 183
posterior wall thickness 219
septal thickness 214
verapamil treatment 214
  dosage of verapamil 216
wall thickness
Hypertrophic obstructive cardiomyopathy
(see also hypertrophic cardiomyopathy)
Beta-blocker-therapy 14, 160, 236, 261
  and cardiac index 254
  and cardiac output 254
  and ECG 264
  effects on heart volume 264
  effects on pulmonary artery pressure 25,
    251
  effects on septal thickness 264
  and exercise capacity 251
  functional results 251, 254, 262
  and heart rate 251
  hemodynamic effects 252
  and prognosis 160
  side effects 263, 265
  operative therapy 238
  and ECG 248
  and exercise capacity 254
  hemodynamic effects 244, 252
  functional results 238, 240, 251
  indications for 239
  long-term results 238, 239, 248
  operative mortality 160, 240, 248
  outflow-tract obstruction 15, 238, 245
  prognosis 15, 160, 243
  septal myectomy and myotomy 12
  surgical procedure 239
  symptomatic improvement 15
  verapamil therapy 160, 161, 208, 237,
    261
  and clinical symptoms 166, 190, 192
  and ECG 207, 264
  effects on coronary artery diameter 173,
    174
  effects on exercise capacity 192
  effects on heart volume 181, 264
  effects on left atrial diameter 183
  effects on muscle mass 173
  effects on septal thickness 173, 195, 207,
    264
  effects on wall thickness 195, 199, 203,
    208, 211
  plasma-levels in responders and non-
    responders 314
  side effects 175, 263, 265

and survival rate 175
verapamil dosage 125, 165, 188, 204

Isoproterenol 115
  and Hydroxy-prolin content of the
    heart 119
  and myocardial calcium content 115
Isovolumetric relaxation 148, 149, 151, 152
  and verapamil 148

Junctional rhythm 196

Metoprolol 188
Mitochondria 65
Mitral valve, systolic anterior movement 33
Myocardial biopsy 58
  electromicroscopy (see also ultrastruc-
    tural findings) 64
  histologic findings in aortic valve
    disease 59
  histologic findings in congestive cardio-
    myopathy 59
  histologic findings in hypertrophic cardio-
    myopathy 59
  value in HCM 58
  and ventricular function 65
Myocardial cell necrosis 118
  isoprotovenol-induced 118
  prevention by calcium antagonists 119
Myocardial hypertrophy
  and calcium antagonisme 285
  distribution in HCM 25
  echocardiographic identification 18
  and functional limitation 31
  isoprotovenol-induced 115, 118, 163
  prevention by calcium-antagonists 119
  quantification of 45, 64
  regression of 244
  and ventricular function 65
Myofibrills 64, 65

Nerve-growth-factor 88
  and myocardial cell diameter 93
  and myocardial hypertrophy 90
  and myocardial norepinephrin-content 89,
    90
  and myofibrillar disarray 93
Nifedipine 115, 175
  antianginal effects 269, 285
  and arterial blood-pressure 139
  and cardial output 139

effect on slow inward current 278
effect on ST-segment depression 271
and filling pressure
and heart rate 139
hemodynamic effects 139
negative inotropic effects 286

Pelhexilene maleat 272
effect on ST-segment depression 272
Pindolol 176
Prenylamine 115, 269
effects on slow inward current 278
propranolol 14, 170, 188 (see also HOCM,
propranolol treatment)

Septal thickness 10, 23, 192, 207, 211, 219
Slow channel inhibition 280
Sudden death 8, 160, 175
and age 9
and arrhythmia 12
and enddiastolic pressure 10
and myectomy 12
and outflow tract gradient 9
risk of 9
and septal thickness 10
and verapamil therapy 229
Syrian-hamster-cardiomyopathy 99
Beta-blocker therapy 104
cell necrosis 103
magnesium aspartate therapy 105
myocardial calcium content 99, 102,
104, 107
verapamil therapy 104, 106

Ultrastructural changes
in aortic valve disease 64
in congestive cardiomyopathy 64
in HCM 64

Verapamil 115, 152
acute hemodynamic effects 140
adverse effects 131
antianginal effects 263, 285

and arrhythmia 171
bioavailability 291
and blood-pressure 126, 143, 151, 168,
197, 209, 216, 227
and carotid-pulse tracing 168
effects of intracoronary infusion 143, 146
effects of intravenous administration 127
and enddiastolic pressure 143, 173
and endsystolic ventricular diameter 171
first pass effect 198, 292, 299
and heart rate 126, 168, 216
and heart volume 168, 181, 182
and hypotension 231
and myocardial hypertrophy 161
negative inotropic effect 286
and outflow tract obstruction 127, 129,
173, 175, 227
pharmacokinetics 291
plasma-clearance 291, 295
plasma-levels 146, 189, 195, 203, 295, 309
and atrial fibrillation 327
and AV-HV conduction 226, 326, 327
and blood-pressure 295
and contractility 228, 326
and ECG 301, 325, 328
and heart rate 327
and heart size 301
and hemodynamic effects 322
interpatient variability 309
methodology of measurement 322
and side effects 316
sinus node recovery 325
and therapeutic effects 298
and PR interval 295
and pulmonary wedge pressure 127
and pulmonary congestion 197
and QRS-amplitude 161, 168
side effects 175, 190, 195, 197, 209, 216,
231, 275
and sinus node automativity 226
and ventricular function 131, 143
therapeutic range 298

Cardiomyopathy and Myocardial Biopsy

Editors: M. Kaltenbach, F. Loogen, E. G. J. Olsen
In cooperation with W.-D. Bussmann
With contributions by numerous experts
Corrected printing. 1978. 203 figures, 56 tables.
XIV, 337 pages
ISBN 3-540-08474-6

Coronary Heart Disease

Clinical, Angiographic, and Pathologic Profiles
By Z. Vlodaver, K. Amplatz, H. B. Burchell, J. E. Edwards
1976. 1252 figures, including 271 LogEtronic scanned radiographs. XV, 584 pages
ISBN 3-540-90165-5
Distribution rights for Japan: Igaku Shoin Ltd., Tokyo

Frontiers in Hypertension Research

Editors: J. H. Laragh, F. R. Bühler, D. W. Seldin
1981. 242 figures
XXXIX, 628 pages
ISBN 3-540-90557-X
Distribution rights for Japan: Igaku Shoin, Tokyo

The Heart in Hypertension

Editor: B. E. Strauer
1981. 187 figures, 55 tables. XVI, 464 pages
(International Boehringer Mannheim Symposia)
ISBN 3-540-10406-8

Hypertension: Mechanisms and Management

Editors: T. Philipp, A. Distler
1980. 72 figures, 17 tables. XVII, 279 pages. (23 pages in German) (International Boehringer Mannheim Symposia)
ISBN 3-540-10171-3

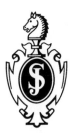

Springer-Verlag
Berlin
Heidelberg
New York

Myocardial Biopsy

Diagnostic Significance
Editor: H.-D. Bolte
1980. 60 figures, 30 tables. XIV, 146 pages
ISBN 3-540-10063-6

Myocardial Failure

Editors: G. Riecker, A. Weber, J. Goodwin
Co-Editors: H.-D. Bolte, B. Lüderitz, B. E. Strauer,
E. Erdmann
1977. 172 figures, 52 tables. XII, 374 pages
(International Boehringer Mannheim Symposia)
ISBN 3-540-08225-5
Distribution rights for Japan: Nankodo Co. Ltd., Tokyo

B. E. Strauer
Hypertensive Heart Disease

Translated from the German
1980. 65 figures, 19 tables. VII, 105 pages
ISBN 3-540-10041-5

Systolic Time Intervals

Editors: W. F. List, J. S. Gravenstein, D. H. Spodick
Editorial Consultant: J. Barden
1980. 159 figures, 46 tables. XV, 303 pages
ISBN 3-540-09871-2

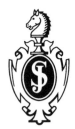

Springer-Verlag
Berlin
Heidelberg
New York

Ventricular Function at Rest and During Exercise
Ventrikelfunktion in Ruhe und während Belastung

Editors: H. Roskamm, C. Hahn
1976. 59 figures, 8 tables. XVIII, 183 pages (77 pages
in German) (International Boehringer Mannheim
Symposia)
ISBN 3-540-07707-3

Printed by Publishers' Graphics LLC USA
MO20120905-305